FEED
YOUR
SKIN
STARVE
YOUR
WRINKLES

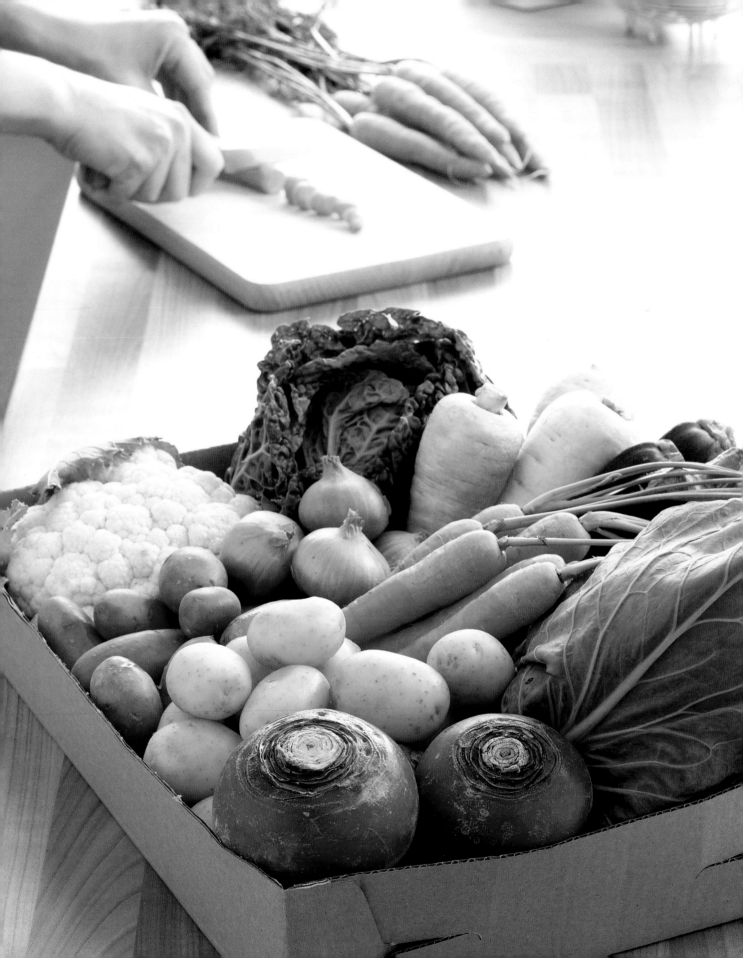

FEED YOUR SKIN STARVE YOUR WRINKLES

Eat Your Way to Firmer, More Beautiful Skin
with the 100 Best Anti-Aging Foods

Allison Tannis, M.S., R.H.N.

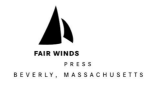

FAIR WINDS

PRESS

BEVERLY, MASSACHUSETTS

First published in the USA in 2009 by
Fair Winds Press, a member of
Quayside Publishing Group
100 Cummings Center
Suite 406-L
Beverly, MA 01915-6101
www.fairwindspress.com

13 12 11 10 09   1 2 3 4 5

ISBN-13: 978-1-59233-342-4
ISBN-10: 1-59233-342-7

Library of Congress Cataloging-in-Publication Data
Tannis, Allison.
    Feed your skin, starve your wrinkles : eat your way to firmer, more beautiful
  skin with the 100 best anti-aging foods / Allison Tannis.
        p.   cm.
    Includes index.
    ISBN 978-1-59233-342-4
    1. Skin--Care and hygiene. 2. Beauty, Personal. 3. Nutrition. I. Title.
  RL87.T36 2009
    646.7'26--dc22

                            2008023265

Cover design: Carol Holtz
Book design: Janine Blackstock
Book layout: Megan Cooney
Food Stylist: Dwayne Ridaway
Food Photography: Madeline Polss Photography p. 6, 188, 193, 195, 199, 205, 213, 227, 231,
233, 241, 249, 255, 259, 261, 263, 267, 269, 271, 275, 281, 285, 287
Getty Images: p. 2 Martin Poole/Getty Images, p. 8 STOCK4B/Getty Images, p. 13
Stockbyte/Getty Images, p. 14 Antony Nagelmann/Getty Images, p. 17 Purestock/Getty
Images, p. 21 Dylan Ellis/Getty Images, p. 26 altrendo images/Getty Images, p. 29 Image
Source/Getty Images, p. 30 Jeff Shaffer/Dawn Smith/Getty Images, p. 32 Sydney Shaffer/
Getty Images, p. 37 Trinette Reed/Getty Images, p. 74 Jerome Tisne/Getty Images,
p. 77 Stockbyte/Getty Images, p. 78 DAJ/Getty Images, p. 96 Tetra Images/Getty Images,
p. 99 George Doyle/Getty Images, p. 123 Image Source White/Getty Images, p. 144
Trinette Reed/Getty Images, p. 147 Martin Poole/Getty Images, p. 171 Photo/Alto/Michele
Constantini/Getty Images, p. 175 Jennifer Levy/Getty Images,
Jupiter Images: p. 120, 148

Printed and bound in Singapore

To my husband, who always
makes me feel beautiful.

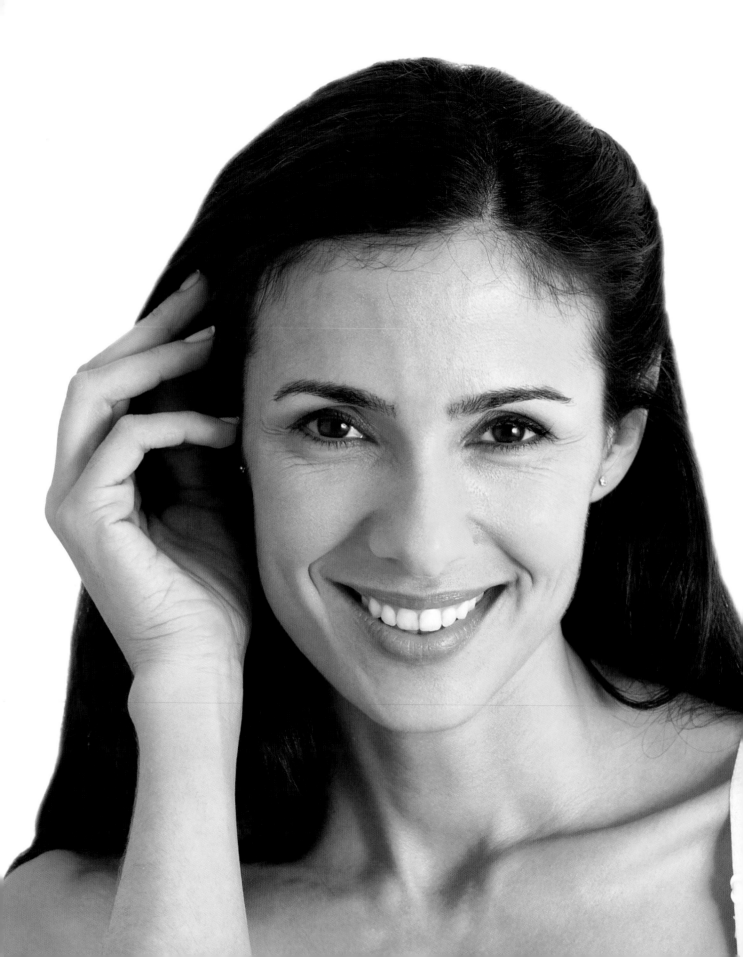

CONTENTS

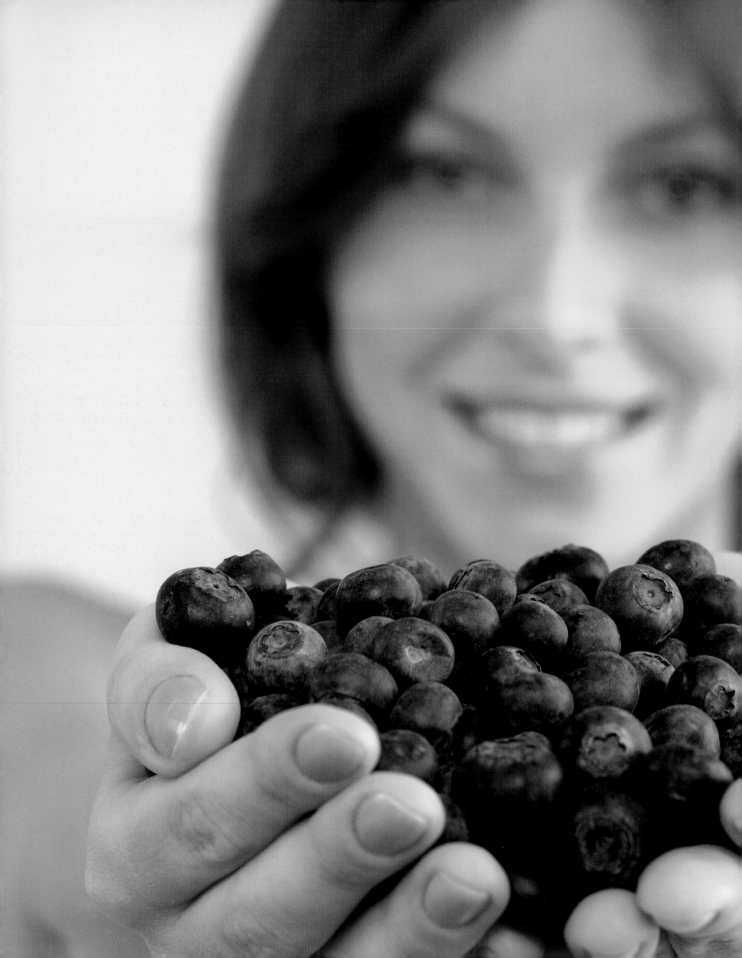

What's Food Got to Do with It?

BEAUTIFUL SKIN IS A MUCH sought-after trait in our society. Regardless of our sex, age, or ethnicity, we all want to feel good in our own skin. This desire, coupled with the growing number of aging baby boomers who are unhappy about their wrinkles, age spots, and sagging skin, has created an ever-growing demand for solutions to prevent the signs and symptoms of aging—including ways to look younger and to keep skin healthy.

The result of our ceaseless desire for smooth, soft, glowing skin has led to an explosion of anti-aging surgeries and cosmetic products on the market. But do you really need to go under the knife or pay hundreds of dollars for special products? Or, can food rescue your skin in the same way and help its natural beauty shine through?

The answer is yes, it can. Not only that, but changing your diet to include foods that support healthy skin is easier and much more cost-effective than any other method out there. Once you learn how skin is built, how it works, what causes skin problems, and what nutrients and foods help your skin look beautiful, you have the ultimate recipe for healthy, radiant skin.

In this book, we'll discuss all of these topics and more, so you will be food-for-your-skin savvy in no time. You'll find information on what skin-beautifying nutrients you need to help get you started on the path to rejuvenation and in-depth features focusing on the 100 foods your skin will benefit from most. Not only that, but you'll also find fifty delicious recipes that highlight these featured foods and show you how to incorporate them into your everyday diet. Having beautiful skin has never been easier!

You Are What You Eat

It's true: You are what you eat. The foods you eat may be the best resource your skin has to help it fight the outward signs of disease and aging. The entire body needs nutrients in order to work properly, and give us the glowing, healthy appearance we all crave. Unfortunately, stress, processed foods, and diets lacking nutrient-rich foods are common elements in most people's daily lives; and the result is faster aging of the skin, a greater number of people suffering from skin conditions such as acne and psoriasis, and more undesirable lines and bags around the eyes. Eating the right foods can arm your skin with all the nutrients it needs to fight disease and damage.

Feed Your Skin and Be Beautiful

Research proves that consuming healthy foods can help your skin have a youthful, plump, radiant, glowing appearance. In 2007, the *American Journal of Clinical Nutrition* published a study done by British researchers that examined whether the food people eat affects the way their skin looks—and the answer was clear. More pronounced wrinkles were found in those with a higher intake of bad fats and processed carbohydrates (such as white bread and packaged cookies and snacks), while a diet rich in vitamin C was found to reduce wrinkling later in life. It's just more proof that food has a lot to do with the beauty of your skin.

Skin: A Unique Organ

The skin is the largest of the body's organs. It functions as a key sensing organ, an oil producer, a detox organ, a temperature regulator, and a protective covering. The skin has to do battle constantly to stay strong and fight the damaging forces that surround it. As the barrier between the body and the environment, it is subjected to a lot of abuse, including:

- Ultraviolet rays from the sun (probably the most damaging factor the skin encounters each day)
- Tanning and other sun exposure damage
- Cleaning-product chemicals, both on clothing and in the air, which interact with the skin, drying it out and causing injury and possible allergic reactions

Your skin reflects your internal health. A healthy person has glowing, radiant, smooth skin. Inflammation, scaling, or puffiness indicates that the body is having health problems. Many skin conditions that leave us with undesirable complexions can be alleviated with a proper diet.

What Does Food Have to Do with It?

The body is made up of more than 100 billion cells, each of which is made up of fats and proteins. Carbohydrates offer these cells energy. These three components are necessary to support your body's basic health.

However, these nutrients alone do not make your body and skin healthy. Your body also needs vitamins, minerals, and phytonutrients to perform optimally and look radiant. These nutrients help the skin repair damage, build support structures, stay moist, and prevent disease. For example, collagen is the skin's main structural component, and the body cannot make it without vitamin C. If you do not eat foods rich in vitamin C, such as oranges, lemons, and strawberries, your skin can lose its tight structure and begin to loosen, sag, and wrinkle.

Nutrients to the Rescue

There are many nutrients that the skin needs to function properly and to look radiant. The table on the next page lists some of the most important nutrients for the skin and describes some of their roles in promoting skin health. Note that because hair follicles live in the skin, your hair's health is related to your skin's health. For that reason, keeping your skin healthy can help your hair regain that smooth, shiny, soft appearance it had when you were a child.

Cosmeceuticals

Along with aging baby boomers, a large market for skin-care products promising to turn back time has emerged, with new anti-aging products appearing on the shelves every day. Some, called cosmeceuticals, are being promoted as more powerful than cosmetics but less powerful than drugs. Cosmeceuticals include creams and lotions that are packed with antioxidants and other wrinkle-fighting ingredients.

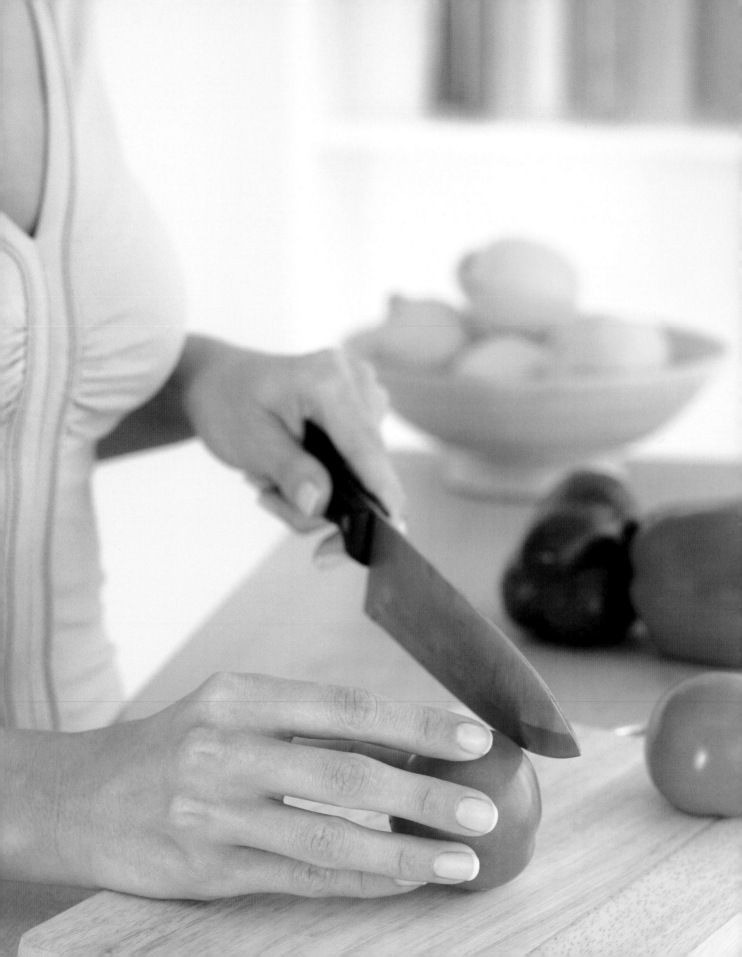

Nutrients That Support Skin Health

NUTRIENT	ROLE
Vitamin A	Fat-soluble vitamin that plays a role in preventing acne, blemishes, and dry skin; May help prevent skin cancer; Deficiency causes dry, scaly skin and an increased likelihood of infection
Vitamin B complex	Consists of all eight water-soluble B vitamins; Essential for the breakdown of carbohydrates, fats, and proteins; Involved in energy production; Deficiency can result in skin conditions such as acne and dermatitis
Vitamin B2 (riboflavin)	Improves oxygen usage by skin cells; Deficiency can result in inflammation
Vitamin B3 (niacin)	Ensures that the skin receives proper blood circulation
Vitamin B6 (pyridoxine)	Required for cell division and protein synthesis
Biotin	Required for skin cells to rapidly divide and grow
Vitamin B12	Used in the treatment of dermatitis
Vitamin C	Water-soluble vitamin that can prevent skin damage and reduce the aging effects of cigarette smoke and sun damage; Required for collagen formation
Calcium	Deficiency associated with eczema and brittle nails
Copper	Stimulates collage and elastin formation
Cysteine	Assists in promoting healthy skin elasticity and texture; Necessary for protein building, cell division, and skin repair
Vitamin E	May help with wound healing
Essential Fatty Acids	Include omega-3 and omega-6 fats; Act as a lubricant, moisturizer, and anti-inflammatory; Reduce the severity of sun damage
Iron	Promotes oxygenation of blood, a healthy immune system, and energy production
Methionine	Plays a role in protein building, cell division, and skin repair
Potassium	Deficiency results in dry skin
Selenium	Preserves elasticity of tissue; Deficiency may lead to premature aging
Silicon/Silica	Promotes tissue firmness; Strengthens hair, skin, and nails; Maintains skin elasticity
Zinc	Helps heal wounds; Needed for cell repair and for production of DNA, RNA (protein blueprints), and enzymes

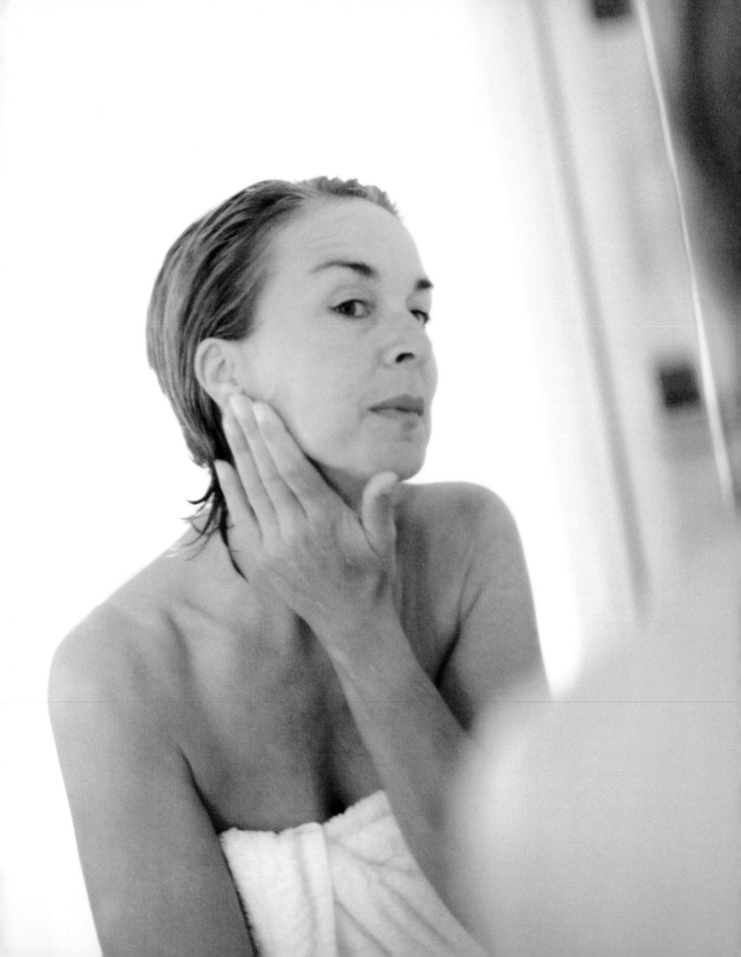

Feed Your Skin at Every Age

No matter your age, eating foods to support your skin is important. Teenagers are commonly scolded for their dietary habits—with fast-food and chocolate frequently at blame for their problems with acne—yet adults actually have a greater need for skin nutrients than do adolescents. The body changes and becomes less able to digest and absorb nutrients as you age, and the result is that fewer skin-healthy nutrients from the foods you eat actually reach your skin. This means that the foods you eat need to have a greater concentration of skin-beautifying nutrients.

Beauty Has Social Implications

The skin is one of the most important components of an individual's physical appearance. In humans, the face has evolved to become one of the most important visual communication tools, with thirty or more muscles controlling facial expressions alone.

Beauty is a visual impression. If a person's skin is damaged or unhealthy, his or her appearance suffers. There are myriad conditions that can affect one's appearance, including:

- Wrinkles. Seen as a sign of age or even frailty by some, others see wrinkles as a sign of wisdom. Regardless of what you think about wrinkles, they affect how you look and how others perceive you.
- Psoriasis. A chronic skin disorder that can have a severe impact on a person's social life and interactions. It is not contagious and should not be seen as a disease or infection; it is simply a skin problem that causes the skin to appear rough, with red patches and even lesions or blisters.
- Acne. Another skin condition that tends to have a major impact on sufferers' social experiences, making them feel self-conscious and embarrassed by their skin. This treatable problem can lead to problems with social and sexual relationships.

Beautifying from the Inside Out

Eating the right foods can help your skin fight acne, reduce redness and inflammation, resolve moisture problems, and even reduce wrinkles. For teenagers, adults, and the elderly, a healthy diet can increase energy levels, lower risks of disease, and make the skin more radiant. Keep reading to discover what foods you can easily include in your day to help your skin look and feel gorgeous.

Feed Your Skin More as You Age

Why does the body digest and absorb fewer nutrients as we age? Well, the longer we live, the more stress and demand is put on the body, particularly the digestive organs. The pancreas, for example, which is responsible for producing the many digestive enzymes required to break down chewed food into absorbable molecules, fatigues with age and can begin to produce fewer enzymes. The end result is fewer nutrients delivered to your skin, which means that the skin can be deprived of what it needs to stay looking youthful. That's why it's important to consciously—and constantly—fuel yourself with the right foods.

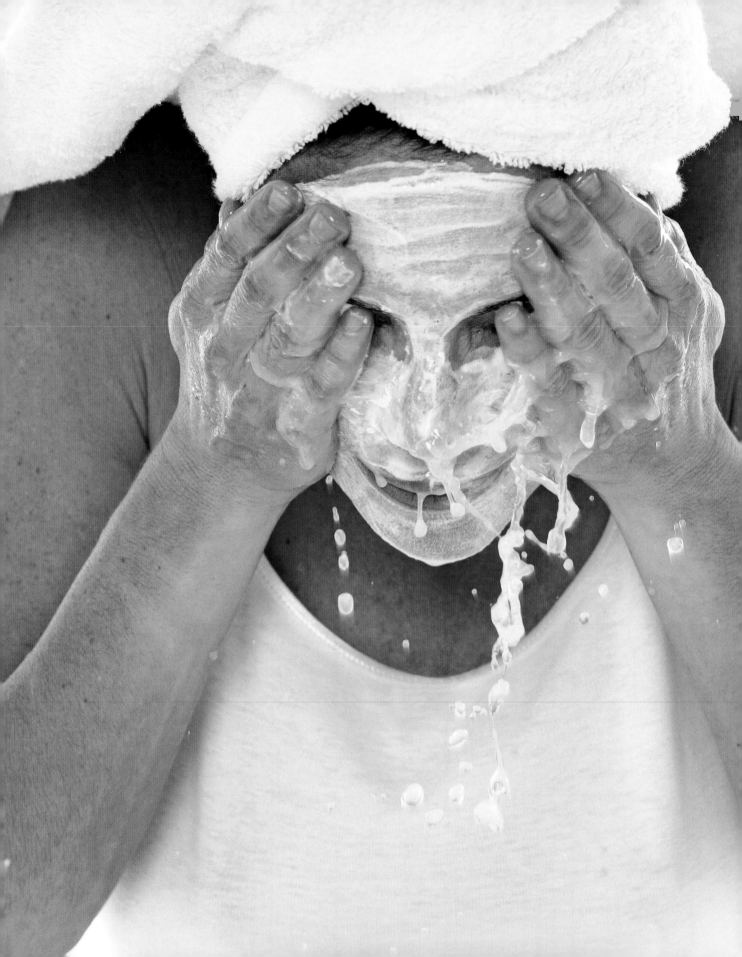

Beauty Is Skin Deep

THE WAY YOUR SKIN looks has everything to do with its design. Certain components in your skin are responsible for giving it its healthy, radiant look. So when something happens to change your skin's health and structure, its appearance changes, too. In fact, the appearance of your skin can tell you and the people around you a lot about your entire body's health. To keep your skin healthy and looking vibrant, you first need to understand the skin's physiology so you can target problems and effectively change your skin from unhealthy to beautiful.

Getting Comfortable in Your Own Skin— and Its Many Layers

The skin is made up of multiple layers, called epithelial tissue. Underneath this epithelial tissue are muscles and other organs. The largest of your body's organs, an average adult's skin has a surface area of up to 21 square feet (6.4 square meters) and a thickness that ranges from 0.01 inches (0.2 mm)—the eye lid—to 0.24 inches (6 mm)—the sole of the foot. Just as the thickness of skin varies, so does its appearance. Skin pigmentation varies among populations and across ages, as does its texture, moisture content, and firmness. Before we dive into how diet can help our skin radiate beauty, let's take a closer look at the skin's structure and functions.

To start with, let's examine each of the skin's three layers: the epidermis, the dermis, and the hypodermis. Each layer plays a role in your skin's appearance.

Layer One: The Epidermis

The top layer of your skin, the epidermis, is made of keratinocytes (discussed below), melanocytes (cells that provide color to the skin), and Langerhans cells (immune cells capable of identifying specific antigens and preventing disease). The epidermis is divided into five layers: stratum corneum, stratum lucidum, stratum granulosum, stratum spinosum, and stratum germinativum (basale).

The outermost layer of your skin, or the stratum corneum, actually consists of dead cells. These cells are flat and composed mainly of keratin, a rigid material that allows the epidermis to perform its primary function: protecting and shielding us from injury and the environment.

How does this layer of dead cells make us waterproof and protect us? Beneath these dead skin cells, there is a layer of actively reproducing cells (keratinocytes). As more cells are produced on this bottom layer, old cells are forced to move up. As the cells move farther away from their blood supply, they die and the normal components of these cells (cytoplasm and organelles) are replaced by a fibrous protein called keratin. The result is the creation of a structural matrix by a process called keratinization. We'll take a closer look at keratin shortly.

Layer Two: The Dermis

The second layer of your skin is called the dermis. It consists of connective tissue and cushions the body from stress and strain. Your ability to sense heat and touch stems from the nerve endings in this area of the skin. The dermis also hosts:

- glands (including sweat, apocrine, and sebaceous), which help keep the skin moist; when they are not functioning properly, however, oily skin can result, and acne can develop.
- fibroblasts, which produce the compounds that make the skin appear smooth and plump, such as collagen and elastin; fibroblasts can be supported by nutrients in food so they continue to give your skin a youthful appearance.
- blood vessels, which ensure that your skin is radiant by delivering oxygen and other nutrients to it; they also remove waste, including harmful chemicals that skin cells are trying to eliminate.
- hair follicles, which are attached to the sebaceous gland.

Layer Three: The Hypodermis

The hypodermis is the innermost layer of the skin and is mostly used to store fat. It also contains fibroblasts, adipose cells (for fat storage), and macrophages, which are immune cells. Macrophages help keep your skin free from infection. Although they can produce inflammation that leads to puffiness, acne, or psoriasis, nutrients can help them work properly and reduce damage caused by the inflammation they stimulate.

As we age, natural loss of fat stores in this layer of the skin can contribute to loose, sagging skin. Nutrients can reduce the visual effects of the hypodermis's loss of fat stores by keeping fibroblasts healthy.

Wrinkle Preventers

There are three key elements in the skin that play a role in preventing wrinkles—keratin, collagen, and elastin. Though we've mentioned them above, let's examine each of these proteins separately to understand precisely how they work in our bodies, and how we can rely on them to promote healthy skin.

Wrinkle Preventer #1: Keratin

Keratin is an extremely strong protein found in the skin, hair, and nails that helps make skin waterproof, while restricting the ability of chemicals and pathogens to gain access to your body.

Along with collagen and elastin, keratin gives skin its strength. It is made by specialized cells in the skin called keratinocytes. If skin is rubbed or pressure is applied, keratin is produced in larger quantities, and calluses develop—as, for example, when the skin of your big toe joint hardens from rubbing against the inside of your shoe. You may not appreciate calluses, but athletes and musicians do because it protects their skin from repetitive rubbing.

What's in an Inch?

The average square inch (25 mm) of skin holds 650 sweat glands, 20 blood vessels, 60,000 melanocytes, and more than a thousand nerve endings.

Perhaps you'll appreciate your keratin more, though, when you realize that it helps prevent sagging and wrinkling. Having too many of these dead keratin cells, however, can dull your appearance. Facial scrubs are designed to remove excess keratin cells so the natural glow of your skin can be seen.

Wrinkle Preventer #2: Collagen

Collagen, which is found throughout the body, is a protein that holds the dermis together and supports the epidermis. It gives skin its strength and durability, and is a vital part of the internal scaffolding responsible for smooth, tight, beautiful skin. Understanding the structure and function of collagen can help you maintain a healthy, youthful appearance.

Collagen is a protein with a triple helix structure that provides a strong framework to support cells. Its tensile strength (the ability to resist force without tearing apart) is greater than that of steel, which explains why your skin is so strong. About one-third of the protein in your body is collagen. It supports your tissues and organs and connects them to your bones. Even your bones are made from collagen, along with minerals like calcium and phosphorus.

Perhaps collagen's most important role is providing the structural scaffolding that surrounds cells and supports cell shape and differentiation, just as steel rods reinforce a concrete block. The mesh-like collagen network binds cells together and provides a supportive framework where cells can develop and function. This framework aids in the healing of tissues and bones, just as scaffolding helps construction workers build walls.

Collagen makes up 75 percent of our skin. Healthy collagen levels give skin a smooth, plump, young, healthy appearance. A breakdown in collagen or a decline in collagen production, however, leads to unwanted wrinkles and the appearance of aged skin. As a result, beauty seekers try to find ways to boost collagen levels and repair collagen damage. Adding nutrients such as vitamin C, which is known to support collagen production, to skin creams is one way to increase collagen synthesis in the skin. Some will go as far as to inject collagen directly into the skin and lips to achieve the desired smooth, plump appearance.

HOW DOES THE SKIN MAKE COLLAGEN?

Collagen is created by fibroblasts, which are specialized skin cells located in the dermis and hypodermis. On the surface of a fibroblast cell are receptors for growth factors, which tell these cells to produce structural proteins such as collagen, elastin, and glucosaminoglycans. Elastin gives skin

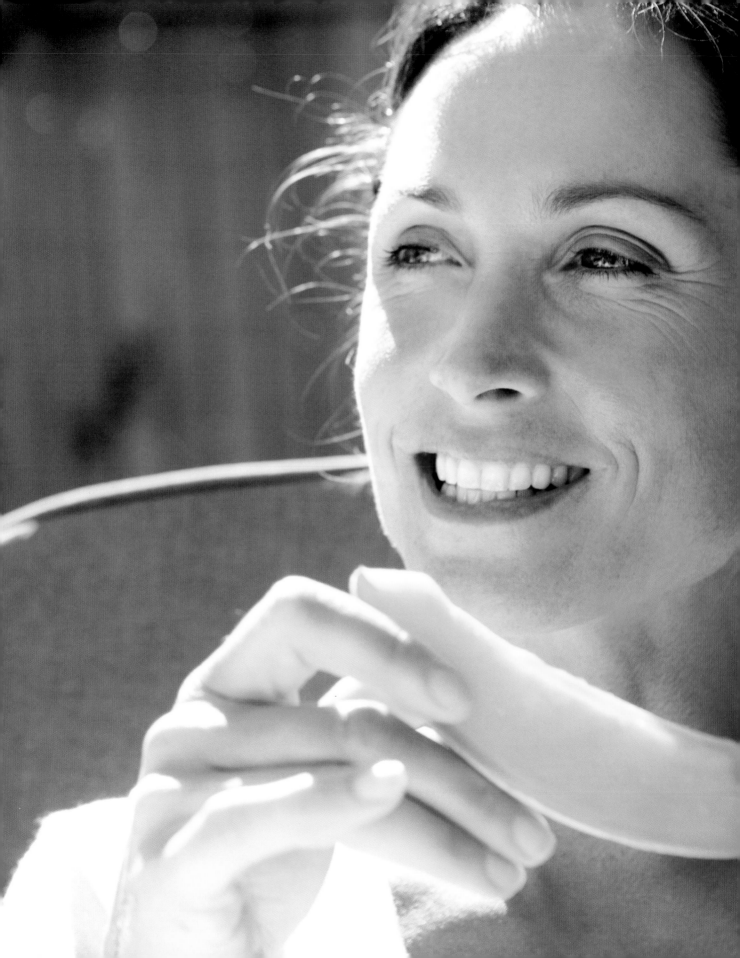

the ability to snap back after being extended (such as when you smile). Glucosaminoglycans make up the ground substance that keeps the dermis hydrated.

Initially, fibroblasts produce short collagen subunits called procollagen. These subunits then leave the fibroblast cell and move into the extra-cellular matrix, where cofactors such as vitamin C bind them together to make collagen. Without a sufficient supply of vitamin C, the subunits cannot be converted into collagen, and the skin begins to lose its structure. In the short term, this leads to weak, loose skin; in the long term, disruptions in collagen synthesis can lead to a variety of disorders, including scurvy. Scurvy is a disease where the body fails to produce collagen, and as a result, the body essentially falls apart as its support structures deteriorate.

Every day, fibroblasts produce collagen to help repair damaged tissue or to build new cellular structures. They also break down and recycle damaged collagen. With age, the level of collagen in the skin drops due to a decrease in collagen production and an increase in its degradation. Preventing this degradation is probably the best way to maintain a healthy, youthful-looking appearance. You can protect your collagen by avoiding radiation from the sun (UVA and UVB), thereby preventing free-radical damage. Wearing wide-brimmed hats and using sunscreen can help reduce your skin's exposure to UVA and UVB radiation.

For battling the exposure you cannot avoid, nutrients are essential. Free-radical damage can be prevented by ingesting antioxidants, which are present in many colorful foods such as berries, tropical fruit, and vegetables. Think of food as a peaceful warrior, ready to protect your collagen and eager to help you look luminous and youthful.

HOW YOU CAN MAKE MORE COLLAGEN

Promoting synthesis of collagen is another way to encourage healthy, plump, smooth skin. This means providing the skin with vitamin C, an important cofactor required to convert collagen subunits into active collagen proteins. Because vitamin C is water-soluble, it cannot build up in the body and form reserves, so consuming vitamin C–rich foods frequently is important to ensure that your skin can make collagen.

Wrinkle Preventer #3: Elastin

Elastin is a coil-like protein that helps the skin resume its shape when poked or pinched. A decrease in elastin can cause the skin to lose its firmness.

With age, the body produces more of a hormone called DHT, which inhibits elastin production. Thus, as we age, elastin production decreases

(Vitamin) C is for Collagen

In 1981, researchers reported that human connective-tissue cells, the same cells that make collagen in your skin, were stimulated to produce eight times more collagen when they were exposed to vitamin C for an extended period of time—proof positive that stocking your diet with vitamin C–rich foods can help your body produce all the collagen it needs.

and the resilience of existing elastin fibers diminishes. This results in areas of decreased firmness, especially along the jawline, along the neck, and around the eyes. In addition, repeated mechanical stress to elastin (from frowning, for instance) can permanently stretch out these fibers and lead to sagging and wrinkles.

Like collagen, elastin can be damaged by ultraviolet light from the sun, as can the fibroblast cells that make both collagen and elastin. Topical creams may claim that they contain elastin and can improve the skin's elastin content; however, there is no proof that topical application of elastin increases elastin levels in the skin.

Because iron has been linked with increased elastin production, eating iron-rich foods like spinach and dried fruits may be the best option for boosting the amount of elastin produced in your skin.

Maintaining Your Skin

Ever wonder how clean your skin really is? Dead skin cells are continually sloughing off the epidermis. Sweat and gland secretions are excreted continually in your skin, and dust, dirt, and other environmental pollutants land on your skin all day long. Together, these create a filthy layer on the skin's surface. Minimizing this layer of grime will help your skin's complexion shine, allow your skin's functions to work properly, and reduce the chance of infection, inflammation, or acne.

A layer of dirt on the skin blocks some of the skin's functions, including the production of antibacterial compounds. Unclean skin is a good environment for the growth of bacteria, which can lead to infection (not to mention an unpleasant odor). Proper hygiene practices can prevent dirt from accumulating on the skin, and wearing season-appropriate clothing can help sweat on the skin properly evaporate. Nutrition can also offer the skin healthy oils (e.g., monounsaturated fats, omega-6 fatty acids) to promote a balanced, healthy moisture level.

Note, however, that none of these practices can prevent the presence of microorganisms on the skin. The skin supports its own ecosystem of microorganisms, including yeasts and bacteria. One square inch (25 mm) of skin holds up to 500 million microorganisms. If this makes you squeamish, you must realize that despite the staggering quantity of microorganisms, their volume is only about the size of a pea.

Not all microorganisms are harmful—in fact, some, known as probiotics, help keep the bad microbes in check and help the skin stay healthy. Stress, travel, changes in diet, and antibiotic use can disrupt the balance of microorganisms on the skin and in the body and can lead to red, puffy skin and even acne and psoriasis. Changes in the skin's balance of microorganisms can decrease the number of helpful probiotics and allow bad microbes, like yeast, to grow and cause great discomfort. A proper diet can contribute to a healthy ecosystem of microorganisms on your skin.

Understanding Acne

When pimples become chronic, the condition is called acne. Acne can result from an overgrowth of certain microorganisms or from too much oil on the skin. Other factors can promote clogging of pores as well, such as an accumulation of dead skin cells in hair follicle shafts.

Propionibacterium acnes is a relatively slow-growing bacteria that is linked to acne. This bacteria lives on sebum, which are the fatty acids in the sebaceous glands at the base of hair follicles. People with acne have more *P. acnes* than do people without this skin condition. This bacteria can generate enzymes that degrade the skin, as well as proteins that elicit an immune response from the body. In other words, the presence of these bacteria on the skin attracts white blood cells to the follicle. White blood cells consequently produce an enzyme that damages the wall of the follicle, allowing the follicle's contents to enter the dermis. The result is the red bump that typically surrounds a pimple.

P. acnes also causes the formation of free fatty acids (a type of fat including triglycerides and phospholipids, typically found in the body at low concentrations) that irritate the skin, thereby increasing the inflammatory process in the follicle and further stimulating the formation of acne.

Understanding Oily Problems

The glands in the skin provide moisture that is necessary for avoiding dryness and psoriasis, but too much moisture can result in oily skin, which is susceptible to clogged pores. Oily skin can appear greasy or rough in texture and have large, visible pores.

This condition is caused by over-active sebaceous glands. The sebum they produce is a natural, healthy lubricant in the skin, but too much of it leads to shininess, blemishes, and pimples—all signs of oily skin. The goal of treating oily skin is to remove excess sebum from the surface of the skin without removing too much moisture. However, oily skin is not all bad; it is less prone to wrinkling and other signs of aging because oil locks moisture into the epidermis. That means that achieving the right level of oil in the skin is important to making your skin look its best. Use careful hygiene and topical moisturizer to achieve this goal. Also note that healthy oils in foods, such as monounsaturates and polyunsaturates, can promote the right balance of moisture in the skin and reduce inflammation, which can cause blemishes and puffiness.

Understanding Dry Skin

The opposite problem of oily skin is skin that becomes too dry. Dry skin is prone to dermatitis, or inflammation of the skin. Over-washing, a lack of proper fats in the diet, and the use of chemicals can cause dry and damaged skin and lead to dermatitis. Inflammation in the skin damages both skin cells and the scaffolding that keeps the skin smooth and tight, leading to sagging, rough, wrinkled skin; blemishes; and an uneven complexion. Infants and the elderly are more sensitive to dermatitis, as their skin's barrier is not as well formed as that of healthy adults. Additionally, people with allergic diseases such as asthma and eczema are more prone to skin inflammation.

Nutrients in the diet, specifically antioxidants, can combat the damage caused by inflammation. Inflammation creates free radicals that damage cells and the skin's structure, and antioxidants neutralize these free radicals and stop them from damaging the skin. Healthy oils in foods can also prevent dryness and inflammation.

Age Got Your Skin?

Your skin reflects a lot about you. It can communicate how you feel, the state of your general health, and your age. You can look aged because of damaged skin, or you can hide your age behind healthy, dewy skin. Learning about where the damage comes from and how to beat it will help you to defy the aging process and achieve the healthy look you want.

The major cause of aging skin, and particularly premature skin aging, is ultraviolet (UVA and UVB) radiation or sunlight. Indeed, sun damage accounts for an estimated 90 percent of the signs associated with aging skin and is sometimes referred to as photoaging.

Ultraviolet light causes pigmentation changes in the skin, such as liver or sun spots; broken blood vessels; dilation of small groups of blood vessels; thinning of the dermis; deep wrinkling; and coarseness of the skin. Most of these cosmetic problems occur because sun destroys collagen fibers, encourages collagen breakdown by enzymes, and causes the accumulation of abnormal elastin. The result is a disruption in the structure of the skin, which prompts wrinkles to form.

The Sun: Aging Culprit Extraordinaire

Sun exposure decreases the number of epidermal Langerhans cells, immune cells that protect the skin from infection and help clean up damaged cells. This in turn decreases the skin's ability to heal itself.

The problem is compounded further because sun exposure also increases the number of mast cells in the skin, and these cells secrete

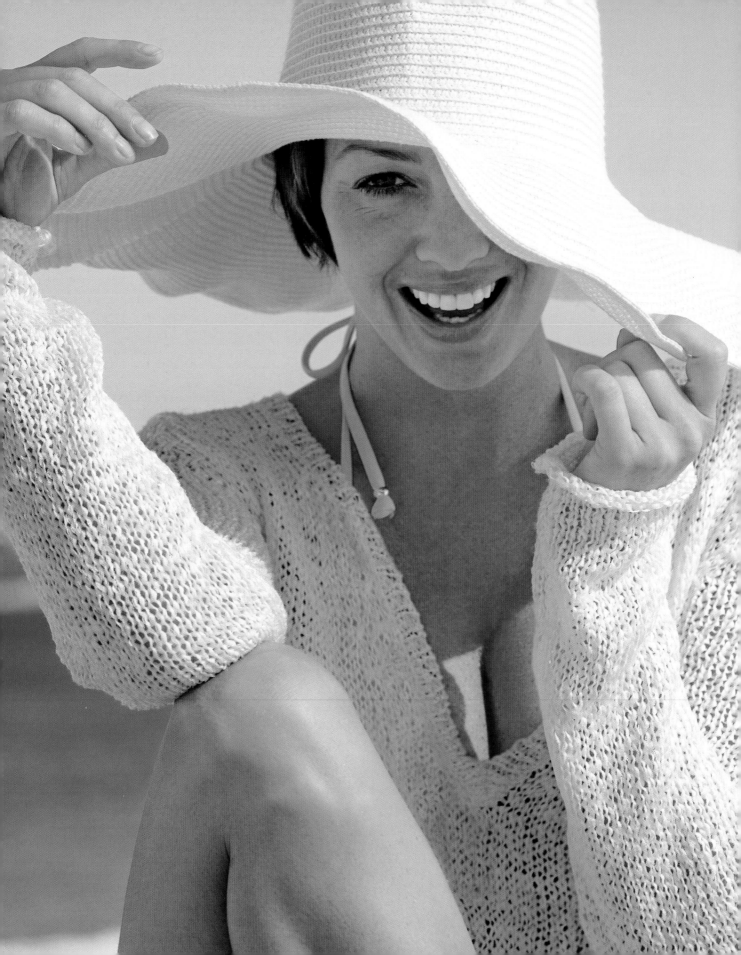

histamine in response to allergens. An increased number of mast cells in sun-exposed areas of the skin increases allergic reactions and inflammation. This combination of a decrease in wound healing and an increase in inflammation-causing cells leads to accelerated skin aging.

Protecting the skin from ultraviolet exposure is vital to your ability to defer aging. Avoiding sun exposure and using sunscreens can help protect your skin from ultraviolet radiation. You can also eat your way to healthier skin by consuming antioxidant-rich foods, which tackle the free radicals your skin produces when exposed to the sun.

Other Aging Culprits at Work

Besides the sun, other factors can damage your skin as well, including cigarette smoke and exposure to chemicals. Toxic chemicals from the environment can damage skin cells, reducing their ability to function properly, and skin that cannot function properly results in increased inflammation, infection, and a loss in structure. For your face, this means puffiness, blemishes, and wrinkles. Avoiding toxins is a great way to defy aging. Nutrients in foods can prevent toxins from damaging cells and promote detoxification processes in the skin, helping you look younger.

Even if you manage to avoid the sun, cigarettes, and other toxins, however, it's impossible to avoid the aging process altogether. There are many physiological changes to skin that occur naturally as we age.

You Can't Run from Aging

As we age, the tight connections between our skin's layers naturally begin to loosen. The structure of the skin's basement membrane changes, weakening the connection between the dermis and epidermis. This weakening increases the likelihood of injuries that can cause the two layers to separate, and wrinkles can form. In addition, the thickness of the dermis decreases with age. Elderly skin has about 20 percent less dermis, which results in less malleable skin, which is more vulnerable to injury. These changes in the dermis are mostly due to alterations in collagen and elastin, the fibrous proteins in the extracellular matrix. Reductions in collagen production and alterations in elastin result in this weakening of the skin and the appearance of wrinkles.

Second, the dermis blood vessels change with age. As the number of small blood vessels in the skin decreases, the supply of oxygen and other nutrients to the skin is reduced. The result is a decline in the skin's ability to repair and regenerate, leading to signs of aging.

Third, sweat glands reduce in functional capacity over time. Moisture in the skin drops, and dryness and inflammation can occur. Despite the

Skin Cancer: Blame It on the Sun

Incidences of skin cancer rise exponentially in people over the age of 30. Almost all skin cancers occur in skin that has been habitually exposed to sun, which suggests that age alone does not predispose skin to cancer. Extrinsic factors—primarily the sun—play a major role.

drop in oil production, however, the skin is not cleaner when it is older. The rate of skin cell sloughing, or shedding, decreases with age, increasing the need for cleaning to allow the skin's natural glow to shine through.

The fourth change to skin tends to be the most unwelcome. With age, subcutaneous fat, found in the innermost layer of the skin, increases in some regions of the body—typically around the waist in males and the thighs in females—and decreases in others. The result is wrinkled skin in some places and plump midriffs and behinds elsewhere. This loss of facial subcutaneous fat explains the facial changes associated with age.

Repeated muscle contractions, reduced estrogen levels, and the force of gravity also contribute to the aging of skin. On the bright side, proper skin care, including a diet rich in nutrients known to promote skin health, can be your best weapon against premature aging.

Nature's Rainbow

If you span the globe, you'll notice differences in skin pigmentation. Dark skin is a trait often linked to African ancestry, while paler skin is often associated with a Nordic or Scandanavian ancestry. Various skin shades between pale and dark can be found in individuals of all ancestries. Whatever your skin pigmentation, it is beautiful—it is nature's makeup.

Ever wonder what makes one person's skin darker than another's? It is due primarily to a pigment called melanin. This pigment is produced by special cells called melanocytes. Melanocytes manufacture melanosomes (packets of melanin), which are transferred to the keratinocytes of the epidermis. Melanocytes are found throughout the skin. An average person's skin, of any shade, has roughly two billion melanocytes. The difference in skin tones is due to the number and arrangement of the melanosomes in the keratinocyte.

There are two types of melanin pigmentation. The first type is called constitutive color, which is the color of melanin that is genetically determined and the color of skin that has not been exposed to sunshine. The other type is called inducible skin color, also known as a tan or the color of skin after sun exposure. Hormones can affect skin color as well. During pregnancy, for example, the skin can darken due to hormones.

Color Spots: Not as Harmless as You Might Think

What about freckles and other spots? Freckles are concentrated spots of color in the skin and are common in people with fair skin. In medical terms, the three main types of freckles are ephelids, lentigoes, and lentigines. They are usually round, flat spots that can be yellow-brown, tan, brown, or black, and they tend to appear on those areas of the skin that

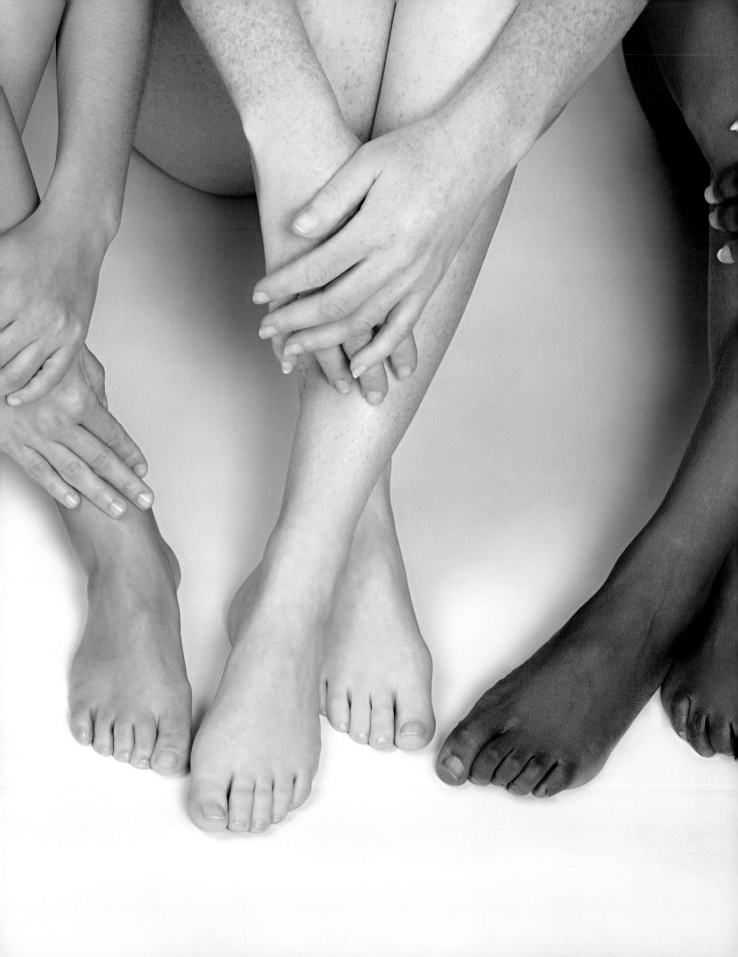

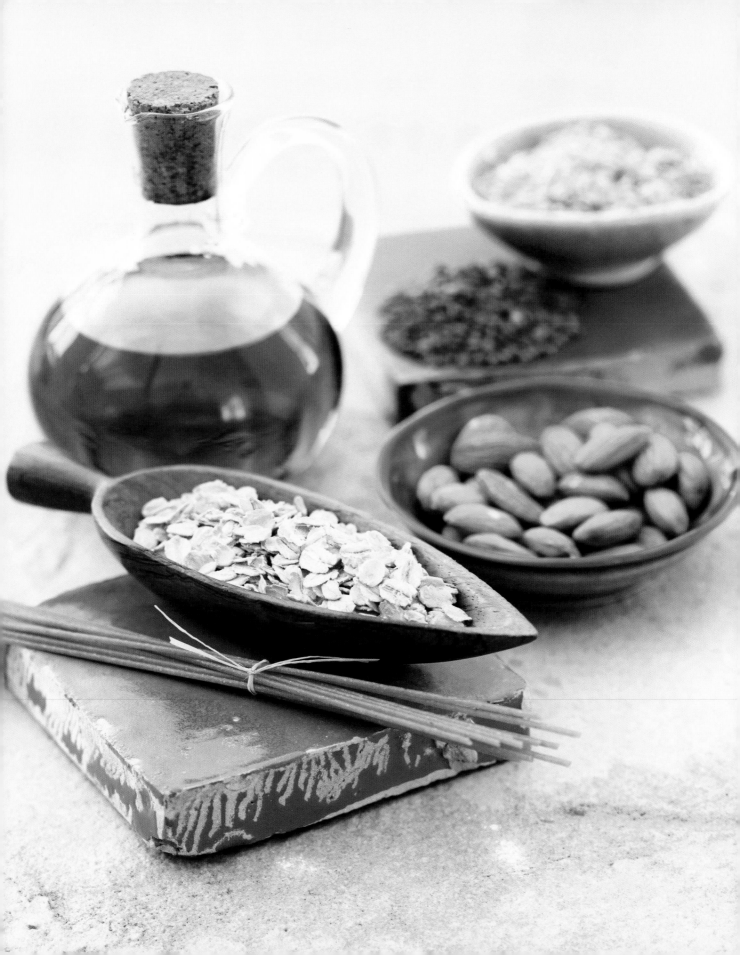

receive the most sun exposure. Even if you think freckles look cute on someone's nose, they are a clear sign of sun damage and can actually be considered a sign of photoaging (skin damage caused by the sun). Using protection against ultraviolet radiation starting at a young age is very important to the health of your skin.

Age spots are another sign of photoaging (skin damage caused by the sun), but these spots are collections of the skin pigment melanin on the top layer of the skin (epidermis). These signs of photoaging can be prevented and potentially reduced with the help of antioxidants. Selenium and vitamins A, C, and E are all helpful antioxidants in the fight against age spots.

Eat Your Way to Beautiful Skin

Nature's makeup not only makes you look beautiful, it also helps protect your skin against the effects of ultraviolet light. Exposure to sunlight increases the amount of melanin in the skin in order to protect the skin from damage. Individuals with greater levels of melanin in the skin, such as those with dark complexions, are better equipped for protecting their skin from the sun, as the darker the skin is, the more melanosomes present. This is why sunscreen is heavily used among pale populations, but is not as necessary for those with dark skin. Darker skin hinders UVA rays from penetrating, and as such, darker-skinned individuals tend to show fewer signs of aging in their skin and have lower risks of developing skin cancer.

A final factor that influences your risk of skin cancer is the presence of DNA repair enzymes in the skin. These enzymes protect skin against damage from free radicals, such as those produced when the skin is exposed to sunlight. Normally, these repair enzymes keep the DNA in good shape. People who lack the genes for these repair enzymes have a higher risk of developing skin cancer. Unfortunately, you cannot improve your DNA, but you can stop free radicals by consuming the antioxidants available in many fruits, vegetables, grains, seeds, and nuts. Eating antioxidant-rich foods can help reduce everyone's risk of skin cancer. In fact, antioxidants protect your entire body from free radical damage. By simply fine-tuning your diet to include healthy, antioxidant-laden foods, you can give your skin the self-defense it needs to fight damage and aging.

What are Moles?

Moles (nevi) are clusters of pigmented skin cells called melanocytes. Although they often appear as small, dark brown spots, they come in a range of colors and sizes. They can be raised or flat and can develop almost anywhere on your body. Moles can be present at birth, unlike freckles, which require sunlight to develop (and therefore are not present at birth).

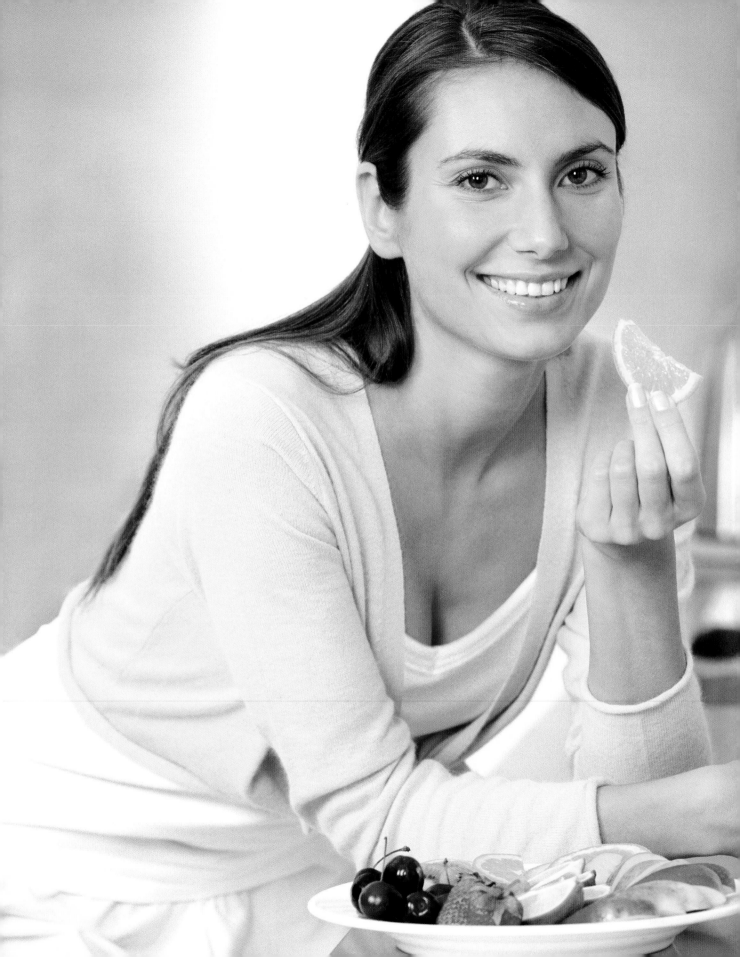

Foods That Fight Wrinkles

WHEN WRINKLES FORM in the skin, many factors are involved, including age, genetics, sun exposure, smoking, and, of course, diet. All wrinkles are a sign of damage, and this type of repetitive damage to the skin may be hard to avoid completely. However, it is possible to reduce wrinkling due to age, which most people wrongly assume is an inevitable part of getting older. This is not to say that you can reach 80 years of age without any wrinkles, but, by avoiding skin damage—from the sun, chemicals, and other sources—you can grow older with noticeably younger-looking skin.

Know the Enemy: What Causes Wrinkles?

Wrinkles emerge and become more pronounced as skin ages. As early as age 25, you can begin to see the signs of aging. The skin is slower in its ability to heal. Small abrasions and cuts take longer to disappear than they did in your teens. Old cells are replaced more slowly. As we reach our mid-forties, we begin to see more drastic changes in our skin as we experience hormone fluctuations. Skin begins to thin and become more fragile and sensitive.

Having strong skin is a key factor in wrinkle prevention. The integrity of collagen and elastin compounds in the skin is most important. Collagen makes up 75 percent of our skin; it is the main structural component that gives our skin strength and elasticity. Elastin helps skin to return to its original position when it is poked or pinched.

An accumulation of environmental factors damages the skin and causes wrinkles. Damage to collagen and elastin coils reduces the elasticity and strength of the skin. The skin will attempt to repair collagen and elastin damage if the proper nutrients are present and the rate of damage is not overwhelming. However, too few nutrients and too much damage can overwhelm the skin, causing wrinkles to form. Add in gravity, which causes jowls and drooping eyelids, and you have age wrinkles.

Enemy #1: The Sun

As mentioned earlier, there are many factors that cause skin damage, but the primary cause of skin damage is excessive sun exposure. Ultraviolet radiation from the sun damages collagen fibers, causing a loss in skin strength and elasticity. Ultraviolet radiation also leads to wrinkle formation by causing elastin to accumulate and clump in the skin.

Ultraviolet radiation enhances wrinkle formation in another way as well. Enzymes called metalloproteinases are produced when skin is exposed to ultraviolet radiation. Metalloproteinases normally remodel sun-injured skin by manufacturing collagen. If, however, an excess of metalloproteinases builds up (from too much sun exposure), the enzyme's function changes from friend to foe and breaks down collagen. This collagen breakdown damages the skin's structure, leaving it loose, weak, and wrinkly.

Enemy #2: Free Radicals

Wrinkles can result from free radical damage as well. Free radicals are unstable oxygen molecules that have only one electron instead of two (like stable electrons). These single electrons will scavenge for another electron, stealing them from other molecules. These "robbed" molecules in turn become unstable and scavenge for a place to find their missing electrons. This cycle can damage cell function and alter genetic material. There are several factors that trigger this cascading process, including exposure to even small amounts of ultraviolet radiation in sunlight, smoking, and exposure to air pollution.

Enemy #3: Hormones

A third factor that may play a role in wrinkle formation is hormones. As we age, we experience fluctuations in our hormone levels. Just as teenage acne is brought on by hormone changes, acne may occur in adult women during pregnancy and menopause. Such shifts in hormones can alter skin metabolism, including the metabolism of collagen and elastin. Changes in this metabolism can result in poor collagen and elastin formation, leading to wrinkle formation.

Menopause is of particular concern when it comes to wrinkles. Menopause involves a decrease in estrogen production in women. It is tough to know which changes in the skin during menopause are due to hormones alone and which are the product of aging or environmental factors. Human research studies have not yet documented which skin changes are specifically caused by a decrease in estrogen, but animal studies show that a lack of estrogen can lower collagen levels by roughly 2 percent per year and reduce skin thickness by roughly 1 percent per year. Thus, it appears that maintaining estrogen levels in the skin may help reduce wrinkle formation during menopause. Foods that contain phytoestrogens, such as legumes and soy, may offer a way to help stimulate collagen formation in menopausal skin.

The combination of environmental damage, free radical formation, and natural skin aging results in the formation of wrinkles. Avoiding smoking and sun exposure may help fight wrinkles. However, there is a better way to fight wrinkles: eat the right foods. We all know that the body's health is influenced quite powerfully by diet. Could your skin's health be improved by eating certain foods? Is food the next wrinkle cure?

The New Wrinkle Cure

Can food really make a difference? Or, like your mother sneaking vegetables into your school lunch box, is this just another ploy to get you to eat well? To find out, let's turn to the research.

From 1989 to 1996, researchers at the International Union of Nutritional Sciences Committee on Nutrition and Ageing conducted a study called Food Habits in Later Life (FHILL), which investigated people over the age of 70 to see whether their diets had influenced

Ultraviolet Light Causes Many Problems for the Skin

Excessive sun exposure eventually damages the skin. It causes the elastic fibers, which normally keep skin resilient, to clump. When the fibers clump, the skin wrinkles and can eventually become leathery. Ultraviolet light also depresses the immune system, which may explain why many people infected with the herpes simplex or cold sore virus are more likely to have an eruption after sunbathing. Over-exposure to the sun can also alter the DNA of skin cells and in this way lead to skin cancer.

Alpha Lipoic Acid: The Ultimate Wrinkle Cure?

One of the most potent antioxidants is alpha lipoic acid. Both fat- and water-soluble, this antioxidant can go anywhere in the cell to neutralize free radicals that cause damage to the skin's strength, structure, and elasticity. This puts alpha lipoic acid among the best wrinkle-fighting nutrients. Best known for helping diabetic patients improve nerve function, alpha lipoic acid is growing in popularity as a wrinkle-fighting nutrient.

Preliminary research has shown that creams with alpha lipoic acid can improve signs of aging, including wrinkles and roughness, in just twelve weeks. It is available in supplements at most health food stores and in some topical creams.

the youthfulness of their skin. Scientists examined the diets of 2000 people from Australia, China, Greece, Japan, and Sweden.

The researchers reported that the elderly Swedish subjects had the least skin wrinkling and that the Australians had the most. Those with the least wrinkling were found to consume a diet with a higher intake of vegetables, olive oil, fish, and legumes, and lower intakes of butter, margarine, milk products, and sugar products.

This groundbreaking research shows us that no matter our ethnic background, eating a healthy diet rich in key foods can help prevent the formation of wrinkles. Avoiding processed foods that are loaded with sugar and trans fats is another important strategy for maintaining youthful looking skin as we age. You need not spend hundreds of dollars at the cosmetic counter; you can avoid wrinkles simply by placing healthy choices on your plate.

Let's discuss a few of the foods mentioned for a better understanding of how they can help—or hinder—our skin's beauty.

Vegetables

Vegetables contain high levels of antioxidants, including vitamin E, vitamin C, beta-carotene, flavonoids, and many more. Antioxidants are compounds that seek out and neutralize free radicals, the unstable molecules in your skin that can cause damage to both your skin's overall structure and the cell's ability to produce collagen and elastin, all of which results in less firm, healthy skin. Antioxidants can neutralize free radicals and thereby prevent damage to your skin that causes wrinkles. It's even possible that antioxidants can help eliminate existing wrinkles. By disarming free radicals, antioxidants may allow your skin time and energy to fix structural issues that create the appearance of wrinkles.

Vegetables can be measured in terms of their antioxidant ability. Scientists have developed an antioxidant value system called ORAC (oxygen radical absorbance capacity). The higher a vegetable's ORAC value, the more wrinkle protection it can offer. Tufts University attempted to list the ORAC value of common foods in the hopes of identifying those that offer the best health benefits. Blueberries were at the top of the list, followed by strawberries, cherries, tea, and bright colored fruits and vegetables. (The creation of this list prompted a search for the food with the highest antioxidant value. Pomegranate emerged as the next big antioxidant-packed fruit, but it was soon replaced by goji berries and açai.)

Nutrients in plants that offer healthy benefits to the body are called phytonutrients. The phytonutrients in vegetables have been associated with a wide variety of health benefits in humans, including prevention

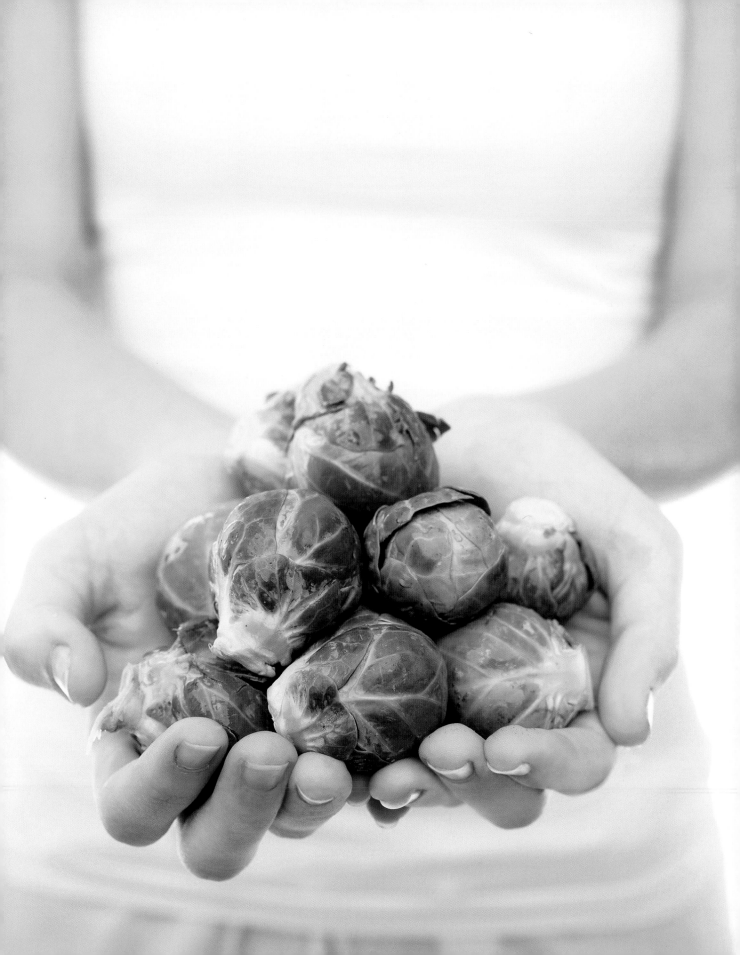

of heart disease and some forms of cancer. It is not surprising, then, that if they can help prevent such major diseases, they may also help prevent wrinkle formation.

The less you do to a vegetable, the more phytonutrients remain intact. Boiling, microwaving, or baking vegetables will lower their phytonutrient value and reduce the vegetables' ability to prevent wrinkle formation. Eating vegetables in a raw or minimally processed state will deliver the greatest phytonutrient boost.

Legumes

Beans may truly be a magical fruit. Legumes are an excellent source of many nutrients, including fiber, magnesium, and protein, and they are a great source of vitamins that produce anti-free-radical effects and protect the skin from damage. Legumes are also a source of phytoestrogens, a compound known to have powerful antioxidant activity. Soy beans, for example, are a rich source of phytoestrogens.

How do these vegetables and legumes protect the skin? The antioxidants in vegetables and legumes are capable of neutralizing the damaging free-radical compounds that exist in cells during times of stress and that result from exposure to ultraviolet radiation. Eating vegetables and legumes in abundance ensures that the skin cells have a steady supply of antioxidants to neutralize any damaging compounds and, thus, prevent skin damage and aging.

Fish

Believe it or not, fish can offer your skin beautiful benefits. Why would fish prevent wrinkles? Fish is a good source of two fats, eicosapentaenoic acid (EPA) and docosahexaenoic acid (DHA), which are both types of polyunsaturated fatty acids (PUFA). These good fats are vital to the health of cell membranes, improving fluidity and structure.

A high dietary intake of fish is also associated with a lower risk of cardiovascular disease, arthritis, and other illnesses—all the more reason to make fish part of your skin-healthy diet.

Olive Oil

The FHILL study found that the elderly subjects whose diets included the regular use of olive oil, as opposed to other forms of fats such as butter or margarine, had fewer wrinkles in their skin.

How can this Mediterranean oil offer these youthful benefits? Olive oil is a good source of monounsaturated fat, which is an important component to healthy skin membranes, helping with cell structure, communication between cells, and the absorption of fat-soluble vitamins such as vitamin E, one of the main antioxidants in your body.

In addition, the monounsaturated fats found in olive oil are less susceptible to oxidation than the trans fats and some polyunsaturated fats found in margarine, making it a much preferred source of fat for wrinkle prevention. (Of note, saturated fat is less susceptible to oxidation than olive oil, but researchers have found that the consumption of foods high in saturated fat, such as butter and meat, is not associated with fewer wrinkles.)

Fruit

Fruits are a major source of wrinkle-fighting antioxidants. In fact, blueberries and pomegranates are two of the richest sources of these nutrients on the planet. Antioxidants neutralize free radicals, which are a leading cause of damage in the skin that results in wrinkles. Eating fresh fruit is a boon for your skin and your overall health. The FHILL study did not include fruit in its investigation; however, as you will soon learn, there are a number of fruits you should include in your diet to feed your skin and guard against wrinkles.

Sugar: Just Say No

Interestingly, the study also found that eating a diet full of high-sugar foods, such as soda, candy, white bread, and processed foods, was associated with greater skin wrinkling. Why? There is a theory among scientists that simple-sugar diets can increase the formation of compounds called advanced glycosylation end products (AGE). (Yes, the scientists thought it was funny to call these compounds AGE, as they are associated with the signs of aging, including wrinkles.) AGE compounds form in collagen, interfering with its ability to keep the skin looking smooth and tight, thereby increasing the formation of wrinkles.

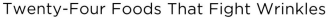

Twenty-Four Foods That Fight Wrinkles

Want to skip the needles and elaborate cosmetics routine? Look to food as your wrinkle-fighting weapon of choice. Here is a list of twenty-four foods that should be the staples of an anti-wrinkle diet:

Wrinkle-Fighting Fruits
- Açai
- Acerola
- Apples
- Apricots
- Blackberries
- Blueberries
- Cantaloupe
- Goji Berries
- Kiwi
- Tomatoes

Wrinkle-Fighting Vegetables
- Bell Peppers
- Brussels Sprouts
- Carrots
- Garlic
- Kale
- Onions
- Spinach

Wrinkle-Fighting Nuts and Seeds
- Almonds
- Flaxseeds
- Sunflower Seeds

Wrinkle-Fighting Foods for Breakfast, Dinner, Tea, and Treats
- Chocolate
- Green Tea
- Oats
- Tuna

WRINKLE-FIGHTING FRUITS

Fruit is an important part of every healthy diet. Because fruit is packed with vitamins, minerals, antioxidants, and other phytonutrients that are beneficial to your skin, it is a vital part of a diet geared toward vibrant skin. Dietitians suggest that adults consume about 8 to 10 servings of fruits and vegetables each day. Choose fresh fruits that are rich in color, which indicates that they are packed with antioxidants. Avoid fruit with added sugar (such as canned fruit), and always opt for fresh fruit over fruit juice.

Açai

Perhaps the best wrinkle-fighting food on earth is açai, a berry which comes from a tall, slender Amazon palm tree native to Central and South America. Açai has one of the highest ORAC (antioxidant) values on earth, making it a true superfood.

Scientists have found that açai actively fights against superoxide, one of the most damaging free radicals. These free radicals can damage molecules in the skin, including the collagen and elastin that keep the skin firm and tight. Açai can stop the source of damage that causes wrinkles, which makes it a super-powered free radical scavenger everyone should have on their side.

Even Better than Blueberries

Açai is also packed with other free radical–inhibiting antioxidants—so many antioxidants, in fact, that the açai is reported to have twice the antioxidant power of its superfood counterpart, the blueberry.

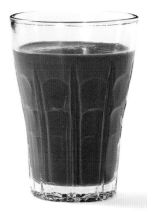

The deep purple of açai berries comes from anthocyanins, a group of plant compounds that are very high in antioxidant value (and found in all red- and purple-colored fruits and vegetables). Twelve other flavonoid compounds are found in açai berries as well, including proanthocyanidins and resveratrol, making them an ideal food to include in your wrinkle-prevention diet.

What's more, scientists have discovered that the antioxidants in açai may be slow-acting, meaning that they have a lasting effect in the body and can help your skin ward off wrinkle-causing free radicals for hours after you eat.

Healthy Heart, Radiant Skin

Beta-sitosterol is present in very high quantities in açai berries. This phytosterol, or plant fat, competes with dietary cholesterol for absorption in the digestive tract and thus reduces the amount of cholesterol you absorb. This reduction is thought to offer cardiovascular benefits such as healthy circulation, which is important to skin health. Good blood supply to the skin ensures that sufficient oxygen, nutrients, and wrinkle-fighting antioxidants reach skin cells.

Açai Fights Inflammation and Supports Healthy Cells

Have you kissed a scientist today? Well, perhaps you should; they have discovered that açai can also prevent inflammation. Açai has been found to inhibit the inflammatory enzymes called COX-1 and COX-2, which play a role in both acute and chronic inflammation. These enzymes may seem familiar, as they are targeted by common pharmaceuticals through non-steroidal anti-inflammatory drugs (NSAIDs).

Inflammation in the skin caused by damage, such as ultraviolet radiation, can release free radical chemicals into the skin, leading to wrinkles and an inability to fix them. By inhibiting inflammation, you can enjoy healthier, younger, and more radiant skin. Perhaps more importantly, if food can help reduce inflammation on a daily basis, you can reduce skin damage and, potentially, the formation of wrinkles. You may even allow your skin the time and resources it needs to repair existing wrinkles.

Oily to the touch, açai is particularly rich in fatty acids and contains high levels of monounsaturated fatty acids. Commonly referred to as plant fats, these fatty acids are known to support healthy cell membranes, which make your skin more resilient to poking and prodding and potentially reduce skin damage and wrinkle formation. Açai also contains the polyunsaturated fatty acids thought to be beneficial to the skin by enhancing skin cell structure and discouraging inflammation.

Fiber-Filled to Fight Toxins

Açai, particularly in powder form, is an excellent source of fiber. A 100-gram serving of the powder provides adults with their total daily recommended allowance. Why is fiber good for your skin? Because it ensures that your colon is functioning optimally and eliminating toxins from your body. Toxins can adversely affect your overall health and the health of your skin. In your skin cells, they can cause damage and divert skin-repairing energy away from wrinkle prevention to toxin repair.

Stay Close to the Source

Unfortunately, açai fruit deteriorates rapidly after harvest, so it is only available as fresh produce in the tropical areas where it is locally grown. North Americans will have to settle for processed versions of the fruit, available at most gourmet shops and health-food stores. You can find açai in purée form, juice blends, smoothies, sorbets, and other products. It can also be frozen, dried, or freeze-dried, allowing it to be consumed in a wide variety of foods.

Fight back with açai. This power-packed fruit is capable of fighting free radicals, and with its anti-inflammatory abilities, it attacks another significant cause of wrinkles as well. Look for açai products that are as pure as possible, since added sugar and preservatives can limit the health benefits of this unusual fruit. For a great recipe idea for açai, check out the Tropical Fruit Smoothie on page 192.

Acerola

This wrinkle-fighting red fruit is also known as a Barbados cherry or West Indian cherry. Acerola contains between 1000 mg and 2330 mg of vitamin C per 100 g, staggering numbers considering the recommended daily allowance (RDA) of vitamin C for males is 90 mg per day and for females 75 mg per day (with the upper intake level set at 2,000 mg). This makes acerola one of the most powerful natural sources of vitamin C, which in turn makes it a great wrinkle-fighting fruit.

Helps Tighten and Firm the Skin

Why is vitamin C helpful in the fight against wrinkle formation? Because your skin requires vitamin C to make collagen, which is one of the the skin's main structural components. When collagen is lost, weakened, or disorganized, the skin looses its shape, and wrinkles form. Natural events in your daily life—including exposure to sunlight, chemicals in cosmetics and the environment, and making repeated facial expressions—result in damage to collagen, so your skin must constantly rebuild it. Acerola offers your skin all of the vitamin C it needs to make sure that collagen formation is happening quickly and, thus, that no wrinkles are forming.

Vitamin C is also a powerful antioxidant that helps your skin neutralize the unstable molecules, or free radicals, that form in your skin due to damage from chemicals, sunlight, and inflammation. Free radicals weaken the skin, so neutralizing them helps prevent wrinkle formation. It also helps regenerate and restore used vitamin E, another wrinkle-fighting antioxidant.

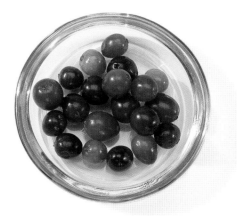

Many Soldiers to Fight the Wrinkle War

In addition to vitamin C, acerola also contains vitamin A, thiamin, riboflavin, and niacin, which help in the battle against wrinkles. Vitamin A is a fat-soluble antioxidant, which can help prevent skin damage that can lead to wrinkles.

Thiamin, riboflavin, and niacin are B vitamins that are essential for proper metabolism, and your skin is one of the most metabolically active tissues in your body. Its cells rapidly divide to maintain a strong barrier between the outside world and your internal organs. To sustain the energy required to produce new skin cells, your skin needs a healthy supply of B vitamins, which also support the skin in repairing damaged cells, making the skin healthier and stronger, and reducing the signs of wrinkles. New skin cells also tend to be youthful and vibrant, and they help reduce the signs of aging.

Where can you find this wrinkle-fighting fruit? Great fresh or made into jam, acerola is gaining popularity in southern climates. For those of you who own a snow shovel, finding fresh acerola may not be easy. Look for it at health food stores in a powdered form that can be added to drinks and smoothies. Powdered extracts of acerola, commonly promoted as sources of vitamin C, are also sold as oral supplements or in specialty skin creams.

Apples

Eating apples may keep not just the doctor away, but your wrinkles as well. At the beginning of this chapter, we discussed a study reporting that food can make a difference in skin wrinkling. In the study, the Anglo-Celtic group consumed more apples, prunes, and tea than the other ethnic groups, and these foods appeared to contribute to favorable skin results.

Quercetin: A Wrinkle-Fighting Powerhouse

Everyone knows that apples are portable, nutritious, and delicious, but you might like to know that apples also have wrinkle-fighting power. Flavonoids, which give apples their color, are great antioxidants—so great, in fact, that they are known to prevent heart disease.

Quercetin, in particular, is a powerful flavonoid found in apple skin and other produce like citrus fruits and onions. Quercetin battles with free radicals to prevent them from damaging cells in your body, including your skin. This and other flavonoids in apples can prevent damage to the skin and fight wrinkle formation.

Skin for Your Skin

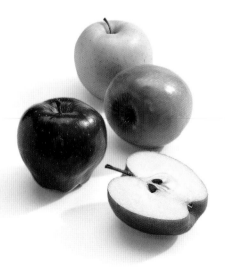

Apple skins protect your skin from the sun. Before picturing yourself with apple peels on your face, though, you should know that these fruits protect you from the inside out. According to a study published in the

Journal of Experimental Botany, the phenols in the skin of certain types of apples may deliver a hefty dose of UVB protection. Granny Smith and Braeburn apples contain quercetin in their skins to protect the fruit against UVB radiation. The theory is that quercetin has the same sunlight-protecting effect on your skin. And because it protects against this radiation, quercetin is also known to prevent damage caused by the wrinkle-inducing free radicals your skin produces during sun exposure. So the next time you plan to spend time in the sun, bring a few apples along as your new must-have beach accessory.

Apples' wrinkle-fighting ability diminishes during storage. After one hundred days, apple skin looses a small amount of its phenolic compounds. Thus, it is best to store apples in the refrigerator and to eat as many as possible while the fruit is fresh.

Farewell, Wrinkles!

There are many ways to enjoy this delicious wrinkle-fighting fruit. Apples are great raw, in juice, as applesauce, or baked in your favorite dish. However, it's important to note that processing apples lowers their phytonutrient content and thus their wrinkle-fighting power. Apple juice may have only 10 percent of the antioxidant activity of fresh apples.

If you have to have a glass, though, apple juice is a better juice choice than most other juices. According to research from the University of Glasgow in Scotland, apple juice ranks second among the best juices in terms of antioxidant activity. While Concord grape juice was number one on the list of twelve (as it has the broadest range of polyphenols and the highest antioxidant capacity), cloudy apple juice, cranberry juice, and grapefruit juice were close behind. It's important to note that in this study, and in another reported in the *Journal of the Science of Food and Agriculture,* cloudy apple juice was found to pack more antioxidant power than clear apple juice, as it contains about four times more protective polyphenols than its clear counterpart.

Go Organic for Healthy Skin

Apples are among the most sprayed produce in North America. According to the Environmental Working Group's 2006 report, "Shopper's Guide to Pesticides in Produce," apples are among the twelve foods on which pesticide residues have been most frequently found. Pesticides are toxic to your body and can certainly affect the health of your skin. Therefore, purchase organic apples whenever possible to avoid pesticide consumption, and if no organic apples are available, try to wash the wax off (with water or a fruit or vegetable wash), as it holds the pesticides to the skin.

Fuji Fighters
What type of apples are the best wrinkle fighters? Out of ten varieties of apples commonly consumed in the United States, Fuji apples have the greatest amount of phenolic and flavonoid compounds, and they are very high in antioxidant activity. Red Delicious apples are a close second.

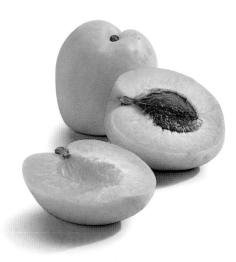

Apricots

Shakespeare may have insisted that apricots are an aphrodisiac, but let's give this fruit its real due by celebrating its ability to iron out wrinkles. For starters, apricots are bursting with beta-carotene, a form of carotene that gives many fruits and vegetables, such as carrots and sweet potatoes, their characteristic orange color. Beta-carotene can turn wrinkle-forming free radicals into harmless compounds. As one of the best sources of beta-carotene on earth, apricots are packed with free radical–scavenging abilities.

Iron It Out

A great source of iron, apricots can also help your skin look more radiant. Your red blood cells need iron to carry oxygen around your body, including to your skin. The skin needs oxygen to complete the metabolic processes necessary to maintain its strength, firmness, and resilience. Apricots also contain vitamin B, potassium, and other important vitamins and minerals, making them a wonderful addition to your wrinkle-fighting diet.

Fight Back with Fat

Fruit is not normally thought of as a source of fat, but apricots contain linoleic and oleic fatty acids. You may know these fats by their more common family names: omega-6 and omega-9. These polyunsaturated fats are healthy fats that play an important role in cell health, including the cells of your skin. Skin cells use these healthy fats in their membranes, and membranes containing healthy fats are better able to absorb nutrients and produce skin-strengthening compounds. Stronger skin means fewer wrinkles.

Although apricot oil is commonly used in the cosmetic industry to improve dry and wrinkled skin, you need not apply these oils topically. Eating apricots and other natural sources of oleic and linoleic fatty acids can help nourish your skin from the inside out.

What's the best way to eat apricots? Fresh is best, as fresh fruit has the most antioxidants and other healthy nutrients. Dried apricots are also a healthy choice as they contain many of the wrinkle-fighting antioxidants found in fresh apricots and are a good source of iron. No matter which way you choose to eat apricots, they will certainly help iron out wrinkles.

Vitamin C for You and Me

Apricots are also a great source of vitamins C, with one little apricot providing more than 5 percent of your recommended daily intake. Vitamin C is the main water-soluble antioxidant in our bodies. This means that vitamin C can attack any free radicals in the watery parts of your skin cells, protecting those areas from damage.

Blackberries

Luscious, dark-purple berries with a mouth-watering tart taste, blackberries are a delicious addition to your wrinkle-fighting diet. The common blackberry is normally available in late spring and early summer, but growing interest in this antioxidant-rich berry means that you can now find supplies at the supermarket almost year round. What is all the hype about?

Packed with Antioxidants

Blackberries are an antioxidant-rich food, making them powerful fighters of free radicals and, thus, excellent wrinkle fighters. Blackberries have an ORAC value (a measurement of antioxidant levels) that is just shy of that found in blueberries, which has one of the highest ORAC values of any food on earth. Blackberries are also particularly high in anthocyanins, a group of flavonoids that are powerful antioxidants, and can benefit your skin by putting these antioxidants to work at reducing inflammation.

Blackberries are also a naturally rich source of bioflavonoids and phenolic compounds, two cancer-fighting antioxidants. A 2004 study examined the effects of fresh blackberry extracts on the proliferation of cancer cells. The findings suggested that blackberry extract is an effective scavenger of free radicals and inhibited the growth of cancer cells. When it comes to wrinkles, the antioxidants in blackberries have a potent ability to prevent free radicals from triggering wrinkle-forming damage.

Finally, blackberries are a good source of vitamin E, one of the most important fat-soluble antioxidants in the body. Your skin contains fats that can be "oxidized," which is science-talk for damaged. Free radicals cause fat oxidation, which in turn causes wrinkles. Blackberries provide a natural source of vitamin E to help keep your skin fats healthy and your skin looking radiant and wrinkle free.

Tall Tales

In the United Kingdom, blackberries are steeped in superstition. Some insist that blackberries should not be picked after the start of October because the devil has claimed them. Suspicions aside, there may be some value behind this legend, as fall's cooler weather allows blackberries to become infected with various molds that can give the fruit an unpleasant flavor. In southwest England, the first blackberry spotted each year is thought to banish warts. Although they have not been proven as a wart treatment, they are packed with antioxidants and should be a staple of your wrinkle-fighting diet.

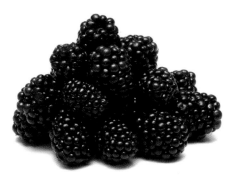

Not that you need more reasons to sprinkle these tart berries on your cereal, dessert, or salad, but blackberries do even more than just fight wrinkles. They contain folate, magnesium, potassium, and copper, which offer your body many healthy benefits. In addition, studies show that blackberries may reduce the risk of heart disease and inhibit colon cancer.

Blueberries

Blueberries may have started the antioxidant superfood revolution, and that certainly isn't a bad thing, since superfoods are known to help fight aging, including wrinkles. Their fame is largely based on the fact that a serving of fresh blueberries provides more antioxidant activity than most other fresh fruits and vegetables.

The Original Superfood

Anthocyanins are the blue-red pigments found in blueberries. These powerful antioxidants protect the integrity of support structures in the skin and veins, which means stronger, healthier skin with fewer wrinkles. It also means stronger, healthier blood vessels, which help improve the nutrient and oxygen supply to your skin, giving it a radiant, healthy glow.

Research has found that anthocyanins stabilize the collagen matrix, the main structure of your skin, by inhibiting enzymes that slice the collagen matrix. They also prevent free-radical damage to the matrix and encourage cross-linking of collagen fibers to form a more stable matrix. A healthy, stable matrix results in firm, youthful-looking skin.

Despite the popular belief that red wine is the ultimate source of anthocyanins, blueberries contain 38 percent more of these free radical fighters—and they're significantly lower in calories, too! Toast your skin's health with a bowl of blueberries and enjoy antioxidant powers that are known to improve your night-vision and to fight heart disease, cancer, and wrinkles.

Which Berry Is Best?

There are approximately 30 different species of blueberries. Choose blueberries that are firm and have a lively, uniform blue color. Here's a great trick when shopping for the best berries: Shake the container. If the berries move freely, buy them; if they do not, they are probably mushy, damaged, or moldy and should be avoided. Ripe blueberries should be stored in a covered container in the refrigerator, where they will keep for about a week.

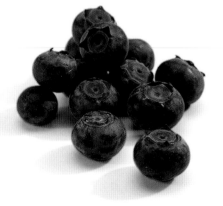

Go wild! Wild blueberries pack more antioxidant power per bite than cultivated blueberries. Organic wild blueberries are even better. If you cannot find either, any blueberry is a better wrinkle-fighting snack than chips, chocolate bars, or candy.

When blueberries are not available fresh, keep some in your freezer and add them to pancakes, smoothies, or your favorite oat or bran baked goods. Anthocyanins can be found in both fresh and frozen blueberries, but not in processed foods, which includes baby foods and canned foods.

Cantaloupe

The cantaloupe belongs to the same family as the cucumber, pumpkin, and squash, three other skin-healthy foods. Bite into this delicious, nutrient-filled snack and say good-bye to wrinkles.

Triple-Powered with Antioxidants

When you think of vitamin C, you probably think of citrus fruits, but cantaloupe is a tremendous source of this wrinkle-fighting vitamin. In fact, just one cup (160 g) of this juicy melon supplies your entire recommended daily amount of vitamin C, which renders free radicals harmless, thus preventing them from damaging the collagen that provides structure to your skin.

Vitamin C is one of the ultimate wrinkle-fighting antioxidants because it not only stops free radical damage but it also regenerates vitamin E, another potent antioxidant in your skin. Why would vitamin E need regenerating? Because after disarming a free radical, vitamin E converts into its inactive form. Vitamin C can reactivate the vitamin E so that it can disarm more free radicals and inhibit wrinkle formation.

Dual Action

Cantaloupe is also an excellent source of vitamin A. Because vitamin A is a fat-soluble antioxidant and vitamin C is a water-soluble antioxidant, cantaloupe offers your skin a dual-action approach to fighting free radicals.

The body can create vitamin A from beta-carotene. A cantaloupe's gorgeous orange color is due to its concentrated amount of beta-carotene, which effectively reduces free radical damage in skin cells.

In addition to vitamins C and E and beta-carotene, this sweet melon also offers you lots of potassium, vitamin B6, and folate, all of which support healthy, beautiful skin.

The Ultimate Tag Team
Anthocyanins have been shown to enhance the effects of vitamin C, which is vital to collagen formation. When it comes to blueberries, you get a two-for-one deal in this regard, as just one cup (145 g) of blueberries provides 30 percent of your daily recommended value of vitamin C and is packed with anthocyanin superstars.

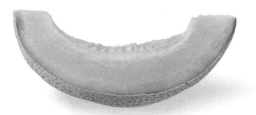

Don't Count the Carbs

Worried about the sugars in melons? Don't be. Cantaloupe contains B complex vitamins, which support energy production by aiding sugar metabolism in the body. In addition, there is a good amount of fiber in cantaloupe, which helps ensure that its sugar is delivered into the bloodstream gradually, thus stabilizing blood sugar levels. Plus, fibrous foods make you feel satisfied after eating them, so you'll be less likely to snack on other, less skin-healthy foods.

The cantaloupe is named after the Italian village of Cantalup, where it was first cultivated in 1700 A.D. Luckily, you won't have to travel there to enjoy this delicious wrinkle-fighting fruit. In the United States, the cantaloupe is the most popular variety of melon. Its North American growing season runs from June through August; however, you are likely to find them widely available throughout the year.

Sliced cantaloupe is a refreshing snack and can be a colorful, sweet addition to many salads. Try adding melon cubes to your next smoothie or to a yogurt parfait. For a cool treat on a warm day, prepare Chilled Cantaloupe Soup (p. 226).

Goji Berries

Goji berries, also known as wolfberries, have anti-aging properties, which makes them an obvious addition to a wrinkle-fighting menu. Used for centuries in Chinese medicine for its beneficial effects on the body, modern technology has now unraveled its therapeutic effects at the biochemical level. Without getting too immersed in the science of it, goji berries have been found to protect the body against free-radical damage.

Goji Berries Keep You Taut

Goji berries contain zeaxanthin, carotene, vitamins, polysaccharides, and other compounds that can help fight wrinkles. A 2007 study reported that goji berries contain natural compounds that inhibit the skin's ability to expand when under mechanical stress. This means that the skin cannot stretch when pulled, such as when you frown. This characteristic may help reduce the formation of expressive wrinkles on the face.

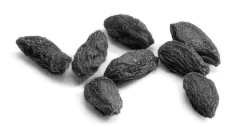

Construction Workers for the Skin

Studies have also reported that when the condition of the skin is not ideal, goji berries appear to promote fibroblast cells, which are responsible for creating a structural framework for tissues in the body, including the skin. Having skin in poor condition can occur when your diet lacks nutrients or when you are exposed to sunlight. The ability of goji berries to promote the health of fibroblast cells can firm up your skin, preventing it from wrinkling. Goji berries also appear to promote cells' formation of collagen, which is one of the main structural components of the skin. More collagen means stronger, tighter skin and a reduction in wrinkles.

The Next Great Superfood

Goji berries are popular in North America because they are bursting with antioxidants. As you age, your body experiences a natural drop in antioxidant levels, and the antioxidants in goji fruit have been shown to compensate for this reduction. Goji berries may increase the skin's antioxidant levels by boosting glutathione, a naturally occurring skin antioxidant. By increasing the levels of antioxidants in the skin, goji berries increase the skin's ability to fight free radicals and thus prevent damage that can cause wrinkles.

Bright red-orange goji berries are typically eaten in their dried form and taste a bit more tart than cranberries, dates, or raisins. There are also several goji fruit juices on the market.

Kiwi

Did you know the kiwi is also called the Chinese gooseberry? Contrary to popular belief, kiwi is not native to New Zealand but rather originated in China. Today, it's commercially grown in both California and New Zealand.

More Vitamin C than Oranges

Kiwi is one of the best wrinkle-fighting foods in the world because it is packed with vitamin C—one cup (175 g) of kiwi offers you 275 percent of your recommended daily allowance (RDA). Vitamin C is water-soluble, which means it can travel all over your body, including to your skin, to prevent collagen damage caused by free radicals.

The human body can store only a certain amount of vitamin C, so it is important to include foods rich in vitamin C in your diet throughout the day.

Peel Off Your Wrinkles
One of the most common ingredients in scrubs and creams for wrinkles is alpha-hydroxy acids. These are acids found naturally in fruits. Sometimes called a natural chemical peel, alpha-hydroxy acids peel off layers of skin and allow the more youthful, healthy skin cells to shine through. Lower concentrations of alpha-hydroxy acids can be found in cosmetic creams, lotions, and solutions. These products seem to be moderately effective at improving the signs of aging skin, including reducing wrinkles. They are generally safe and well-tolerated when used appropriately in the short term.

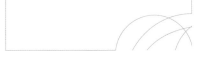

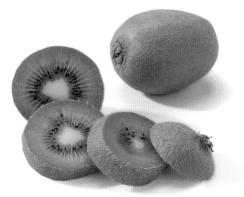

Make Collagen Twice as Quickly

Need another reason to include kiwi in your skin-beautifying diet? Researchers have found that kiwi fruit can double collagen synthesis in the skin. To a lesser degree, it can also stimulate fibroblast growth, all of which translates to stronger skin with better structure that is less likely to show wrinkles.

Kiwi fruit also helps your skin rejuvenate. Polysaccharides in kiwi fruits have been found to stimulate skin cell proliferation (formation) by up to 30 percent. This means that more young, healthy skin cells are being manufactured to help you maintain a glowing complexion.

Sliced kiwi is a refreshing and delicious snack. Add kiwi to your fruit salad, include it in a spinach salad, or eat it for a low-calorie dessert. For the best wrinkle-fighting results, select kiwi that is firm with no signs of decay.

Tomatoes

Tomatoes are one of the most popular fruits on earth. That's right, a tomato is a fruit—packed with disease-fighting, wrinkle-curing nutrients.

For the Love of Lycopene

Tomatoes contain a powerful plant chemical called lycopene, which is one of the best scavengers of skin-damaging free radicals. Lycopene is twice as effective at fighting wrinkles as vitamin A (beta-carotene), and because it is fat-soluble, lycopene appears to be particularly effective in tissues, like the skin, that have a high fat and lipid content.

In addition to protecting cells from free radicals, lycopene improves the functioning of cell-to-cell junctions, the main communication tool of tissues like the skin. Theoretically, this chemical's ability to regulate these junctions may improve skin texture and firmness. Lycopene also improves some functions of cell metabolism and helps cells work more effectively. More efficient metabolism means better collagen repair and fewer wrinkles.

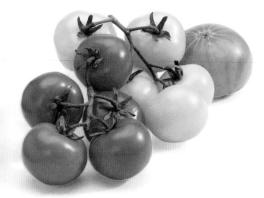

Slather It On

Tomatoes may be the new sunscreen. Lycopene can block the UV light that causes your skin to produce free radicals. In fact, tomatoes have an SPF of about 3, and although this amount is insufficient to protect the skin from direct UV exposure, it is enough to reduce the effects of indirect sunlight, such as the sun exposure you get through the glass in your car. So how do you reap the benefits? Simply make eating tomatoes a tasty addition to your daily routine.

Research has also shown lycopene to reduce skin cell damage and redness. This can result in a more youthful, radiant complexion. Most importantly, reducing skin cell damage means wrinkle prevention. It's also worth noting that lycopene offers a range of other health benefits, including reducing the risk of cancer and heart disease.

Heat Them Up

Here's the catch: In raw tomatoes, lycopene is tightly bound to indigestible fiber. As such, eating raw tomatoes provides relatively low amounts of lycopene. Cooked tomatoes, however, whether in stews or sauces, provide an excellent dietary source of lycopene. To be most fully absorbed, however, lycopene needs to be in the environment of a healthy fat, so adding extra-virgin olive oil to your tomato sauce is a great way to enhance your lycopene absorption. Roasting is also a marvelous way to cook tomatoes and bring out their concentrated, rich flavor. Make a batch and use them in our Roasted Tomato Soup (p. 224) or Quinoa Pilaf with Roasted Tomatoes and Pine Nuts (p. 254).

WRINKLE-FIGHTING VEGETABLES

Eat your vegetables. They are good for you. (It's worth repeating.) Choose raw vegetables over cooked ones, as cooking can damage and extract nutrients from vegetables, rendering them less effective. Dietitians recommend that adults eat 8 to 10 servings of fruits and vegetables every day. What is a serving? One cup (30–70 g) of leafy vegetables, like kale or spinach, or a half cup (50–75 g) of other vegetables, like green beans, bell peppers, carrots, or Brussels sprouts. It's easy to get four servings into your diet. A salad is typically 2 cups (110 g) of lettuce and ½ cup (50–75 g) of vegetables. That's three servings! To get plenty of wrinkle-fighting nutrients, aim for four or more servings of vegetables each day.

What Is the RDA?
The recommended dietary allowance (RDA) is a suggested level of vitamins and minerals that your body needs to prevent deficiencies. Is it safe to exceed the RDA? Yes. Many vitamins and minerals are known to prevent disease and slow aging at higher dosages. In Canada, the RDA equivalent is the recommended daily intake (RDI).

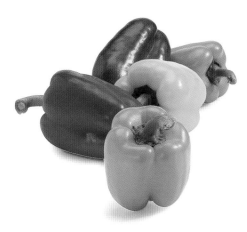

Bell Peppers

A pot of gold may lie at the end of this rainbow of nutrients. The best wrinkle-fighting bell pepper is the sweet red variety, but whether it's green, red, yellow, or orange, these brightly colored vegetables have great effects on the skin.

Dual-Action Vegetables

Bell peppers are a rich source of vitamins A and C. Vitamin A is fat-soluble and attacks free radicals in the fatty part of your cells making them harmless. Vitamin C is water-soluble and attacks free radicals in the watery parts of your cells. Therefore, bell peppers defend your skin by launching a dual attack on free radicals (which can damage your skin's structural integrity by weakening the collagen).

Smooth Skin and Healthy Arteries

Did you know that free radicals are also major players in the build-up of cholesterol in your arteries? This build-up can lead to nerve and blood vessel damage. Proper blood vessel and nerve health is important to healthy, beautiful, youthful skin, because without healthy blood vessels near your skin, the skin cannot get the wrinkle-fighting nutrients it needs from the blood to prevent signs of aging. By providing vitamins A and C, two potent free-radical destroyers, bell peppers not only prevent the skin from aging by stopping free radical damage, but also ensure that the supply route to the skin—the blood vessels—is functioning properly.

Like tomatoes, red bell peppers contain lycopene, a newcomer to the world of skin-healthy compounds. This fat-soluble substance appears to be particularly effective in tissues with high fat and lipid content, such as the skin, and works to disarm free radicals, leaving them harmless and unable to cause damage to the skin.

Protects Like Sunscreen and Increases Skin Firmness

Red bell peppers also contain lutein and zeaxanthin, antioxidants that help your skin maintain its youthful appearance. In 2003, the Journal of Investigative Dermatology reported that lutein and zeaxanthin, when present in the skin before exposure to UVB radiation, protect it from inflammation and damage. Such inflammation and damage are known to lead to the formation of wrinkles.

Lutein also increases skin elasticity, which plays a vital role in wrinkle prevention. Continual bending of the skin, such as when you frown, weakens skin and can result in the formation of wrinkles. By increasing the skin's elasticity, lutein can help it bounce back and reduce the risk of wrinkle formation.

Some research also suggests that lycopene can tighten junctions between cells as well. As such, lycopene also may be able to increase skin firmness, further aiding in the battle against wrinkles.

A Wrinkle Cure with a Crisp Taste

Known for their crispy, refreshing taste, bell peppers are also a great source of water, which helps hydrate your skin cells and ensure that they work properly. Dehydrated skin cells are less able to repair damage to skin. Moreover, water is essential to keeping your skin looking firm, moist, and healthy.

Fight wrinkles with these crispy peppers. Chop them into small pieces and add them to salads, nachos, pizzas, pasta sauce, or chili. Slice them into snack-sized treats and include them in your veggie-trays. An essential ingredient in Ratatouille (p. 270), bell peppers also show up in our Black Bean and Spinach Soup (p. 222). They are a colorful addition to any meal and a delightful, delicious way to fight wrinkles.

Did You Know?
Bell peppers are a staple in central Europe, where they are dried to make paprika. This spice is a necessity for Louisiana Creole dishes and an integral ingredient in Mexican and Portuguese cuisines.

Brussels Sprouts

Although they are definitely not one of my nephew's favorite foods—and probably not one of yours, either—Brussels sprouts are a must on your list of wrinkle-fighting foods. Despite their small size, they're packed with amazing antioxidants, which disarm free radicals and reduce damage to collagen, thus reducing the formation of wrinkles.

Layers of Protection Against Wrinkles

Your body has built in detoxification processes that remove compounds, such as free radicals, that cause skin damage. Some plant nutrients, called phytonutrients, can work at an even deeper level in our bodies by signaling to your skin to increase production of these detoxifying enzymes.

All cruciferous vegetables, including Brussels sprouts, contain phytonutrients and optimize your skin cells' ability to disarm and clear free radicals and other toxins. Today, researchers have concluded that eating cruciferous vegetables frequently (3 to 5 times per week) lowers the risk of prostate cancer, colorectal cancer, and lung cancer. If these miniature cabbages can help remove toxins that cause cancer, one can just imagine how many wrinkle-causing toxins they are able to remove as well.

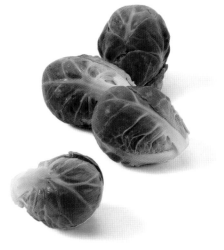

Bursting with Vitamins

Brussels sprouts contains ample amounts of both the fat-soluble antioxidant vitamin A and beta-carotene, both of which play important roles in promoting supple, glowing skin. Brussels sprouts also contain about 160 percent of your daily recommended amount of vitamin C, the body's primary water-soluble antioxidant, which supports the manufacture of one the skin's main structural components: collagen.

Steaming Maximizes Their Power

What's the best way to eat your Brussels sprouts? Well, my nephew would say covered in melted cheese. The best way to eat Brussels sprouts for wrinkle prevention, however, is to lightly steam them. This method of cooking has been shown to retain the most phytonutrients and maximize their availability. Alternatively, Brussels sprouts make a lovely sauté, like in our Brussels Sprouts with Mustard and Spicy Maple Pecans (p. 240). They can also be scattered around a chicken during roasting for a richer, more caramelized flavor.

Brussels sprouts are available year round, although they are at their best from autumn through early spring, when they reach the peak of their growing season. If possible, choose organically grown varieties, as they contain higher levels of phytonutrients than their conventionally grown counterparts.

Carrots

This vegetable is not just for rabbits. And they're not all orange, either—carrots also come in white, yellow, red, and even purple varieties. The orange-colored carrot that's so common and abundant in North America emerged in the Netherlands in the fifteenth or sixteenth century. The struggle for independence by the Dutch, who are well known for their patriotic orange color, helped to popularize this orange vegetable. And they should be proud—the orange color in carrots is what makes it a wrinkle-fighting food.

Improve Vision, One Carrot at a Time

Eating carrots is thought to be good for your eyes because carrots contain a good amount of beta-carotene, an orange-colored nutrient that is converted to vitamin A in the body. A lack of vitamin A can cause poor vision, particularly night vision, and eating more carrots or other vegetables that are rich in vitamin A can help restore your eyesight.

In one cup (130 g) of raw carrots, you'll find roughly 685 percent of the recommended daily value for vitamin A. This vitamin will not only help you admire your reflection in the mirror, however; it will help smooth away those wrinkles, too.

Carotenoids Prevent Wrinkles

Every day our skin comes in contact with environmental factors like sun radiation and toxins that cause the formation of free radicals in our skin. These free radicals damage the DNA, proteins, and lipids in our skin cells, causing them to become weak and fragile and to display unwanted signs of aging. Antioxidants, cartenoids included, are your protection against free radicals and the skin wrinkling they cause.

Eating carotenoid-rich foods every day is important as stress, illness, and ultraviolet radiation can reduce the concentration of carotenoids and other free-radical-fighting antioxidant substances in the skin. To help your skin stock up on carotenoids, be sure to include carrots and other orange fruits and vegetables in your diet.

Avoid a Carrot Buffet

Try not to let your wrinkle-fighting desires go too far with carrots. Massive over-consumption of carrots can cause hypercarotenemia, a condition in which the skin turns orange. You'd need to ingest 20 mg of carotene per day (about three eight-inch carrots) to begin to run the risk of developing hypercarotenemia. The resulting effect is not pretty, and it goes against what we're trying to achieve.

Also be wary that vitamin A can lead to toxic symptoms, including birth defects, liver abnormalities, and central nervous system disorders, if consumed at high dosages. Vitamin A is a fat-soluble vitamin that can accumulate in your tissues, which is helpful when you're exposed to sunlight (as the pool of vitamin A can help protect your skin against the wrinkle-causing damage of free radicals), but dangerous if taken in excess. Daily consumption should not exceed 10,000 IU (most multivitamins only contain 5,000 IU). You could never actually eat this many carrots, but some supplements contain high amounts of vitamin A, so be sure to read your labels carefully.

Easy to Add to Your Dietary Repertoire

Raw, chopped, or diced carrots make a good snack. Take your salad from boring to bright with the simple addition of grated carrots. Carrots are very versatile; they are quite at home in soups, stews, salads, roasts, pasta sauces, or wraps. Never thought of pickled carrots? Give it a try with our

Smokers Beware

A note of caution for readers who smoke cigarettes: Smokers should not consume vitamin A, in its form of beta-carotene, in high amounts reaching 8,000 to 10,000 IU. Research has indicated that smokers increase their risk of developing lung cancer when they consume large amounts of beta-carotene.

recipe on page 246. Carrots are easy to include in your diet, and because they are a root vegetable that stores easily, these wrinkle-fighting vegetables can be a year-round treat.

Garlic

Garlic has a mighty reputation to match its mighty flavor. This member of the lily family, whose cousins include onions, leeks, and chives, has been revered for thousands of years for its healthy, beneficial effects. It was given to slaves building the pyramids to enhance their endurance and strength, eaten by athletes in ancient Greece to improve their health and ability, and used for therapeutic purposes in India and China as early as the sixth century B.C. Today, thanks to research that validates its health benefits, garlic has gained unprecedented popularity.

Inflammation Inhibition

Acne, injury, or exposure to toxins can cause skin inflammation, which causes a cascade of issues for the skin, including the presence of free radicals and other damaging compounds. Damage to the skin can reduce its resilience and destroy collagen that keeps it firm, leading ultimately to the formation of wrinkles. Reducing or preventing inflammation can reduce the risk of wrinkle formation.

Garlic can prevent inflammation. It contains compounds that can inhibit the enzymes lipoxygenase and cyclooxygenase, which generate inflammatory messengers. These messengers emphasize inflammation in the skin and can cause more damage. Indeed, cyclooxygenase is targeted by common pain medications called non-steroidal anti-inflammatory drugs (NSAIDs). Garlic also targets cyclooxygenase, effectively curbing inflammation and reducing wrinkle formation.

Your Guardian: Vitamin C

Your skin will appreciate the vitamin C in garlic. This water-soluble antioxidant can help prevent damage in your skin and also boosts the levels of other antioxidants, making it all the more useful and powerful. One ounce of garlic contains roughly 15 percent of the recommended daily value of vitamin C.

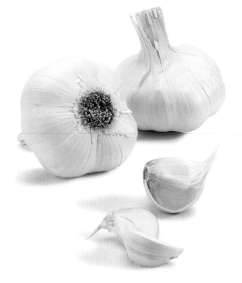

Protects Against Wrinkles, Vampires, and Cancer

Garlic contains a compound called ajoene, which researchers have found might be useful in treating skin cancer. A study in the Archives of Dermatology Research reported that ajoene, when applied topically, helped shrink skin cancers in a majority of the patients. Could eating garlic have the same effect?

Eating garlic introduces ajoene to your body, although it may not have as direct an impact as a topical application. It is clear, however, that eating garlic offers a number of health benefits to your skin and the rest of your body. One of these benefits, for example, is garlic's ability to boost the immune system.

Kitchen Tricks for Garlic

Off-white cloves of garlic are arranged in a head, called the bulb. Both the cloves and the entire bulb are encased in paper-like sheathes that can be difficult to remove. A chef's trick is to place the bulb on a cutting board and crush it with the heel of your palm to loosen the cloves. For ease in peeling them, use the side of your knife to place pressure on them. These two tricks can save you a lot of preparation time in the kitchen.

The taste of garlic is like no other: It hits the palate with a hot pungency and a subtle sweetness. There are probably a thousand ways you can add garlic to your diet, from salad dressings and sauces to roasted vegetables and spreads. Just a few of the garlic-friendly recipes we offer include Roasted Garlic and Mustard Vinaigrette (p. 234), Whole Wheat Pasta with Clams and Toasted Bread Crumbs (p. 264), and Asparagus with Anchovy, Garlic, and Lemon Sauce (p. 244).

Choose garlic that is plump and has unbroken skin, and be sure to check that it feels firm and not damp. Avoid garlic that is soft, shriveled, or has begun to sprout. For maximum flavor and nutritional benefits, always purchase fresh garlic. Store garlic in an uncovered or loosely covered container in a cool, dark place to help maintain freshness.

Not All Garlic Is Created Equal

There are several different types of garlic, including elephant garlic, which has oversized cloves. This type of garlic, however, is closer to a leek and does not offer the same range of wrinkle-fighting benefits found in regular garlic.

Kale

This leafy-green vegetable is well known as a healthy food. In fact, nutritionists suggest that we eat leafy-green vegetables like kale every day, probably because they are full of antioxidants that fight skin-damaging free radicals.

Repairs and Rejuvenates

Kale is a source of vitamin A, a nutrient used in topical prescriptions to help the skin. Vitamin A changes the structure of the skin, stimulating the formation of blood vessels and collagen—the main structural component of your skin. Increasing the creation of collagen with vitamin A helps keep the skin strong, firm, and wrinkle-free. Blood vessels bring oxygen and nutrients to your skin cells, ensuring that they can regenerate and repair. Regeneration and repair of skin cells enables the skin to maintain a strong, firm appearance.

Clinical trials of the vitamin A derivative used in many prescription cosmetics have shown that it improves the overall appearance of skin. It improves skin tone and smoothness while reducing pore size, dark spots, and wrinkles. Like many prescriptions, however, there is a downside: Its effects are short-lived. Once it is discontinued, the skin returns to the aged appearance it had before the regimen was started. Luckily, vitamin A is available in many healthy foods that can be included in your diet consistently, without a downside.

Gets Old Skin Growing Again

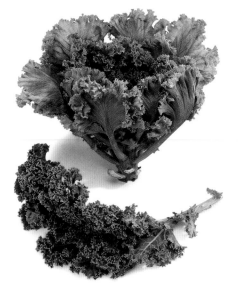

Ingesting foods rich in vitamin A, like kale, can help stimulate collagen and blood vessel formation, endowing the skin with a youthful, firm appearance. Vitamin A also stimulates growth of the base layer of skin cells—which means more beautiful, youthful-looking skin—and helps cells differentiate, a process in which they mature into strong, wrinkle-resistant cells. One cup (130 g) of boiled kale contains approximately 192 percent of your recommended daily value of vitamin A.

Kale is also a particularly good source of manganese, vitamin C, and vitamin K. Manganese is required to activate the enzyme that allows the body to use vitamin C, one of the most important antioxidants in the skin.

Kale is a great addition to any wrinkle-fighting menu. For your next vegetarian dinner, try our Mushrooms Stuffed with Barley, Kale, and Feta (p. 248). Finely shredded, the leaves are a vibrant addition to salads, or you can steam or sauté larger pieces for a deliciously nutritious side dish.

Onions

Onions may bring a tear to your eye and pungency to your breath, but they will also bring beauty to your skin. They contain vitamin C and quercetin, great antioxidants that can protect your skin from the wrinkle-forming damage caused by free radicals, which form in the presence of inflammation and sunlight.

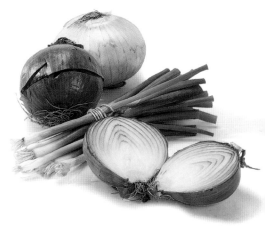

Keeps Inflammation at Bay

The base of many recipes, onions and garlic do not just share space in the kitchen pot; they also share family genes and offer your skin similar healthy benefits. Like garlic, onions inhibit lipoxygenase and cyclooxygenase, which are enzymes that generate inflammation. By reducing inflammation, onions promote beautiful, wrinkle-free skin.

There are even more compounds in onions that help fight inflammation. Vitamin C, quercetin, and isothiocyanates have anti-inflammatory effects on the skin, helping to stop damage to collagen and other structural components of your skin that keep it tight and strong.

Acne Warriors

There is yet another way that onions support beautiful skin. In one cup (160 g) of onions, you get 20 percent of your recommended daily intake of chromium, which is important in the battle against acne. Bacteria is a common cause of acne, and chromium helps reduce skin bacterial infections and thus helps battle acne. Let onions help your skin look glowing and beautiful by including this vegetable in your diet.

Onions can be brown, white, yellow, or red. Thanks to Christopher Columbus, who brought onions to the West Indies, their cultivation has spread throughout the western hemisphere. Today, the leading producers of onions include China, India, the United States, Russia, and Spain.

What's the best onion to eat? That is difficult to answer. There are many different types, including Maui Sweet onion, Vidalia, Spanish, and Walla Walla, to name a few. There are also smaller onions like scallions and pearl onions. Each offers unique culinary advantages, but all offer similar nutritional compounds known to support the health of your body and your skin. Like garlic, onions show up in an endless variety of dishes, from soups (see our Tortilla and Avocado Soup on p. 220) to salads (Avocado, Grapefruit, Pomegranate, and Red Onion Salad on p. 230) to stews (Pumpkin and Chickpea Stew with Couscous on p. 268).

Onions for Colds?

The same compounds in onions that help prevent wrinkle-causing free radical damage—quercetin, vitamin C, and other flavonoids—also help kill harmful bacteria, making onions an especially good addition to soups and stews during cold and flu season.

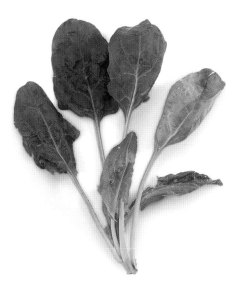

Spinach

One of the original superfoods, spinach was first made popular by Popeye, who ate his can of spinach to give him superior strength. Just one cup (100 g) of boiled spinach contains more than 1000 percent of your daily value of vitamin K and about 300 percent of vitamin A. Plus, one cup gives you most of your daily requirements of manganese, folate, magnesium, and iron. It may not make your muscles stronger, but it sure will help you fight wrinkles.

Cheat Aging by the Dozen

There are more than a dozen different flavonoid compounds in spinach that function as antioxidants, which prevent damage caused by free radicals. In fact, the antioxidant properties of these flavonoids in spinach are so amazing that researchers have created specialized spinach extracts. These extracts have been used in many clinical studies, and have been found to lower free-radical damage associated with aging and cancer.

Spinach is also packed with nutrients that can help with conditions in which inflammation plays a role, including asthma, arthritis, and wrinkles. Vitamins A and C, both found in spinach, have anti-inflammatory properties and thus help prevent free-radical formation.

Breathe Deeply and Nourish Your Skin

Iron is one of the most important minerals in your body. Red blood cells carry oxygen from your lungs to the tissues in the rest of your body, and iron is an integral component of the compound in red blood cells, hemoglobin, that transports oxygen.

Hemoglobin is also part of key enzyme systems that produce energy and promote metabolism. Your skin is a rapidly regenerating tissue, so its needs for energy, oxygen, and metabolism are particularly high. Without proper iron, your skin cannot repair and regenerate properly, and it cannot create sufficient collagen and elastin, the key elements in skin that keep it firm and tight.

Eating spinach can offer your body the iron it needs to provide sufficient oxygen to your skin to keep it healthy and firm. Iron is particularly important for menstruating women who are at risk for iron deficiency. Spinach is the best source of iron for your skin because the other most popular source, red meat, contains wrinkle-promoting compounds. In one cup (100 g) of boiled spinach, you'll get 36 percent of your daily value for iron.

Eat Your Wrinkles Away

How can you get this wrinkle-reducing vegetable into your diet? When dining at a restaurant, order dishes with "à la Florentine" in their name, as this means they are prepared on a bed of spinach. The name originated from the Italian Catherine de Medici, who, in the sixteenth century, married the King of France but brought along her own cooks to prepare her food. To honor her native city of Florence, she reportedly dubbed any dish containing spinach "Florentine."

There are many ways to prepare this vegetable, which belongs to the same family as chards and beets and thus has a similar taste profile. Spinach and baby spinach are delicate additions to salads and offer the best nutrients when eaten raw. Lightly steaming spinach offers a more robust and acidic flavor, without too much loss in wrinkle-fighting nutrients. There are three different types of spinach commonly available at the market: savoy (or curly leaf), smooth leaf, and baby spinach, all of which are worth trying. For maximum wrinkle-fighting power, choose leaves that are a vibrant green with no signs of yellowing. Store fresh spinach loosely packed in a plastic bag or in your refrigerator crisper for no longer than five days, or its ability to prevent wrinkles will diminish.

WRINKLE-FIGHTING NUTS AND SEEDS

Nuts and seeds are excellent sources of many nutrients, particularly minerals, which tend to get overlooked in favor of vitamins C and E. Your best choice is raw or toasted seeds and nuts because they do not contain the added salt, sugar, and fat found in the salted, roasted, and chocolate- or yogurt-covered versions. Research supports including nuts as part of a healthy diet, and a handful each day is all you need. A great source of protein and fiber, nuts offer a hearty, satisfying snack while you're at work or on the go. Seeds are equally delicious for snacking, and they can be added to salads, desserts, breads, and more. For your skin's sake, keep these tasty, convenient, wrinkle-fighting treats within easy reach.

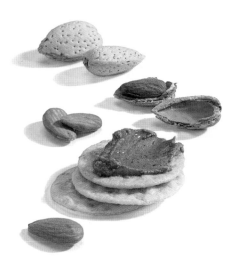

Almonds

The Chinese consider almonds a symbol of female beauty, and for good reason. Edgar Cayce, regarded by some as the father of holistic medicine, recommended the consumption of almonds to improve complexion. Today, we think of almonds as a great wrinkle-fighting food.

Two Heads Are Better than One

Almonds are a source of wrinkle-fighting antioxidants, natural compounds that help your body fight free radicals. Research has revealed compounds in almonds have strong antioxidant activity. A Canadian study, for example, examined the skin of almonds and found high levels of four different types of flavonol glycosides, known to have positive antioxidant effects.

The glycosides in almonds work hand-in-hand with vitamin E, in an action referred to by scientists as synergy. These two antioxidants work together to fight free-radical damage, one of the main factors known to cause wrinkle-forming damage to the skin.

Vitamin E is a well-known antioxidant that acts like a free-radical scavenger, searching your skin cells and guarding them against wrinkle-causing damage. Almonds are one of the best sources of this skin-protecting antioxidant. Plus, vitamin E combats the damaging effects of cigarette smoke on the skin.

Neutralizes Free Radicals and Fights Inflammation

There is yet another way that almonds may offer your skin wrinkle-fighting benefits. Because inflammation causes wrinkles, and studies show that almonds have an anti-inflammatory effect—due to their high omega-3 fatty acids content—they can stop one of the causes of wrinkles before it starts.

No Dieting Here

Do not be concerned with rumors that almonds are fattening. A study in the *British Journal of Nutrition* reported that eating up to two one-ounce (28 g, or 20 to 25 almonds) servings of almonds per day increases satiety—that is, it helps you feel full and satisfied. Consequently, almonds may actually play a role in weight management. When you eat this satisfying, nutritious, wrinkle-fighting snack, you feel satisfied and choose to eat less of those other, not-so-healthy snacks. This is in part because almonds are a great source of fiber.

There are lots of ways to incorporate these wrinkle-fighting nuts into your diet. Sprinkle them on salads, eat them as a snack, or include them in your favorite trail mix or muesli (see recipe on p. 194). To add texture and richness, we even added almonds to our recipe for Romesco Dipping Sauce (p. 212).

When storing almonds, remember that air, heat, and humidity can affect them. Those in shells have the longest shelf life. When buying almonds from a bulk bin, make sure that the store has quick product turnover. Look for almonds that are uniform in color and not withered or limp. Almonds should smell nutty and sweet—a sharp or bitter odor indicates that they have turned rancid. Choose "dry roasted" almonds over "roasted," as the former have not been cooked in oil, and check that the label does not include sugar, preservatives, or syrups, all of which counter-act the healthy aspects of this wrinkle-fighting food. Eat whole almonds for the best wrinkle protection, as the skin of almonds is particularly full of antioxidants.

Almonds are also ground into flours and used to make milks suitable for vegans and anyone with lactose intolerance. For people with peanut allergies, almond butter is a delicious alternative.

Flaxseeds

Flaxseeds are one of the most popular health foods because of their unique nutritional content. Known for their ability to reduce hot flashes during menopause, flaxseeds are also packed with healthy compounds that can help fight wrinkles.

Mega-Wrinkle Protection
Flaxseeds are best known for their fatty content in the form of omega-3 fatty acids, which can reduce skin-damaging inflammation. Flaxseed is one of the few vegetarian sources of omega-3 fatty acids (fish is the other great source). One omega-3 fatty acid found in this seed is alpha linoleic acid, and it acts as an antioxidant in the skin.

Adding flaxseeds to your daily routine can help your skin fight the inflammatory damage that causes wrinkles. Where does this inflammation come from? Every day your skin does battle against toxins and ultra-violet radiation (sunlight) in the environment, which injure your skin cells and triggers inflammation. Inflammation involves white blood cells that produce free radicals that damage the skin. By reducing inflammation, omega-3 fatty acids can inhibit the production of free radicals by white

A Hearty Snack
Researchers recommend that almonds be included in most diets, as studies have connected almond consumption with heart-healthy effects. They are thought to elevate the good cholesterol in the blood (high density lipo-proteins, or HDL) and lower the levels of bad cholester-ol in the blood (low density lipoproteins, or LDL). Also, the fact that they improve circulation in your body means oxygen and wrin-kle-fighting nutrients like vitamin E can reach your skin cells.

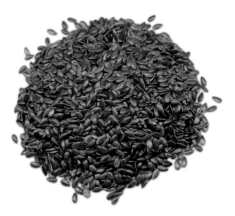

blood cells. Because inflammation leads to damage to the skin and damage to your skin means wrinkles, omega-3 fatty acids have clear wrinkle-fighting power.

Keeps Your Hormones in Check

Because hormones play a role in skin appearance and aging, changes in the skin are obvious at times of hormone fluctuations, such as in adolescence and menopause. As such, phytohormones (substances in foods that mimic the actions of hormones in the body) have become an area of interest by skin researchers.

In 2002, date palm kernel was investigated as a rich source of phytohormones. Application of date palm kernel to the skin around the eye reduced surface wrinkles by almost 30 percent and reduced the depth of wrinkles by 3.5 percent, likely due to phytohormones. Other foods with phytohormones, such as flaxseeds and soy, may also help fight wrinkles in a similar way.

Flaxseeds also contain a high concentration of a type of phytohormone called lignan, a good fat. Lignans are phytoestrogens; they mimic some effects of estrogen because they have a similar structure to estrogen. As such, they offer women a natural way to fight symptoms of lower estrogen levels, like the hot flashes associated with menopause.

Low estrogen levels are also known to have detrimental effects on your skin, including a decreased ability to correct skin damage like wrinkles. Therefore, phytoestrogens in foods like flaxseed might help keep your skin beautiful and youthful as you hit menopause. They also offer your skin additional antioxidant protection from wrinkles.

When eating flaxseeds, be sure to mill or grind them, as most of these wrinkle-fighting nutrients are found inside the seed. For added texture and crunch, sprinkle organic milled flaxseed on cereal, yogurt, oatmeal, and smoothies (we've included it in both our smoothie recipes on pp. 190 and 192). Just remember to keep it in the fridge to prevent its skin-beautifying oils from going rancid.

Sunflower Seeds

Sprinkled on salads, added to your nut mix, or eaten on their own, sunflower seeds are a fabulous food that can help you fight wrinkles. Sunflower seeds contain lignans, phenolic acids, vitamin E, and omega-6 fatty acids, all of which can help your skin look youthful and radiant.

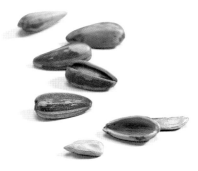

Blooming with Antioxidants

Like flaxseeds, sunflower seeds also contain lignan phytoestrogens, which are known to help fight wrinkles. Phytoestrogens have antioxidant abilities, which means they can reduce free radical damage to your skin's structure. Such damage makes skin less firm and ultimately leads to wrinkle formation.

Another antioxidant compound in sunflower seeds is called phenolic acid. One type of phenolic acid is chlorogenic acid, a potent antioxidant. And more antioxidants mean more wrinkle-fighting power in every bite.

Cure Wrinkles: Eat Fat

Although it may sound strange, certain fats are good for you and can help your skin fight wrinkles. Good fats such as linoleic acid, an omega-6 fatty acid, play an important role in skin health. Fats make up the majority of your skin cells' outer membranes, which are very important to the health of your skin. A cell's membrane controls what enters and leaves the cell. A healthy cell membrane allows all the important nutrients to enter a cell, such as those nutrients needed to prevent wrinkle-causing oxidation. Linoleic acid is present in high quantities in sunflower oil, which means that it can help your skin cell membranes get all the wrinkle-fighting nutrients they need to look youthful and radiant.

Sunflower oil is a good omega-6-containing oil to use in high-heat cooking, such as sautéing. It does not smoke at high temperatures. Of note, other omega-6 containing oils cannot be heated. Olive oil, which has a better fat profile, is good for medium-heat cooking only because it will begin to smoke at higher heats, indicating that the oil has spoiled.

Snack Up

Sunflower seeds are a source of phosphorus, copper, manganese, and selenium, all of which are important minerals for your bones and skin and for supporting your immune system. High in protein and fiber, sunflower seeds make a perfect snack. We added them to our Tamari-Flavored Snack Mix (p. 204) for a treat that blends chewy sweet raisins and dried cranberries with the savory crunch of peanuts and sunflower and pumpkin seeds.

A Necessary Nutrient

In its oil form, sunflower seeds are an outstanding source of vitamin E, the most important fat-soluble antioxidant in your body. It has the ability to both protect your skin from ultraviolet light and prevent cell damage from free radicals.

Sunflower seeds will make you feel full and stave off cravings for less skin-healthy foods like potato chips and donuts. Sprinkle sunflower seeds over a salad or in a stir-fry for a delicious crunch and vitamin E boost.

In all forms, sunflower seeds offer potent wrinkle-fighting power to your skin. Go ahead and use sunflower oil in your next culinary creation or enjoy the crunchy seeds in their natural form—both are winning ways to cure your wrinkles.

WRINKLE-FIGHTING FOODS FOR BREAKFAST, DINNER, TEA, AND TREATS

A wrinkle-fighting diet consists of more than fruits, vegetables, nuts, and seeds. You can also fight wrinkles with a cup of tea, a morsel of meat, or a bite of chocolate. Other comfort foods can help you fight wrinkles as well, like a bowl of oatmeal on cold winter mornings. One bowl a day is recommended for heart health, and will offer your skin loads of iron and other vitamins.

You've no doubt heard that green tea fights cancer, but you may not know that green tea is packed with nutrients that fight wrinkles. Meat is also a very important part of your skin's health. And two to three servings of fish a week is part of any healthy diet, including a healthy diet designed to fight wrinkles. Enjoy the following nutrient-packed foods throughout your day and you're sure to boost your wrinkle-fighting power.

Chocolate

Chocolate comes from cocoa beans, which are a terrific source of many antioxidants. In fact, cocoa has more antioxidants than red wine or green tea. These antioxidants help your skin neutralize free radicals before they damage the structures in your skin that keep it tight and youthful looking.

Dark Is Best!
Before you load your purse with a dozen chocolate bars, however, you need to know that not all chocolate is created equal. When cocoa beans are converted into chocolate bars, they can lose a lot of their antioxidants. That means that the best source of these wrinkle-fighting antioxidants is a cup of cocoa or a dark chocolate bar. Milk chocolate bars are not a great

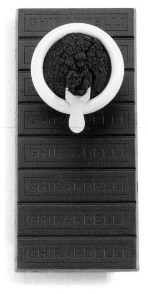

choice because they contain added saturated fat that can reduce the ability of the antioxidants in the chocolate to benefit your skin.

A cup (235 ml) of hot cocoa made with skim milk may be the best choice of all, in fact, because of its low amount of fat—about one-third of a gram of fat per one-cup (235 ml) serving, compared with eight grams of fat in a standard-size 1.5 oz (40 g) milk chocolate bar—and its high amount of antioxidants. In a 2002 study published in the American Chemical Society's *Journal of Agricultural and Food Chemistry,* researchers found that a cup of cocoa is twice as rich in antioxidants as a glass of red wine, up to three times richer than a cup of green tea, and up to five times richer than black tea.

Fights Wrinkles and Inflammation

Chocolate has been linked to improved heart health because it combats inflammation, and it is thought to improve your skin's ability to fight wrinkles for the same reason. When damage caused by free radicals triggers an inflammatory response, the result is redness and puffy skin. Enjoying a warm cup of cocoa in the evening or eating a piece of dark chocolate after dinner may help you avoid having puffy eyes the next morning.

The purist will reach for a bar of dark chocolate, but if you're looking for other ways to enjoy chocolate's skin-healthy benefits, try our Tropical Flavors Snack Mix on page 206, which includes dark chocolate chips, or the Chocolate Yogurt Mousse on page 278, a low-fat dessert that is guaranteed to wow your dinner guests.

Green Tea

Green tea has become one of the world's most popular beverages. It has been proclaimed one of the most antioxidant-rich drinks on earth and has gained popularity as an anti-aging superfood. But people aren't just drinking it; green tea extracts are showing up in all sorts of food and cosmetics, including dietary supplements, snack bars, and skin care products.

One of the World's Best Antioxidants

The healthy compounds found in green tea have outstanding antioxidant abilities—in fact, green tea is among the top ten most antioxidant-rich foods on earth. Antioxidants stop free radicals from damaging collagen, elastin, and skin cells.

Epigallocatechin-3-gallate (EGCG) is the active compound in green tea thought to be responsible for its amazing antioxidant ability. It appears to

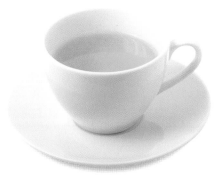

prevent the movement of white blood cells into the skin, protecting skin from the damaging oxidizing products that they release and thus preventing wrinkle formation.

EGCG is also a powerful anti-inflammatory agent, as it inhibits the expression of a key gene involved in the inflammatory response. Because inflammation increases the presence of free radicals and other damaging compounds in the skin, which can ultimately lead to wrinkles, green tea is an ally you truly want to have on your side.

Enjoy the Sun Again

Sunlight contains a particularly harmful ultraviolet radiation called UVB. Exposure to UVB rays causes free radical stress, a type of injury to the skin, as well as photoaging (skin damage caused by the sun), all of which leads to wrinkle formation. Research conducted in 2001 confirmed that the antioxidants in green tea help reduce damage to the skin and DNA cells from sunlight. Green tea helps the skin stay on top of regeneration, which is required to reduce the signs of wrinkles and aging.

Green tea also improves the skin's elasticity. In a 2005 study published in the journal *Dermatologic Surgery,* researchers found that the women taking green tea supplements showed improvement in their skin's elastic content. Increasing the elasticity of the skin helps it rebound after repeated movement and retain a smooth, wrinkle-free appearance.

Drink Up for a Longer, Healthier Life

Green tea can do more than reduce wrinkles, too—researchers have found that consumption is associated with reduced mortality. They also determined that green tea consumption helps humans maintain their brain power as they age. In 2006, the American Journal of Clinical Nutrition reported that people who drank more than two cups (475 ml) of green tea per day had a 50 percent lower chance of having cognitive impairment, compared to those who drank less than three cups (710 ml) per week.

Oats

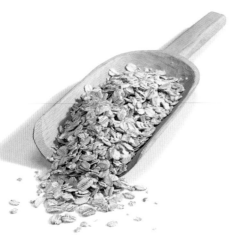

Grown throughout the world, oats are used in many food products. You can find them in bread, porridge, snack bars, cookies, and even beer—in England, an oat stout is made using oats in the brewing process. When it comes to your skin, eating oats—in their healthier forms—provides numerous benefits, including wrinkle-fighting power.

A Superfood That Irons Out Wrinkles

Made popular in the 1980s, when reports linked them to a decreased risk of heart disease, oats still hold a dominate spot in the cereal aisles today. They are also a good source of dietary fiber, magnesium, phosphorus, and manganese, which are all needed for optimal health. And oats are, most importantly, excellent wrinkle fighters.

One cup (80 g) of oats provides you with 41 percent of your recommended daily intake of iron, which plays a key role in oxygen movement in your body. When the skin receives proper oxygen supplies, regeneration and repair of skin cells can occur, creating skin that is thick, strong, and wrinkle free. The result is a youthful, glowing appearance. A lack of oxygen to your skin cells, however, slows skin metabolism sufficiently and reduces the skin's ability to regenerate and repair.

Note that many women suffer from an iron deficiency, which can make them feel sluggish and have a grey complexion. A physician can help determine your iron status.

Cysteine Fights Damage and Inflammation

Perhaps one of the best reasons to include oats in your wrinkle-fighting diet is that they contain the amino acid cysteine, a super-powered, multi-leveled, wrinkle-fighting nutrient.

Cysteine is necessary for the formation of keratin, a protein in the skin that, along with collagen and elastin, helps keep it firm and strong. Keratin also makes this outermost layer of the skin almost waterproof.

Cysteine also plays a role in restoring the natural pool of antioxidants in the body, including glutathione, an antioxidant that protects cells from toxins. Antioxidants like glutathione prevent free radicals from causing damage to the skin that can reduce its strength and lead to wrinkles. Thus, cysteine prevents wrinkles by supporting skin structure and promoting keratin production, and it prevents damage to that structure by restoring antioxidants.

Finally, cysteine protects the skin against wrinkles by reducing the production of inflammatory chemicals. Inflammation creates free radical products that can cause damage to the skin, which can compromise the skin's integrity and lead to the formation of wrinkles.

Revitalizes Skin

Oats are a rich source of thiamin, a B vitamin, important to cells because it plays a role in energy production. Every cell in your body needs B vitamins to help produce energy required for maintenance, growth, and repair. Skin cells are among the most active cells in your body because

N-acetyl Cysteine (NAC)
NAC is a popular supplement derived from cysteine. NAC is not present in food, but rather is created by the body from cysteine. Studies suggest that the supplement may play a helpful role in the immune system, heavy metal detoxification, and breaking down mucus buildup.

they regenerate quickly, and without sufficient B vitamins, the process slows down. Slow regeneration of skin cells is associated with signs of aging, including wrinkles. Your skin cells also need thiamin to help make the necessary energy to repair damage caused by wrinkle-causing free radicals.

There are so many tasty ways to include oats into your daily diet. Rolled oats can be added to your muesli (see p. 194 for our recipe) or a favorite cookie or bread recipe. Oat bran is easy to include in your daily diet by sprinkling it on yogurt or cereal, or adding it to salad dressings. No matter how you choose to add oats to your diet, the thiamin, cysteine, and iron they contain can help fight wrinkle formation and minimize existing wrinkles.

Tuna

Tuna is known for its brain-boosting benefits, but it's also a great cure for wrinkles. Cold-water fish, such as salmon and tuna, are rich sources of omega-3 fatty acids necessary for beautiful looking skin. Thanks to new scientific research noting tuna's ability to fight heart disease, cancer, and arthritis, and improve brain functioning and skin appearance, it's become an increasingly popular food.

What's the Fatty Deal?

Tuna contains the omega-3 fatty acids docosahexaenoic acid (DHA) and eicosapentaenoic acid (EPA). DHA is known to boost mental energy and increase brain activity. EPA is one of the best anti-inflammatory nutrients on earth and is particularly effective at protecting against inflammation due to injury from chemicals or sunlight. Such inflammation makes the skin's structure less strong and rigid, which in turn encourages it to fold or wrinkle.

Scientists have also identified fat compounds made from EPA in our body called resolvins, which have been shown to reduce inflammation in animal studies by inhibiting the production and movement of inflammatory messengers, thus reducing inflammation.

Tuna Sunscreen

If you were to use tuna as a sunscreen, you may not smell good, but your skin would love you. The omega-3 fatty acids in tuna can protect your skin from sunburns. Research from the University of Manchester, UK suggests that eating more omega-3–rich fish, such as tuna, can lessen the

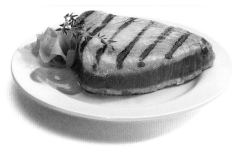

inflammation caused by exposure to UVB radiation. Reducing inflammation from sunburns can help prevent not only the pain of sunburns, but also their damaging effects, like sun spots and wrinkles.

Packed with Nutrients That Help Skin Repair

Tuna is packed with nutrients that support skin health. It is a source of selenium, niacin, and vitamin B6, all of which are essential to proper cell metabolism. The skin is a rapidly dividing tissue that requires these and other nutrients to support its quick cell turnover. Without proper turnover, our skin cannot maintain its firmness and wrinkles can form.

Where should you get your dose of wrinkle-fighting tuna? Look for whole, fresh tuna buried in ice at the market or fishmonger. Tuna fillets and steaks should be placed on top of ice. Stay away from tuna with dry or brown spots or a fishy smell, as these indicate that the fish is not fresh. At home, your refrigerator is a little too warm for storing fish, so to maintain optimal freshness, place crushed ice in a baking dish in the refrigerator and lay your fish on top or in it, just as you found it at the market.

If fresh tuna is not available, the next best choice is canned tuna. Tuna can be packed in oil, broth, or water. Opt for water-packed tuna because tuna packed in oil has added vegetable oil, which is high in omega-6 fatty acids. This type of fatty acid is commonly over-consumed in the Western diet, while omega-3 fatty acid consumption is often too low. An imbalance between the two can lead long-term diseases such as heart disease, cancer, asthma, arthritis, and depression.

Your skin will thank you if you consume fish three times a week. Salmon, anchovies, sardines, tuna, and mackerel are the best sources of wrinkle-fighting omega-3 fatty acids.

Fresh Fish or Capsules?

Distilled fish oil in supplement form offers a mercury- and PCB-free alternative to fresh fish, and guarantees that you consume enough omega-3 fatty acids to support your skin health. Enteric-coated pills are best for avoiding fishy burps.

Fresh fish is, on the other hand, a great source of protein and many other nutrients, however. As such, most dietitians recommend a combination of supplements and fresh fish.

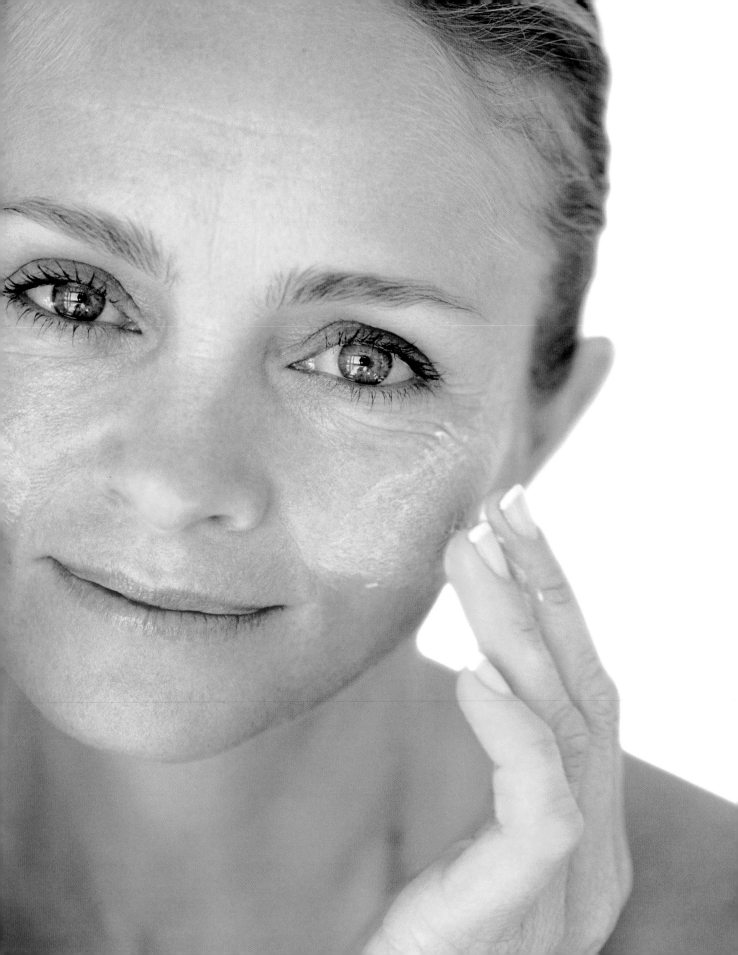

Foods That Moisturize

ACHIEVING THE PERFECT moisture balance allows the full beauty of your skin to shine through. If it's too dry, skin can appear tight, red, and flaky, and can accentuate the signs of wrinkles. If it's too oily, skin can look shiny and have blocked pores and acne. Finding the perfect moisture level for skin to emit a radiant glow can be a challenge—which might explain why moisturizer sales have been growing at rates of up to 25 percent around the world—but it's a challenge that can easily be overcome by paying attention to diet and the foods that pass through your lips.

How Our Skin Maintains Moisture

The skin contains many layers. The outermost layer of the epidermis, known as the stratum corneum, is responsible for regulating water loss and retention. Many factors influence the level of hydration in the stratum corneum: fat (intracellular laminar lipids); the natural moisturizing factor, or NMF, which is comprised of the components that make sure the structure of the epidermis is intact; and the structure of the skin layer itself. Additional components that help maintain proper moisture are hyaluronan, a compound involved in tissue repair and natural humectants, such as glycerol, that draw water from within the skin to the surface. (Many cosmetic products contain glycerol because it helps skin appear well hydrated.)

Conversely, the body's ability to create NMF and intracellular laminar lipids depends on the moisture level in the stratum corneum. This means that if the skin is dehydrated, it is less able to produce the hydrating compounds that inhibit water loss from the skin. It becomes a vicious cycle. Therefore, keeping the skin hydrated is of utmost importance.

As the temperature rises in the summer, for example, be sure to drink more water and eat more fruits and vegetables to protect your skin from dehydration. In the winter, eating foods with high water content and drinking lots of water is equally important, particularly if you live in regions of the world where most of your day is spent in furnace-heated buildings, which can be dehydrating to the skin.

Keeping your skin moisturized is important not only for having a desirable glow but also for proper wound healing, particularly with acute injuries. The health and beauty of your skin requires that these injuries be repaired properly and quickly, and moisture is a must for that to happen. Without it, skin can become dry, crack, and break. Sunlight can further damage and burn skin cells.

There are multiple ways we can eat our way to moist, beautiful skin. Water is the most obvious way to hydrate the skin, but what else can help?

Luscious Lipids

Lipids are the oily components within the skin that provide a barrier to slow the loss of moisture; they are critical to healthy skin appearance. Many nutrients are lipids, including lutein, vitamin E, linolenic acid, and lecithin.

Lutein can improve the moisture content of the skin and is sometimes added to topical skin products to help moisturize. It can also help moisturize the skin from the inside out. In a human clinical trial, daily consumption of 10 mg of lutein increased skin hydration. Plus, lutein has been found to improve the skin's elasticity and to help fight signs of aging.

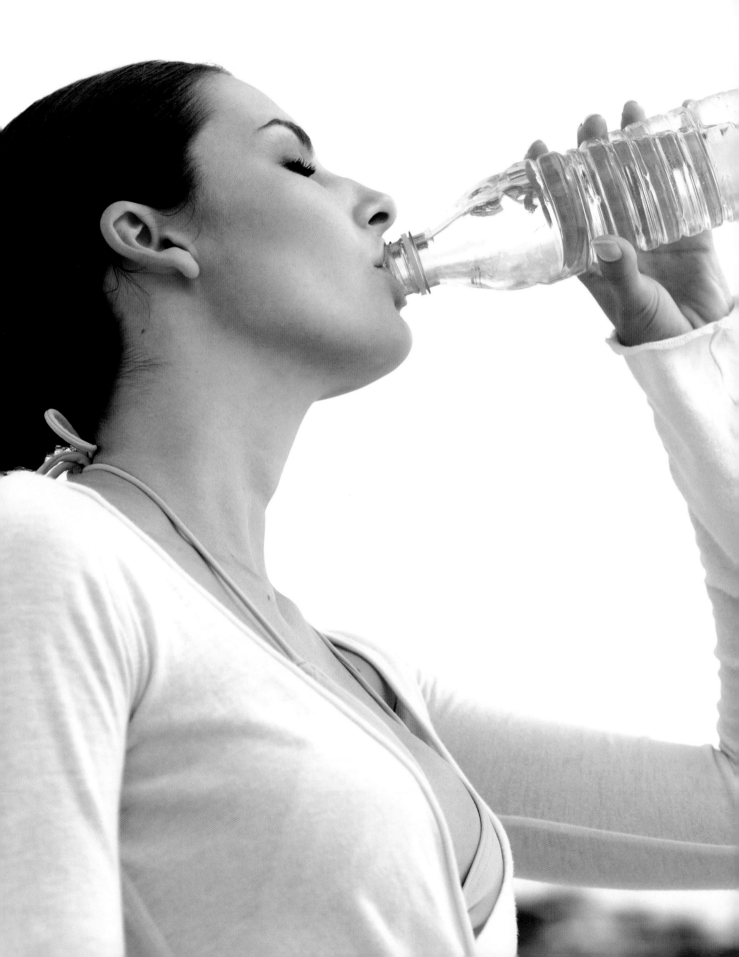

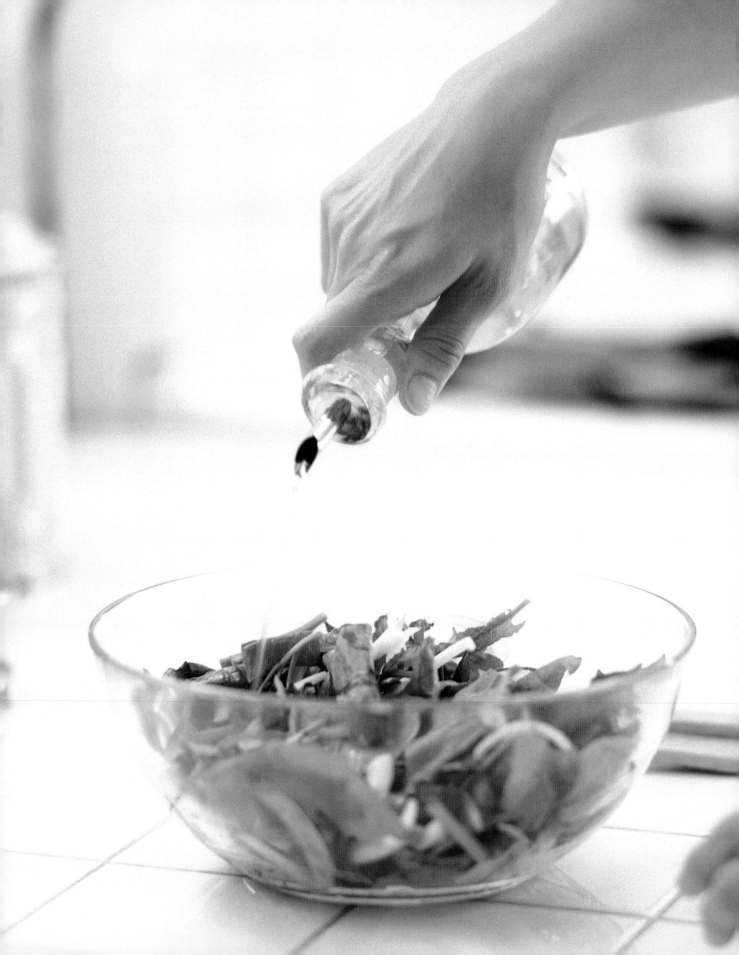

Vitamin E is a very popular antioxidant in topical skin products. This fat-soluble vitamin can improve skin moisture, increase smoothness, and provide mild protection from ultraviolet sun damage. There is no need to slather on this antioxidant, however; instead, you can moisturize your skin by eating foods that are high in vitamin E, such as nuts, seeds, and green leafy vegetables.

Linolenic acid, an omega-6 fatty acid, is a well known moisturizer of the skin. Borage oil and evening primrose oil are the richest sources of linolenic acid and are very effective moisturizing oils. They can be added to food or used topically to improve the moisture of the skin by improving its lipid content.

Lecithin, a type of fat, is found in soybeans and eggs. Lecithin contains fatty acids, primarily omega-6 fatty acids and a small amount of omega-3 fatty acids. Because these fats are liquid at room temperature, we call them oils. Lecithin is commonly found in topical hydrating products. It acts as a humectant that draws water from within the skin to the surface layer.

Don't Wither Away

Is it true that dry skin causes wrinkles? No, but dry skin can make wrinkles more pronounced. Drinking sufficient water and eating foods that contain moisturizing fats and a high water content can keep your skin properly hydrated and prevent wrinkles from becoming more visible. Cosmetic products containing moisturizers can temporarily puff up the skin with water and reduce wrinkles; however, this effect is only temporary, so it makes little sense to waste hundreds of dollars on these products—especially when diet can do a great deal to improve moisture content and the aging appearance of skin.

With age comes a natural drying of the skin. In women, this is partly due to the natural drop in estrogen levels after menopause. Estrogen prevents skin from aging, increases the skin's thickness, and improves skin's moisture content. Following menopause, when women no longer produce estrogen, the results in the skin become obvious and include a decrease in skin moisture content. Some nutrients in foods, however, can mimic the effects of estrogen in the body and may help reduce the dryness associated with age-related drops in estrogen levels. By reducing the dryness of the skin, the appearance of wrinkles decreases, giving the appearance of youthful, radiant skin.

In a study published in the October 2007 issue of the *American Journal of Clinical Nutrition,* researchers used data from the National Health and Nutrition Examination Survey to examine the relationship between the appearance of the skin in older age and the consumption of nutrients.

They found that people who ate more foods containing vitamin C and alpha linoleic acid (an omega-3 fatty acid) were less likely to suffer from dry skin in their later years. Those who consumed higher amounts of fatty foods and processed carbohydrates had less beautiful skin.

Thirteen Foods That Moisturize

To improve the texture of your skin and reduce fine lines, increase your intake of nutrients like the ones mentioned above and make sure your system is properly hydrated. Try to avoid drinking dehydrators such as alcohol and coffee. Instead, aim for 6 to 8 glasses of distilled water or herbal tea daily.

Following is a list of thirteen nutritious foods that will help moisturize your skin from the inside out:

Luscious Lipids
- Avocado
- Borage Oil
- Coconut Oil
- Grape Seed Oil
- Olive Oil

Hydrating Heros
- Tea
- Stevia
- Water
- Watermelon

Dryness Disrupters
- Kelp
- Lentils
- Pumpkin
- Zucchini

LUSCIOUS LIPIDS

Eating fat is good for you! But it's important to remember that not all fats are created equal. Good fats, such as those found in the following foods, are beneficial to your overall health and your skin's appearance. The recommended daily allowance of fat is 65 g per day. Of that, only 20 g should be saturated fat, a so-called bad fat, which means that most of your daily intake of fat should come from polyunsaturated and monounsaturated fats, two types of unsaturated fat. These healthy fats are found in fish, nuts, seeds, and oils from plants. So ditch your fat phobia and remember these words—healthy skin needs healthy fats.

Avocado

Whoa, hold your horses. Have you been avoiding avocados because they contain 15 percent of your recommended daily amount of fat? Time to stop. Fats are among the most important skin-moisturizing nutrients you can have in your arsenal. If you want radiant, smooth, glowing skin, all you have to do is start peeling.

Fatten Up? Not a Chance!

Avocados will not increase your waist size. Let's compare an avocado with butter: First off, in two tablespoons (28 g), an avocado has 50 calories, while butter has 240 calories. The real difference, however, is the type of fats in these two foods. Avocados contain lots of skin-healthy polyunsaturated and monounsaturated fats, which help control skin's moisture level. By contrast, butter is full of saturated fats, which are known to increase inflammation and compromise skin health.

Mean Green Moisturizing Machine

Keeping skin moisturized helps ensure that you have a smooth, consistent complexion. A loss of moisture in the skin can lead to a reduction in healing, which can promote signs of wrinkles, as well as inflammation, redness, and puffiness. Luckily, avocados contain more of the carotenoid lutein, a fat that helps moisturize the skin, than any other fruit. Avocados are also rich in B vitamins, which help with metabolism and energy. These vitamins need to be metabolized constantly to ensure that the skin's moisture stays balanced.

There are many other nutrients in avocados that promote beautiful, moist skin. Avocados have 60 percent more potassium than bananas;

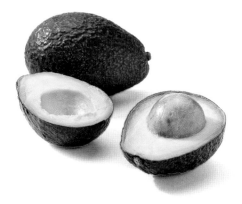

one cup (150 g) of avocado slices provides you with roughly 25 percent of the recommended intake. Potassium plays an important role in fluid balance in the body, including the moisture content in the skin.

Finally, avocados contain the skin healthy nutrients vitamins E and K. Vitamin E is the most important fat-soluble antioxidant in the skin; as fats are a major component of the skin's moisture, it's essential to have sufficient vitamin E to prevent cell damage from free radicals. Vitamin K is another fat-soluble vitamin, which plays a role in both blood clotting and bone health.

Absorb More Nutrients with a Slice of Avocado

Enjoying a little bit of avocado along with carotenoid-rich vegetables and fruits is an excellent way to improve your body's ability to absorb skin-healthy nutrients. In a study published in the March 2005 issue of the *Journal of Nutrition,* researchers tested the theory that since carotenoids are lipophilic (meaning fat-loving or soluble in fat), consuming monounsaturated-rich avocado along with carotenoid-rich foods like vegetables might enhance carotenoid absorption in the body. And the theory proved true. They found that adding even a small amount of avocado (e.g., 2 ounces/57 g) to a salad of carrot, lettuce, and baby spinach, or to salsa, greatly increased the body's ability to absorb the carotenoids alpha-carotene, beta-carotene, lycopene, and lutein, all of which protect the skin.

Not sure how to incorporate this skin-moisturizing food into your diet? Add diced avocado to your next salad. Make guacamole by mashing a ripe avocado with garlic and lemon (two other skin-healthy foods) and enjoy it with whole-grain tortilla chips. Or spread avocado on toast and top with slices of ripe tomato and crumbled goat cheese. Whichever way you choose to eat it, your skin will radiate beauty thanks to avocado's many moisturizing nutrients.

Borage Oil

Borage oil is a little-known secret for keeping your skin healthy. Able to be applied topically or taken internally, it is the ultimate skin hydrator, restoring moisture and smoothness to dry and damaged skin.

From Flower to Seed to Oil

Borage is a wildflower commonly called the starflower. Grown throughout the world, it is a relatively large plant, with star-shaped, bright blue flowers. There's no need to go digging in ditches for it, however, because borage oil—cultivated from the seeds of the plant—can easily be found at your local health food store. The oil is very beneficial to the skin and is the richest known source of gamma-linolenic acid (GLA), an essential fatty acid that helps moisturize the skin.

Scientists believe that borage oil helps restore the intracellular moisture barrier of skin that is either chronically dry or has been environmentally damaged. In a clinical trial, subjects with dry skin were given a cream containing borage oil to apply topically to their skin for a period of two weeks. The results indicated that borage oil is effective at restoring moisture and smoothness to dry skin. Additional research conducted on the effects of supplement form of borage oil has suggested that the oil can also be taken internally as a means of promoting healthy skin in people with dry skin conditions.

Gives You the Fatty Acids You Need

GLA is produced in your body from linoleic acid, another essential fatty acid, which is found in many foods such as nuts, seeds, and most unrefined vegetable oils, like sunflower oil. In a healthy person, linoleic acid is converted to GLA through enzymes in the body, and in turn, GLA converts to a hormone-like substance called prostaglandin E1 (PGE1), which acts as an anti-inflammatory. As such, PGE1 is useful in the treatment of rheumatoid arthritis, Raynaud's disease, atherosclerosis, and skin conditions.

Borage oil is unique in that it provides the body directly with GLA, rather than providing linoleic acid alone, which would then have to be converted by the body into GLA; essentially, borage oil cuts out the dirty work. It's also important to note that as we age, our bodies become less efficient at converting linoleic acid to GLA, so obtaining this fatty acid directly is the most surefire way to stay out of inflammation's way.

Clinically Proven

GLA is essential to skin health, as a deficiency in GLA has been detected in sufferers of skin disorders. Research has found that people with skin disorders characterized by dry skin and inflammation, such as eczema and psoriasis, have an increased level of linoleic acid and low levels of GLA. This suggests that something is blocking the conversion process of linolenic acid to GLA. The outcome is a decrease in PGE1, and this decrease is associated with dry skin and trans-epidermal water loss.

Moral of the story? Supplement the diet with GLA from borage oil or apply borage oil topically to the skin. Researchers have found that even serious skin problems can be improved by borage oil's ability to support the skin's moisture and reduce inflammation.

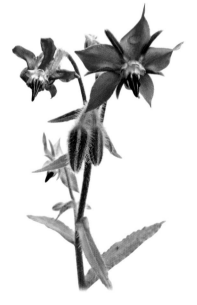

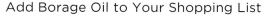

Add Borage Oil to Your Shopping List

Look for borage oil at your local health food store. Moisturize your skin from the inside out every day by sprinkling borage oil on your foods; add it to salad dressings or smoothies. Know that borage oil should not be heated, as heat will change its composition and make it a poor source of GLA.

You can also buy borage oil in capsule form. Because it has a higher concentration of GLA (23 percent) than any other oil, evening primrose and black currant included, less needs to be consumed in order to achieve the required dosage. Follow label instructions carefully.

Coconut Oil

If you can't take the heat, get out of the kitchen. Many oils used for cooking at high heats are a problem for your health. Canola, safflower, and sunflower oils, for example, contain rich amounts of omega-6 fatty acids, which are highly susceptible to heat damage—that is, they become oxidized and unhealthy to consume when brought to high heat. Opting instead for coconut oil—an oil that can take the heat—is a much healthier choice for both the skin and body.

Protects Your Skin's Natural Fats

Coconut oil is derived from the dried fruit of the coconut palm tree and is known for its long shelf-life—it can last up to two years due to its high saturated fat content. In the health arena, it has gained popularity for its resistance to oxidation, which can wreak havoc on the body and skin. Oxidized fats can increase damage to the skin and, as a result, compromise the skin's moisture barrier.

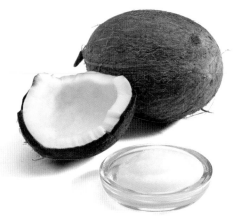

Coconut oil is a topical agent well known for improving the skin's texture, leaving it soft and smooth. It has been used successfully by people with psoriasis because it acts as a skin emollient. Emollients prevent dryness and protect the skin by acting as a barrier against outside forces. Coconut oil can also help in healing keratosis pilaris—a genetic condition in which the skin has many rough bumps—by moisturizing the affected area.

Whether consuming coconut oil is as beneficial for the skin as using it topically is not yet known. However, populations in the South Pacific that have used coconut oil in their cooking for hundreds of years are known to have beautiful skin. Moreover, populations that rely heavily on this oil in their diet are not known for having a high risk of heart disease, despite the oil's high saturated fat content. Scientists believe that this is because most of the saturated fat it contains comes in the form of lauric acid, a healthy fatty acid known for its antimicrobial and antiviral properties.

Approximately 52 percent of the saturated fats in coconut oil are characterized as medium chain fatty acids (which include lauric acid). These fatty acids are sometimes called MCTs in advertisements and are thought to promote fat loss. Lauric acid, for example, is believed to increase the thyroid hormones, thus stimulating metabolism. Some companies have touted coconut oil as the next weight-loss miracle, although no research studies have yet confirmed these claims.

Not All Are Created Equal

Whether you slather it on your skin or use it as a healthier alternative to butter, coconut oil is a good choice for health. Please note, however, that there are different types of coconut oil. Hydrogenated coconut oil is used in food products as a preservative and may promote heart disease. Extra-virgin coconut oil is a healthier form of coconut oil that is not thought to cause heart disease.

And a final note of caution: A diet rich in coconut oil may result in a deficiency of polyunsaturated fatty acids, particularly essential fatty acids known to support the health and moisture level of the skin. So be sure to include fish, flaxseed, borage oil, and evening primrose oil (all of which contain these fatty acids) in your diet along with coconut oil if you plan on consuming it regularly.

Frying Pan Conditioner
In India and Sri Lanka, coconut oil is commonly used for conditioning and styling hair. There, it is known for restoring hair's moisture, softening it and giving it shine, and is also thought to treat dandruff and damaged hair.

Grape Seed Oil

For thousands of years, the grape plant has been appreciated for its medicinal and nutritional value. European folk healers developed an ointment from the sap of grapevines to cure skin and eye diseases, and grape leaves have been known to stop bleeding, inflammation, and pain brought on by hemorrhoids. Now add to the list that grapes are wonderful healers of the skin, and you've got a fruit that truly deserves its star status.

Protects Your Moisture Barrier

Although the nutritional benefits of grapes tend to focus on their skins, the seeds are packed with skin-beautifying nutrients. Vitamin E, flavonoids, linoleic acid, and compounds called procyanidins (e.g., tannins, pycnogenols, proanthocyanidins) are highly concentrated in grape seeds. These active compounds have antioxidant properties; in fact, a study of healthy volunteers found that supplementing the diet with grape seed

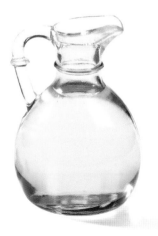

extract substantially increased levels of antioxidants in the blood. Because free radicals are believed to contribute to the skin's aging process and the development of skin conditions, including dryness, the antioxidants found in grape seeds may reduce or even help prevent some of the damage free radicals cause.

Thanks to the abundance of grape seeds available after wine making, grape seed oil is also easy to come by at your local market. Toss grape seed oil in your salad dressing recipe and marinades, or use it topically as a moisturizer. No matter which way you choose to use it, your skin will enjoy a lovely, moisture-rich glow.

Olive Oil

In response to the enormous popularity of olive oil as a healthy oil, more than 750 million olive trees are harvested each year. A major component of the Mediterranean diet, olive oil is known to improve the health of your heart, but it can also improve the moisture level of your skin and much more.

Fights Photoaging

Olive oil has a high concentration of monounsaturated fat, which comprise about 25 percent of the fatty acids in the skin. The monounsaturated fat in olive oil positively influences the fluidity of cell membranes, and when skin cells are more fluid, cell membranes can function more optimally, promoting an appearance of smooth, beautiful skin. In addition, a higher content of monounsaturated fat has been shown in research studies to help the skin reduce oxidative damage, as the fat acts as an antioxidant. This fact may explain why the *Journal of the American College of Nutrition* reported that population studies link higher intakes of olive oil with less photoaging (skin damage caused by the sun).

Offers Vitamin E

This luscious liquid also contains vitamin E, which is potentially the most important fat-soluble antioxidant in the body. One tablespoon (15 ml) of extra-virgin olive oil provides nearly 9 percent of the recommended daily value for vitamin E.

In the skin, vitamin E protects lipids from oxidation, which can damage the skin and lead to a dry appearance. It is also commonly found in topical skin products as it is well known to be an effective skin moisturizer.

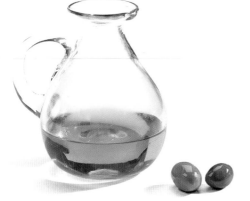

More Powerful than Green Tea

The main polyphenol in olive oil is hydroxytyrosol. This little known nutrient is a silent powerhouse of protection for the skin: It has one of the highest free-radical scavenging abilities of any nutrient on earth. (Quick Refresher: Free radicals are the unstable compounds that form in response to sun damage or inflammation, and they wreak havoc in the cells and damage the cells' structures and DNA. Antioxidants neutralize free radicals and prevent them from causing damage to skin cells, thus helping the skin stay healthy and strong.) Hydroxytyrosol has three times the antioxidant power of epicatechin—found in green tea—and two times that of quercetin—found in apples. In other words, olive oil not only tastes good on bread and salads, but it is also packed with antioxidant power.

Additionally, olive oil contains oleocanthal, an anti-inflammatory nutrient. Reducing inflammation in the skin can promote a healthy, moist complexion by preventing damage to the skin's moisture barrier. In addition, reducing inflammation can prevent puffiness and redness in your complexion.

When incorporating this beautiful, skin-healthy oil into your diet, note that it can be heated to medium heat. It has a higher smoke point than other healthy skin oils, such as borage oil, but it should not be overheated. (For cooking at high heat, use canola oil or coconut oil.)

When purchasing olive oil, keep in mind that there are different types; the best is extra-virgin olive oil, which is the oil extracted from olives on the first press. It has a low acidity and thus offers the best flavor profile. Virgin olive oil has a bit more acidity. Pure olive oil is usually a blend of virgin and refined oil and is not a smart choice for your skin because the refining process can remove some of the oil's healthy nutrients.

Olive Oil's Many Benefits

Oleuropein, the compound responsible for giving extra-virgin olive oil its bitter, pungent taste, is an olive leaf extract with antiviral, antibacterial, and antioxidant properties. The low incidence of heart disease associated with Mediterranean-style diets may be partially due to this compound's effects. Oleuropein's anti-inflammatory action also discourages redness, puffiness, and skin damage.

DRYNESS DISRUPTERS

As we've learned, with age comes a natural drying of the skin. In women, this is partly due to the natural drop in estrogen levels after menopause, which causes a decrease in the skin's moisture content. Luckily, some nutrients in foods can mimic the effects of estrogen in the body and may help reduce dryness. By reducing the dryness of the skin, the appearance of wrinkles decreases, giving the appearance of youthful, radiant skin.

Kelp

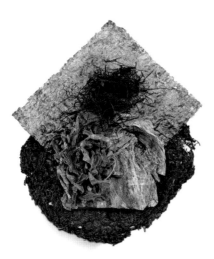

Kelp is a large, leafy, edible seaweed that tends to grow along colder coastlines and is rich in vitamins and minerals. Kelp is an excellent source of iodine, a major component of the hormones thyroxine and triiodothyronine. Maintaining proper levels of these hormones in the body ensures that skin cells can rebuild and repair damage, including damage to the moisture barrier. Kelp also contains vitamin B12, another vitamin that supports skin cell metabolism.

Two-Way Moisturizing Power

Lutein, a lipid found in kelp, supports the skin's moisture barrier in two ways. First, it reinforces the moisture barrier; and second, it is an antioxidant that prevents free radicals from oxidizing and damaging fats in the skin.

Kelp also contains vitamin E and vitamin C. Vitamin E is a fat-soluble antioxidant that protects the fats in the skin's moisture barrier from free-radical damage. It is a common ingredient in topical skin products, as it is well known to support a healthy moisture level in the skin.

Vitamin C is a water-soluble antioxidant that protects the skin from free-radical damage, which may explain why studies have found that people who consume higher amounts of vitamin C are less likely to suffer from dry skin. Vitamin C's ability to improve the moisture content of the skin may also be due to its role in lipid metabolism, as lipids are a major component of the skin's moisture barrier.

It is not recommended that you harvest seaweed off the beach and add it to tonight's dinner (this source can be contaminated or spoiled). Instead, you can find kelp in many specialty stores or as a common ingredient in Japanese restaurants. In addition, kelp powder (available at health food stores) can be sprinkled into smoothies or on cereal or yogurt as a skin moisture-boosting treat.

Lentils

Like other types of beans, lentils are a member of the legume family. Nutrient-dense, they help your skin preserve its radiant, moisturized glow. Lentils contain B vitamins, beta-carotene (vitamin A), and zinc, all of which contribute to maintaining healthy skin.

Caution: Repair Work Ahead

Lentils grow in pods that contain either one or two lentil seeds that are round-, oval-, or heart-shaped disks, and often are smaller than the tip of a pencil eraser. Inside these small seeds you will find the B vitamins folate and thiamin, which are involved in metabolism. The skin is a place of very active metabolism, and if it slows due to a lack of B vitamins, the skin cannot maintain its moisture barrier or repair damage. Healthy skin can hold moisture, but damaged skin cannot. Folate is also particularly supportive of cell production in the skin, making these little seeds an all-around superb food for skin health.

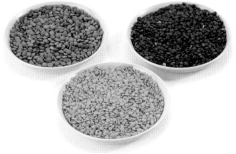

Lentils are also a good source of zinc, which is needed for enzyme production and for cell repair for DNA and RNA. Zinc's ability to promote cell repair makes it a helpful agent against skin dryness. As an added benefit, zinc also plays a role in strengthening the immune system.

The New Comfort Food

Lentils are available in prepackaged containers as well as in bulk bins. As with all food purchased in bulk, make sure that the bins are covered and that the store has good product turnover to ensure maximum freshness. Generally speaking, canned food is not the best choice for your skin, but canned lentils deliver a nutritional value similar to that of dried lentils cooked at home.

There are various ways to add lentils to your diet. The easiest is simply to add them to your favorite soups, pasta sauces, and salads. We combined braised lentils with eggplant and mushrooms (see p. 250 for recipe) for an earthy, satisfying side dish that could easily serve as a hearty dinner when paired with a slice of multigrain bread.

Pumpkin

A pumpkin's bright orange color is your signal that it is loaded with beta-carotene, a powerful antioxidant. Beta-carotene is one of the plant carotenoids that gets converted to vitamin A in the body. Vitamin A acts as an antioxidant to neutralize harmful free radicals in our skin, thereby helping to prevent wrinkles, resist infection, and keep our skin moist and youthful. Without enough vitamin A, our skin becomes dry.

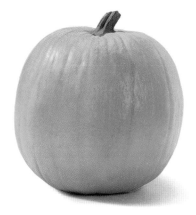

Beautiful Beta-Carotene

The antioxidant abilities of beta-carotene can fight aging in other parts of your body as well. Research indicates that a diet consisting of beta-carotene–rich foods may reduce the risk of developing certain types of cancer and may also protect against heart disease.

Beta-carotene is your body's potent ally for warding off the degenerative aspects of aging. And when it comes to canned pumpkin, you'll find all the beta-carotene you need—one cup (245 g) of canned pumpkin provides more than 400 percent of your recommended daily value. That same serving also provides nearly 20 percent of the recommended daily value for iron, which plays a vital role in the formation of the collagen scaffolding that keeps your skin tight, strong, and smooth.

More Vitamins to Round Out the Pack
Pumpkin also provides you with vitamin C—17 percent of your daily value in one cup of the canned stuff. Vitamin C is an antioxidant that defends your skin against the free radicals that can destroy collagen. Because free radicals are made naturally in your skin, and because vitamin C cannot be stored in your body, it is really important to make sure that your daily diet is stocked with this vitamin.

Not Just for Pie
Not sure how to include pumpkin into your diet other than by baking it in a pie? Here are some quick ideas: Try roasting pumpkin for a delicious spin on winter squash, or pair it with chickpeas and curry in a fabulous fall stew (see p. 268 for recipe).

Abundant in the autumn months, fresh pumpkin is a great skin-healthy food. Canned pumpkin is also fine if that's all that's available. Perfect for soups, breads, and muffins, canned pumpkin is stocked on shelves year round, and it gives you most of the health benefits of fresh pumpkin (plus, it is easier to work with).

Zucchini

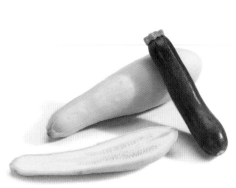

Zucchini, also known as summer squash, is a relative of the melon and cucumber. This vegetable contains many nutrients that can help your skin protect itself from the damage that restricts its ability to retain moisture.

Care for Your Skin with Carotenoids
Green and yellow vegetables are good sources of carotenoids like lutein and zeaxanthin. These carotenoids are not converted into vitamin A in the body like beta-carotene, but they are powerful antioxidants. That means that they neutralize free radicals, which would otherwise steal electrons

from another part of the skin and damage it. The antioxidants found in zucchini can help prevent free-radical damage to the moisture barrier and help promote beautiful skin.

Mighty Lutein Protects

With healthy eyes, you can better see your skin's beauty. Lutein is most known for its ability to protect the eyes from light-induced damage and aging, and it may also protect the skin from damage and aging in the same way it protects the eyes.

Research trials have determined that the lutein found in zucchini promotes skin health by reducing inflammation responses. When the skin is exposed to ultraviolet light (sunlight), lutein reduces the inflammation response. This ability of the lutein in zucchini to reduce inflammation means that exposure to sunlight will produce less damage to skin structure, including the moisture barrier. The result is more beautiful, moist skin.

HYDRATING HEROS

Drinking sufficient liquids and eating foods that contain moisturizing fats and a high water content is vital for keeping your skin properly hydrated and preventing wrinkles. Instead of wasting money on pricey cosmetic products that offer only temporary fixes, try incorporating the following foods into your diet to naturally improve moisture content and beautify your skin.

Tea

It's tea time. Take a break in the afternoon—or morning, or evening—and reap the benefits of this skin-smart beverage. Tea's water content alone is reason enough to make you reach for a cup and drink to your skin's health—without water, your body becomes dehydrated and your skin turns dry and can appear flaky, red, and irritated. Tea's benefits, however, extend far beyond its water qualities.

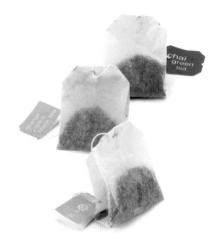

Cup of Protection

Almost one quarter of tea is antioxidants, which prevent free-radical damage to a cell's DNA. If the lipids or DNA of the moisture barrier are damaged, the result is compromised water control and dry skin. Tea delivers a host of antioxidants called phenols, which are also present in berries and grapes, to keep the skin healthy and hydrated.

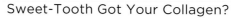

Quercetin: Fit for a Queen

Tea contains antioxidant compounds called flavonoids, which include catechins, epicatechins, thearubigins, rutin, and quercetin. Rutin is a very strong antioxidant: Research studies in animals have found that rutin can prevent damage to skin cells and therefore has a healing effect. Quercetin has also received rave reviews for its ability to prevent free radicals from causing damage to cells.

Tea's many antioxidants are water-soluble, so brewing your tea bag in hot water speeds the release of these antioxidants from the tea leaves. Once in your glass, the antioxidants can travel throughout your body, spreading health and vitality.

Which type of tea is best for your skin? Green and black teas are loaded with antioxidants. Herbal teas have relatively fewer antioxidants, but they will moisturize your skin as they hydrate your the body, unlike alcohol and soda (which have dehydrating effects).

Avoid adding sugar to your cup of tea, since sugar is not healthy for your skin or your body—it speeds up your natural aging process, making your skin look older than it otherwise would. Plus, eating sugar replaces other calories in your diet that are healthier for your skin. If you prefer a sprinkle of sweetness, try adding stevia or honey to your tea. These natural sweeteners are not as bad for your skin as white sugar.

Stevia

When asked "One lump or two?" skip the sugar and use stevia instead to help you nourish your skin for a beautiful, moist, wrinkle-free appearance. Stevia, a cousin of the chrysanthemum plant and a sibling of the sunflower, is a sugary tasting plant that does not raise your blood sugar levels, which makes it popular with diabetics, dieters, and anyone interested in skin health. Stevia extract is 300 times sweeter than sugar, though, so you will only need a very small amount of it to sweeten your cup.

Sweet-Tooth Got Your Collagen?

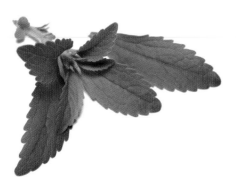

Too much sugar is bad for your skin, your teeth, and your general health, yet refined sugar consumption continues to rise in the United States. According to the Center for Science in the Public Interest, sugar consumption rose by 25 pounds (11 kg) between 1986 and 1998 to 152 pounds (69 kg) per person per year.

When sugar starts to replace nutritious calories in your diet, obesity and numerous other health problems result. Eating more sugar than necessary can speed up your body's natural process of glycation, in which sugar and protein gang up on other parts of your body. They particularly gang up on collagen, which is one of the major structural components of your skin. Collagen damage from glycation can make your skin less elastic, more wrinkled, and more vulnerable to sun damage.

Save Your Skin from Sugar

Stevia is native to Paraguay, and the people of both Paraguay and Brazil have used it for centuries to make a sweet herbal tea. Unlike sugar, it does not increase your blood sugar levels. It is a sensible sweetener for anyone trying to protect the skin's collagen, for diabetics, and for people on carbohydrate-controlled diets.

The safety of stevia has been under question for many years. There have been more than 900 studies investigating its properties, and according to the United States Food and Drug Administration, nineteen of these studies pointed to safety concerns. In particular, the media tends to refer to a 1960s study in which unrealistically high levels of stevia were given to rats and they became infertile. In 2006, the World Health Organization (WHO) evaluated the stevia studies and concluded that stevia is not toxic and that there is no evidence that it causes cancer. The study also reported that the health benefits of stevia are substantial, including the potential to help people with hypertension or type-2 diabetes.

Despite the WHO findings, lingering health and political controversies have limited the use of stevia in many countries. It is widely used as a sweetener in Japan and some South American countries, but the United States, Australia, New Zealand, and Canada, it is not yet available as a food additive—it is only available as a dietary supplement sold through health food stores and some specialty grocery stores. Millions of Japanese have been using stevia for over thirty years with no reported or known harmful effects. Perhaps in time, stevia will be approved for use in more products in North America and will become a more standard part of a healthy skin regimen.

Water

Drink up! Water is involved in a great number of body functions, including digestion, absorption, circulation, and excretion. It also helps flush toxins from the body, particularly from the skin. Without a sufficient water supply, toxins can build up, causing damage and reducing the beauty of

Sugar-Free Mask for Beautiful Skin

Stevia concentrate has traditionally been used to help a number of skin complaints, and has proved effective in the treatment of seborrhea, dermatitis, and eczema. You can apply a drop to any blemish, acne outbreak, lip or mouth sore, or cut or scratch to speed up the healing process. You can also apply it as a facial mask to soften and firm the skin and smooth wrinkles: Spread the dark liquid over the entire face, allow it to dry for 30 to 60 minutes, then rinse.

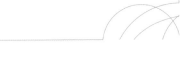

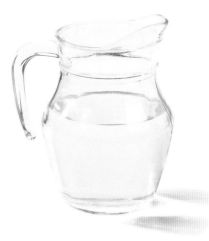

the skin. Hydrating the skin by drinking lots of water is absolutely crucial to keeping you your most beautiful.

A Healthy Sailor is a Hydrated One

Another of water's primary roles is to carry nutrients into skin cells, which are very active and therefore have a high demand for nutrients. In addition, skin cells need water to stay hydrated and firm—dehydrated skin cells are flaccid and contribute to a loose, wrinkled, unhealthy appearance. Water within the cells plays an important role in many metabolic pathways, including energy production. Both you and your skin will feel more energized if you consistently drink plenty of water.

Drinker Beware

Drinking a lot of water helps promote proper skin structure and overall health, but you can still have dry skin even if you drink a lot of water. This is because dry skin is caused by outside elements, such as wind, sun, dry conditions, and other skin irritants, which cannot be remedied through the intake of water (moisturizers would do a better job on these outmost skin surfaces).

People with eczema and similar diseases can drink an abundance of water but still suffer from dry skin because it has been caused by underlying problems, including inflammation and fat imbalance.

Skip the Java

Caffeinated drinks, alcohol, sweating, and dry environmental conditions can dehydrate the skin and body. In addition, using soaps and other oil-removing chemicals on the skin can dry it out. A diet rich in water and skin-moisturizing nutrients, such as essential fatty acids, can help combat these dehydrating factors. Feeling thirsty yet?

Watermelon

Although it's the official "vegetable" of Oklahoma, the watermelon is, in fact, a fruit. (It was declared a vegetable by Oklahoma due to its status as a member of the cucumber family, though the dictionary declares it a fruit.) Watermelon is commonly red or pink, but it can also be yellow or orange. This delicious fruit is packed with water and nutrients that help moisturize the skin.

A Candy-Flavored Defender

A slice of watermelon contains fewer than 50 calories—about the same as a single stick of licorice. While both are tasty, licorice offers your skin no benefits, while watermelon is packed with some of nature's most effective antioxidants, including vitamins A and C. These antioxidants are fat- and water-soluble, respectively, which means that together, they can neutralize free radicals—unstable compounds that damage skin cells—in every part of the skin.

Fight Water Loss

Red or pink watermelon is a source of lycopene, another potent antioxidant. Concentrated amounts of lycopene are found in tomatoes, but watermelon offers a hefty dose of this antioxidant as well. Lycopene is fat loving, which means it can help prevent damage to the lipid aspect of the skin's moisture barrier. It is also thought to improve the connections between skin cells, called cell junctions. When loose, cell junctions are unable to retain moisture, but lycopene can tighten them and reduce water loss from the skin. Tighter cells mean smoother, more youthful looking skin.

Kick Start Your Skin

Watermelon provides significant amounts of vitamin B1 (thiamin) and B6 (pyridoxine). These B vitamins are necessary for energy production in the skin. Energy is required by skin cells to maintain the skin's structure, including the barrier that keeps in moisture. Watermelon's B vitamins can help generate energy in the skin and sustain a healthy moisture barrier.

Did you know that watermelon is 92 percent water by weight? So besides the many nutrients it provides that support the skin's moisture, watermelon hydrates the skin with its sky-high water content, guaranteeing that it works properly.

You could certainly find other foods that offer the same nutrients, so what makes watermelon special? It has a very low calorie count per cup. That means that a cup of watermelon delivers more nutrients per calorie than almost any other food. Any way you look at it, watermelon is an outstanding nutrient value for the skin. So whether it's summertime or snowing, treat yourself to a big slice of watermelon or a refreshing glass of watermelon punch (see p. 274).

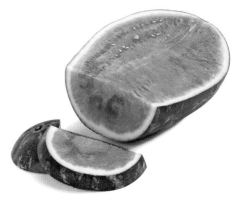

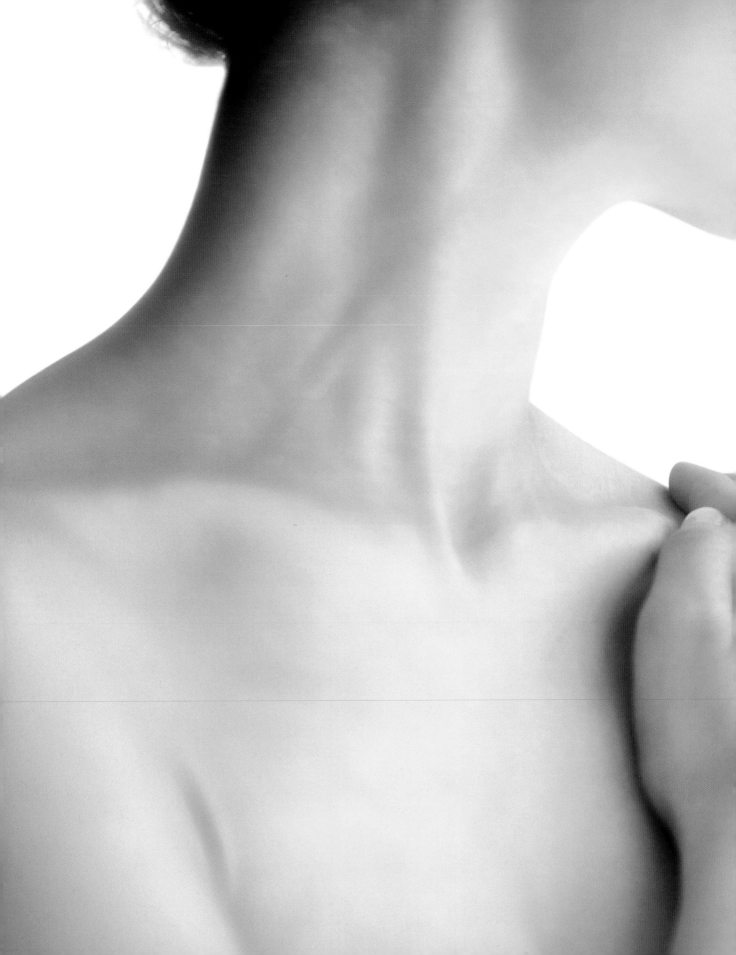

Foods That Tighten, Smooth, and Fight Sag

DOCTORS' NEEDLES and scalpels and hundred-dollar creams are various methods to tighten, smooth, and fight sagging—but it's much more simple (and fun) to eat your way to beautiful skin. Some of your favorite foods, such as peanuts, cheese, and mango can help you do this. In this chapter, we'll cover these and a slew of other foods that contain nutrients to help you buff and firm your way to a rejuvenated look. Your new face-lift is only a few bites away!

Does Food Really Alter Skin Roughness and Elasticity?

Let's turn to the research: In a 2004 study published in the *Journal of Dermatological Treatment,* sixty-two women (45 to 73 years old), were each given either a placebo or supplement with nutrients known to support skin health. The supplements included vitamin E, vitamin C, carotenoids, selenium, zinc, and pycnogenol (an antioxidant found in bark). The researchers reported that those who took the nutrient supplement significantly increased the elasticity of their skin—by 9 percent—after just six weeks (those who took the placebo experienced no significant increase). In addition, the roughness of the skin in the nutrient-supplement group decreased by 6 percent after 12 weeks treatment compared with the placebo-control group. Now that's strong evidence.

Natural Face-Lift

Consuming nutrients is the equivalent of giving yourself a natural face-lift. Let's examine some of these nutrients more closely to see how they work.

One of the best nutrients for the skin is vitamin E. This fat-soluble antioxidant fights many signs of skin aging and damage by neutralizing free radicals, the harmful compounds in the skin caused by sunlight and environmental chemicals. Antioxidants can neutralize free radicals, putting an end to their damaging rampage, which means less damage to the skin's structure. In particular, vitamin E is known to improve skin moisture, softness, and smoothness.

The skin's structural components include collagen and elastin. These molecules can be damaged by free radicals or mechanical manipulation, such as repeated frowning. Many nutrients, including vitamin E, vitamin C, and beta-carotene, can protect elastin and collagen molecules from free-radical damage. In addition, nutrients such as selenium, iron, copper, CoQ10, and silica can promote the formation of collagen and elastin. The carotenoid lutein can also help tighten skin. According to clinical research trials, just 10 mg of lutein daily can increase the skin's elasticity.

A diet rich in foods with these antioxidants can prevent the skin from sagging and losing its baby-smooth appearance—consider it your natural nip and tuck.

Say Good-Bye to Sagging

Sagging skin, a sign of aging is due to several environmental factors and certain internal factors such as hormones, which fluctuate during menopause especially. Changes of the skin that appear during menopause suggest that a drop in estrogen accelerates the aging process, as estrogen prevents oxidative damage that is caused by free radicals in the body.

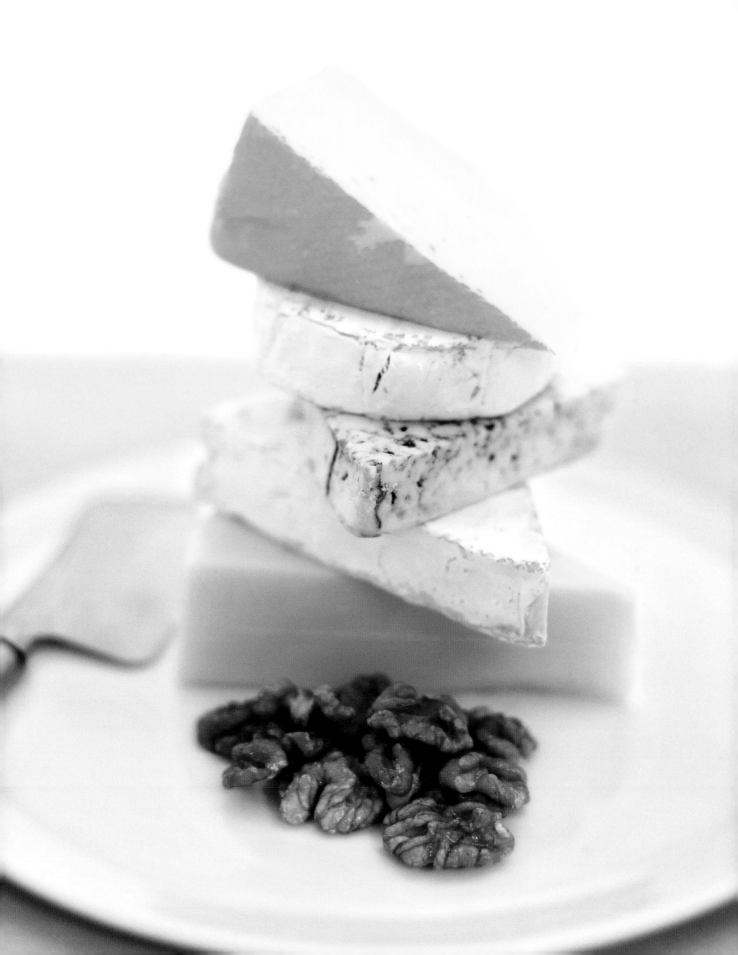

Thankfully, antioxidants have the ability to take over where estrogen leaves off, and help menopausal women (and everyone else) prevent skin damage. In particular, the B vitamins, vitamins C and E, and beta-carotene are thought to help prevent the free-radical damage that causes skin to age. Scientists suggest that antioxidants, when included in the diet or applied topically, may have favorable effects on the health of skin in women of menopausal age.

Eighteen Foods That Tighten, Smooth, and Fight Sag

Many foods work like a natural face lift because they are full of nutrients that prevent damage to the skin and promote repair. A general recommendation is that adults eat at least eight servings of fruits and vegetables each day, about two servings of dairy products, and two to three servings of protein, such as nuts, eggs, and soy. You can easily fulfill these requirements—and enjoy beautiful, healthy skin—by choosing the foods that follow in this section (and elsewhere in the book).

Tasty Tighteners
- Asparagus
- Black-Eyed Peas
- Celery
- Cheese
- Dried Fruit
- Peanuts
- Rhubarb

Savory Smoothers
- Papaya
- Soy

Sag Soldiers
- Brazil Nuts
- Chickpeas
- Clams
- Dates
- Eggs
- Green Peas
- Mango
- Raisins
- Rosemary

TASTY TIGHTENERS

Beautiful, tight, and youthful looking skin is just a few mouthfuls away. Try incorporating these seven delicious foods into your diet and let the nutrients they contain help your skin look tighter. Nutrients like silica, iron, and B vitamins can help your skin maintain that youthful, taut appearance. Even the good microbes that live in your body and in some foods, called probiotics, can help tighten your skin. Take a bite into these healthy choices and feed your skin right.

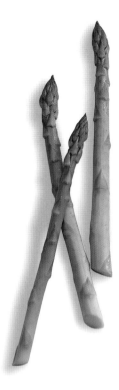

Asparagus

Tighten up your skin's appearance with a few stalks of asparagus. Native to northern Africa, western Asia, and most of Europe, asparagus is now grown throughout the world and is considered a culinary delicacy. It can also offer you a natural face lift—giving you all the more reason to add it to your shopping cart.

Strengthen Your Skin

Silica is a trace mineral rich in asparagus that strengthens the body's connective tissues, such as the muscles, hair, tendons, nails, bone, and skin. In your skin, a deficiency in silica can compromise elasticity and reduce your ability to heal wounds. This deficiency also makes the tissue weak, inflexible, and unstable, which can lead to sagging. Modern food-processing techniques reduce the amount of silica we get in our diet. Therefore, to tone and tighten your skin with silica, you need to seek out foods rich in the mineral, such as rice, oats, lettuce, cucumber, and, of course, asparagus.

Wash It Down with a Glass of Water

Asparagus has been used in cooking for thousands of years; you can even find it in recipes from the oldest surviving cookbook, which was compiled in the third century. Its uses extend beyond cooking, as well: It has been used in the treatment of urinary tract infections, kidney and bladder stones, and is considered an aphrodisiac. Today we know that asparagus is also a diuretic, which means that it can increase your loss of water. To prevent your skin from losing precious moisture while taking in asparagus's nutrients, be sure to enjoy the veggie with a glass of water.

Does Size Matter?
No. The tenderness of asparagus has to do with how fresh it is, not the size of its spears. Fresh asparagus will snap easily while older spears will bend. Choose the freshest asparagus—they have more nutrients that nip and tuck.

Black-Eyed Peas

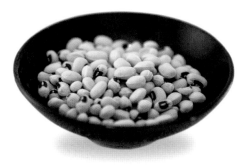

Black-eyed peas might be the name of a popular rock group, but they are also your ticket to beautiful skin. These adorable two-colored peas contain iron, fiber, and an assortment of other nutrients that help your skin's health, giving it a beautiful, tight, smooth appearance.

Packing a One-Two Punch

The tightness of your skin's appearance on your face is affected by the health of your facial muscles. Iron and protein, two nutrients found in rich amounts in black-eyed peas, can help these muscles stay strong, toned, and healthy, giving your skin a tighter appearance.

In just one cup (250 g) of black-eyed peas, you get 23 percent of your daily recommended value of iron. Your red blood cells use this iron to carry oxygen from your lungs to your skin and facial muscles. The protein in black-eyed peas—13 g in one cup of cooked peas—offers your skin amino acids, which are the building blocks for enzymes, hormones, and muscles. Your face muscles contract and relax more than 30,000 times a day—that's a lot of work! Without amino acids, your facial muscles cannot properly repair and rebuild after its daily workout of smiles and frowns. Keep your skin looking tight by ensuring that your facial muscles are well nourished.

Black-eyed peas also contain calcium, magnesium, phosphorus, potassium, zinc, vitamin C, thiamin, riboflavin, niacin, pantothenic acid, vitamin B6, folate, and vitamin A. These nutrients are not present in great quantities, but every little bit of these skin-nourishing nutrients helps your skin look even more beautiful.

These low-in-fat, high-in-fiber peas are a perfect food for your waistline, heart, and skin. Pick some up on your next visit to the market and try the delicious Smokey Black-Eyed Peas recipe on page 252.

Celery

Crisp and delicious, celery is not just a healthy snack; consider it your new facial specialist. Like asparagus, celery is rich in silica, a mineral that is important to the tone and firmness of your skin. It is also a source of vitamin C, another nutrient known to give you a natural face lift. Finally, celery has a very high water content, which helps hydrate your skin cells, giving them a plump, firm appearance.

Abundant Wrinkle Cure is Tough to Absorb

Silicon is used in surgical implants to enhance beauty, but the silicon in celery offers you a natural way to beautify your skin. Silicon is a structural part of your skin, hair, nails, and bones and thus forms the body's scaffolding, giving the skin a tight, firm appearance. Silica is a source of the mineral silicon, and it is found in good amounts in celery.

Even though silica is the second most abundant element on earth, humans commonly suffer from a deficiency in it and have weak, saggy skin as a result. It also doesn't help that, as you age, you become less able to absorb silica because your stomach acids weaken, making it difficult for your body to digest the mineral properly. For these reasons, it's all the more important that you incorporate celery into your salads, soups, snacks, and anywhere else you can.

Vitamins and Minerals

Celery is also rich in potassium and sodium, the most important minerals for controlling fluid balance in your body. Celery was used traditionally as a diuretic and can help you get rid of excess fluid, such as the puffiness that can build up under the eyes. Once you've relieved the puffiness, you'll want to tighten and firm the skin. Celery's silica and vitamin C can help with this too.

Celery is an excellent source of vitamin C—one serving provides roughly 15 percent of the recommended daily value. One of the most important vitamins in your skin, vitamin C helps fight free radicals that cause damage to the structure of your skin, making it loose and saggy.

Call in the Troops

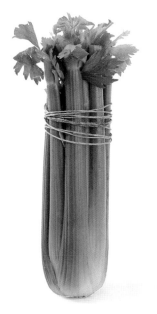

Celery contains compounds called coumarins that help prevent free radicals from damaging cells, thus decreasing the mutations that can lead to cells becoming cancerous. Coumarins also stimulate the activity of certain white blood cells, which serve as immune defenders, targeting and eliminating potentially harmful cells, including cancer cells. Celery also contains compounds called acetylenics, which have been shown to stop the growth of tumor cells.

A Versatile Vegetable

Chop, dice, and slice celery into your diet and enjoy toned, tight, and beautiful skin. Slice celery to make veggie sticks, fill them with natural nut butters, or add diced celery to any of soup (such as the Corn, Squash, and Lima Bean Soup on p. 216) or salad recipes to reap the beautifying benefits of its toning and tightening nutrients.

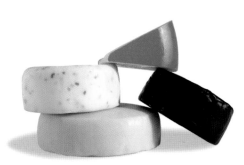

Cheese

Cheese is a source of probiotics, which are beneficial microbes (i.e., bacteria and yeast) that live in your body. Probiotics offer a wide array of health benefits, including improving your ability to digest and absorb nutrients, boosting your immune system, preventing bad microbes from multiplying and causing disease, and improving the overall look of your skin.

Hyaluronic Acid Gives Structure to Skin

Hyaluronic acid is one of the chief components of the extracellular matrix (the material outside the cells that gives tissue its structure and support), making it an important component in maintaining the strength and tightness of the skin. With age, there is a natural loss of hyaluronic acid in the skin, which results in sagging. This is because hyaluronic acid is involved in skin tissue repair. Skin that can no longer repair itself through cell proliferation and migration will lose its smooth, even appearance. But here's the good news: Preliminary studies suggest that probiotics may actually enhance the production of hyaluronic acid, so it's high time you serve up some probiotic-rich dairy!

B-Happy

Probiotics in cheese and other dairy products supply many healthy benefits by improving the body's ability to digest and absorb nutrients. In particular, probiotics manufacture B vitamins in the gut. Once absorbed, these vitamins promote proper metabolism in the skin cells and are involved in energy production (and since the skin is a high energy-using tissue, these vitamins are greatly needed here). Increasing the ability of the body to absorb nutrients is probably the most effective way you can promote the health of your skin.

Soft or hard, all types of cheese contain probiotics that are healthy for your skin. Before you devour a grilled cheese sandwich, however, know that the bacteria in probiotics can be destroyed by heat, so keep cheese away from the stove for beautiful skin.

Dried Fruit

Dried fruit is a healthy, sweet snack that can help tighten your skin and deliver a radiant complexion. Almost all fruits have a dried counterpart, with the most common varieties being raisins (grapes), currants, apricots, figs, and dates. For more on raisin and dates specifically, see pages 113 and 117.

Collagen Building Block

Dried fruits are a terrific source of iron, which plays a vital role in the formation of the collagen scaffolding that keeps your skin tight, strong, and smooth. Apricots and figs have the most iron per ounce of all dried fruits, each providing roughly 7 percent of the daily recommended iron intake per serving. (One serving of dried apricots is eight; one serving of dried figs is four.)

Dried fruits are also rich in other dietary minerals, including calcium, magnesium, phosphorus, potassium, sodium, copper, and manganese, and in vitamins A and B.

Sun-Kissed Nutrients

Though the fresh version of fruit typically contains higher amounts of vitamin C, dried fruit also provides a steady supply. Vitamin C is an antioxidant that defends your skin against the free radicals that can destroy collagen. Since free radicals are made naturally in your skin, and because vitamin C cannot be stored in your body, it is important to make sure that your daily diet is stocked with this vitamin, so that your skin can protect itself from the damage that leads to sagging.

Dried fruit is a great way to get vitamin C into your diet when you're on the run. Mix dried fruit with Brazil nuts for a great snack with a natural nip and tuck effect on your skin. Eat dried fruit like raisins right out of the box or use them to make tasty sauces, baked goods, and more. It's luscious any time of the day, from sweetening a breakfast cereal (try our Breakfast Bulgur with Dried Cherries, Apples, and Apricots on p. 196) to pepping up a lunch-time salad, to adding a tangy flavor to a dinner dish. For an elegant dessert that's low in fat and high in potassium and beta-carotene, serve prunes that have been soaked in maple syrup and Armagnac (see p. 282).

The Many Faces of Dried Fruit

Raisins are produced from unseeded or seeded white or black grapes. Sultanas, a type of raisin, are juicy, sweet, and amber in color and are produced from a seedless white grape, mostly the Thompson grape. Currants are dried, black, seedless grapes. All currants derive from the same variety of grape, known as the Zante grape, which originated from Corinth—hence the name "currant"—in Greece.

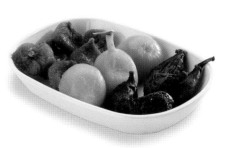

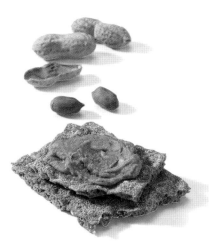

Peanuts

From baseball games to bar snacks, peanuts are a popular nut—well, legume, technically. Packed with nutrients that promote beautiful skin, such as protein, monounsaturated fat, vitamin E, resveratrol, and CoQ10, peanuts are like mini estheticians for your skin.

Beauty Is in the Shell

According to archaeologists, peanuts have been around for more than 7,600 years. Today, most people eat peanuts in the form of peanut butter, salted peanuts, and peanut brittle. Sadly, none of these forms is good for your skin. Commercial peanut butter can be a source of trans fat, a very unhealthy fat for your skin and your heart, and salted peanuts are usually roasted in oil, a process that destroys the helpful fats and vitamin E they contain. Additionally, peanut brittle is high in sugar, which can trigger inflammation in your skin. For these reasons, the best way to enjoy the health benefits of peanuts is to skip the processed forms and shell or grind them yourself.

Free Radical Fighters

Peanuts contain monounsaturated fats, good fats that are very stable and not easily damaged (oxidized) by free radicals. When your diet contains this fat, free radicals that form from sunlight and toxins are less able to damage your skin cells.

Free radicals are also targeted by the vitamin E in peanuts and other nuts. Vitamin E can help neutralize free radicals and prevent damage to your skin, which prevents signs of aging like wrinkles, spots, and sagging. The B vitamin niacin, also found in peanuts, helps in this arena as well, by helping skin cells make energy.

Better than Apples—and Carrots, Too

Roasted peanuts rival the antioxidant capacity of strawberries and black-berries and actually have more antioxidants than carrots and apples. Researchers at the University of Florida have also found that when peanuts are roasted, their level of p-coumaric acid—a potent antioxidant that helps your skin fight free radicals—increases.

Peanuts are also a good source of resveratrol, an anti-aging nutrient normally associated with red wine. Touted for its ability to lower the risk of heart disease, resveratrol is also effective at neutralizing free radicals, which means less damage for your skin to fix and a tighter, smoother appearance.

Energizes to Tighten and Smooth

Peanuts are one of the few ways to add the vitamin-like substance CoQ10 to your diet. CoQ10 is a nutrient found in the body that aids mitochondria, the powerhouses of cells, in the complex process of transforming food into energy. Our bodies are able to produce some of the CoQ10 we need on their own, but this natural supply decreases with age—and this decline can lead to signs of aging. It is therefore imperative that we consume foods containing CoQ10, like peanuts, fish, and spinach (all of which are featured in this book) so that our bodies have enough of the nutrient for synthesis.

Peanuts are an easy addition to make to any diet. Toss them into soups and salads, or incorporate them into a snack mix (such as the Tamari-Flavored Snack Mix on p. 204) for quick afternoon, evening, or anytime treat.

Rhubarb

Rhubarb is a delicious pink vegetable used like a fruit in pies and jams. It is a great addition to any skin-beautifying diet, full of nutrients that naturally tone and tuck your skin for a more youthful appearance.

Two Nutrients to Protect and Build Firm Skin

In this delicious vegetable, you'll find both vitamin C and silica. These nutrients protect and fortify your skin's structure, giving it a tight, toned, and beautiful appearance. Vitamin C is a powerful antioxidant that fights free radicals, disarms them, and stops them from damaging collagen, elastin, and other skin structures.

Silicon (silica) may be the second most abundant mineral on earth, but it is very difficult for your body to absorb (a problem further compounded by the fact that we excrete between 10 and 40 mg of it every day). Because silica gives your bones, hair, nails, and skin their strength, you need to make sure your diet is full of foods rich in this mineral, as a deficiency can lead to inelastic, dry, itchy, and sagging skin.

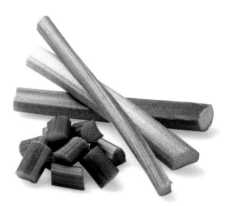

Silica also helps your skin retain water. More water in your skin gives you a more toned, tight, and youthful appearance. Silica binds 300 times its own weight in water, so it is not surprising that rhubarb has the ability to hydrate your skin cells and make it easier for them to transport healthy nutrients.

Rhubarb is a tasty tool that supports the firmness of your skin and keeps it from sagging. Try stewing it with strawberries for a wonderful yogurt or ice cream topper you can feel good about.

SAVORY SMOOTHERS

Two exotic solutions for more beautiful skin—papaya and soy—may not be foods commonly found in North America, but they are delicious and very nutritious. From vitamin C to isoflavones, these two powerhouses are packed with nutrients that will help you skin appear more smooth in no time, so dig in and enjoy!

Papaya

You can spend your money on an exotic vacation instead of paying for an expensive face lift, thanks to this tropical fruit. Papayas offer the luscious taste and sunlit color of the tropics while delivering an abundance of nutrients, including carotene, vitamin C and flavonoids, folate, pantothenic acid, potassium, magnesium, and fiber. This wealth of nutrients supports the health of your skin and gives you ample reason to skip the surgery and head to the refrigerator.

Tropical Antioxidant Powerhouse

Papaya contains a number of antioxidants, including vitamins A, C, and E. Eating one papaya provides you with one third of your daily vitamin C needs.

Along with the carotenoids and flavonoids found in papaya, vitamin C is an inhibitor of free radical damage. Free radicals damage your skin's collagen and elastin, the fibers that support your skin's structure, and that damage leads to wrinkles and other signs of aging.

Naturally Exfoliate

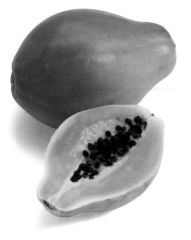

Removing dead skin cells is a necessary step to giving your skin a smoother appearance. Look no further than papaya: It contains papain, a natural enzyme that helps slough off dead skin cells. Papaya is commonly added to topical creams and lotions that claim to reduce the signs of wrinkles. It works like an exfoliant and helps tighten the skin.

Originally grown in southern Mexico, Central America, and northern South America, papaya is now cultivated in most countries with a tropical climate, including Brazil, India, South Africa, Sri Lanka, and the Philippines. The ripe fruit is usually eaten raw, with the skin and seeds removed, and makes a great addition to any fruit salad. Although it has fewer skin-smoothing nutrients, the unripe green fruit of papaya can also be eaten (typically in salads or cooked in curries or stews).

Soy

Soy and soy beans are a natural way to nip and tuck your skin to a tight, toned, and beautiful appearance. Native to Asia, soy can be found in many forms, including (soy) milk, (soy) beans, and tofu. All of these forms can offer your skin a host of healthy benefits.

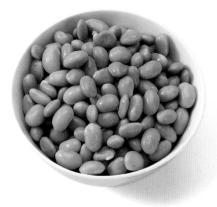

Rebuild It with Collagen

Our skin ages as we do. The appearance of aged skin has a lot to due with changes in the metabolism of the tissue. In particular, the metabolism of collagen decreases in activity over time, producing less and less as you get older. The effect is skin that looks loose, bumpy, and sagging.

Can you counteract the changes in collagen metabolism to regain tight, smooth skin? Researchers believe that soy may help. In laboratory studies, fibroblasts (the cells that produce collagen) produced more collagen and hyaluronic acid (a structural component of the skin) when they were treated topically with a soy extract. In clinical trials, soy-based topical creams have also improved the look of skin. Soy seems to flatten the junctions between the skin layers, making the skin appear tighter and reducing sagging.

Which compound in soy is thought to be anti-aging? Isoflavones, a class of very strong antioxidants known to have many beneficial effects on the body, including the skin. Soy's high concentrations of these super nutrients can beautify the skin and make it appear more youthful.

Soy Any Way You Like It

Soy milk and tofu are terrific sources of protein. Your body depends on protein in order to produce enzymes, which are required for every reaction in your skin, including the production of structural components that help your skin look youthful and beautiful.

Women will enjoy soy's many other health benefits as well, including reducing the risk of breast cancer and improving bone strength. To incorporate soy into your diet, try soy milk (even in hot cocoa—see p. 276 for recipe), miso soup, or tofu. Tofu is fairly bland on its own, but it absorbs flavors from other ingredients and is a lovely complement to any number of side dishes. Cubed tofu is a wonderful addition to a vegetarian stir fry or layered into lasagna.

Fermented Soy Is Best
The typical Japanese diet includes fermented soy, which is thought to offer superior health benefits. A study published in the *Journal of the American Dietetic Association* compared the effects of consuming fermented soy to consuming unfermented soy. The findings showed that fermented soy increased the availability and absorption of the isoflavones found in soy. For better health, choose fermented soy products such as miso and tempeh.

SAG SOLDIERS

When your skin is attacked by damaged ultraviolet radiation, chemicals in cosmetics, and the environment, you need an army on your side. But where can you find soldiers for your skin militia? In foods like nuts, peas, dates, eggs, and others, which contain nutrients that make them excellent sag-fighting soldiers. Many of these foods contain protein, a vital nutrient that keeps your face muscles (and all muscles) strong, giving your skin a sturdy structure to hang on to.

Brazil Nuts

Eating nuts may seem like a strange way to give your skin a natural face lift, but Brazil nuts are one of the most effective foods for tightening up your skin. They contain selenium and vitamin E, two powerful tools for endowing you with a beautiful, tight, and toned appearance.

Best Source of Selenium

Brazil nuts are enriched with selenium, a mineral that your body and skin need for optimal health. This antioxidant stops free radicals—unstable compounds that steal electrons from your skin's structures (collagen and elastin)—from causing damage to your skin. Selenium is also responsible for the elasticity of your skin. Just 3 to 4 Brazil nuts a day can provide you with enough selenium to help fight sagging skin.

In addition to being rich in selenium, they are a good source of magnesium and thiamin, nutrients that support skin health. Vitamin E is also found in Brazil nuts. This antioxidant is an effective weapon against free radical damage that can weaken your skin and is known to help reduce the appearance of wrinkles. Used topically to smooth the skin, vitamin E is a smart part of a skin-saving diet.

Toss Brazil nuts onto salads, add them to your trail mix, or eat a handful for a protein-rich snack. No matter which way you enjoy these delightful nuts, your skin will benefit.

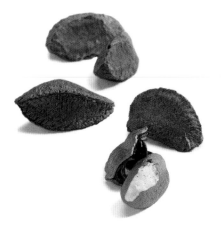

Chickpeas

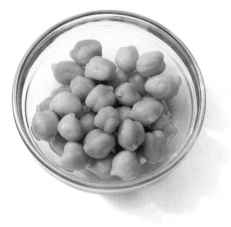

Also known as garbanzo beans, chickpeas are used to make some Middle Eastern favorites like falafel and hummus. They are also great in salads, soups, and pastas. With all their versatility, you'll find it easy to add them to your diet—and beneficial to your skin, too, because chickpeas offer your skin nutrients that tighten, smooth, and rejuvenate for a more youthful appearance.

Minerals Against Sag

Chickpeas are a fantastic source of manganese—just one cup (240 g) contains 85 percent of your daily recommended value. This trace mineral is required for energy production and also functions as an antioxidant, fighting free radicals that cause your skin to sag.

The more toxins in your skin, the more likely it is to sag. Luckily, another trace mineral in chickpeas, molybdenum, can help. Molybdenum is an important part of sulfite oxidase, an enzyme responsible for detoxifying (removing) toxins called sulfites, which cause damage that reduces the smooth, tight appearance of your skin.

Think there aren't any sulfites in your skin? Think again. Sulfites are a common preservative found in prepared foods, particularly premade salads. Make sure sulfites do not pull your skin down by making fresh salads with chickpeas instead.

Folate and Fiber: Working for You

You will also find lots of folate in chickpeas. This B vitamin has many important roles in your body. Folate is needed for energy production, and your skin needs lots of energy to keep up with daily repairs caused by exposure to the sun and toxins. Just ½ cup (120 g) of chickpeas provides you with 35 percent of the recommended daily allowance for folate.

We have all heard that we should make fiber our friend, as it helps keep us regular and controls blood levels of cholesterol and sugar. Fiber is also a friend to your skin. Healthy cholesterol and blood sugar levels keep your blood vessels working optimally, thus ensuring that your skin receives a good supply of nutrients. Your beauty is not skin deep— a healthy, glowing appearance is a sign of overall health. Lucky for us, fiber is not hard to come by, especially in chickpeas. Just one cup (240 g) provides half of your daily fiber requirement.

Chickpeas are my favorite bean. With a subtle taste and meaty texture, chickpeas are a great substitute for meat in many dishes. Plus, they are very easy to use: Open the can, rinse, and enjoy! We included them in our recipe for Pumpkin and Chickpea Stew with Couscous (p. 268) and roasted them for a crunchy snack (p. 202).

Clams

Clams are a storehouse of nutrition; they contain many B vitamins, vitamin C, vitamin A, zinc, copper, and many other minerals. Moreover, they are a low-fat source of protein. Serve up some clams and enjoy beautiful skin.

Clam Up

Vitamins A and C are among the most important antioxidants in your body. Vitamin A is the primary antioxidant in the fatty parts of your skin, and vitamin C is the primary antioxidant in the watery parts of your skin. In combination, these two can protect all of your skin from free-radical damage that can cause a reduction in collagen and elastin, the main compounds that keep skin tight and smooth and resist sagging.

Fights Sluggish Skin

Your skin needs a lot of energy to keep up with the repair jobs left by free radical damage, and when the skin fails to repair itself, it can look dull, dry, and saggy. Clams are a tremendous source of energy. They contain thiamin, riboflavin, and niacin, three B vitamins that are involved in many functions in your body, including energy production. Plus, clams are packed with protein, which energizes your skin.

Creatures of the sea, clams are full of minerals that support your skin's natural moisture levels and enrich your diet with some of the less common minerals like zinc and copper. Minerals are important to many of the enzymes that allow your skin to grow, repair, and look radiant.

You do not need to eat a whole bucket of clams to get healthy skin benefits. As little as one ounce (28 g) of clams can offer your skin the nutrients it needs to look its best.

Raw or Cooked?

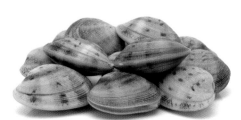

Clams and oysters offer the most nutrients when they are eaten raw. Be cautious when purchasing shellfish, however; when we eat clams, we are also eating the contents of their stomachs, which can be harmful to humans because shellfish are filter feeders—that is, they obtain nutrients by pumping large quantities of water across their complex gill systems. By obtaining nutrients this way, they also take in any bacteria, viruses, chemical contaminants, and other toxins in the water. Shellfish can contain the bacteria that cause cholera and the virus that causes Hepatitis A. In most developed nations, however, there are government programs that protect the shellfish supply from contamination—just be sure to purchase your shellfish from qualified sellers.

Dates

Do you love candy? Then try some of nature's candy—dates. Delicious, sweet, and full of nutrients, dates are a great addition to any diet. Like all fruits, they contain antioxidants, which help fight the damage in your skin that can cause it to lose its resilience. You'll find lots of antioxidants in dates, making this sweet treat a dessert with sag-fighting power.

Filled with Fiber

With more than half of your daily recommended intake of fiber in one cup (178 g) of dates, this nutritious candy helps fight sagging in more ways than one. Eating a diet high in fiber can help you maintain healthy cholesterol levels, which keep your blood vessels healthy, strong, and able to provide your skin with all of the nutrients, oxygen, and antioxidants it needs.

Fiber can also help reduce toxins in your skin. It traps toxins in your intestines and prevents them from getting into your blood, where they could hitch a ride to the fatty layer and cause damage.

Different Kinds of Sweet

Different sweet foods react differently in your body. Naturally sweet foods, like fruit, are not as bad for you as artificially sweet foods, like candy and soda. We know eating sugar is not good for your skin, but when you absolutely must tackle that sweet tooth, foods with natural sugars, such as dates, are the best choice.

You can measure how quickly a food breaks down into energy in your body using the glycemic index, a scale from 1 to 100 that tells us how good or bad a sweet food is for our skin. Too much sugar promotes inflammation, which damages your skin. Thus, foods with high values on the glycemic index are bad for your skin. White sugar, found in soda, baked goods, and candy, has a glycemic index of 100, whereas fruits tend to have a much lower glycemic index. Choosing foods with a lower glycemic

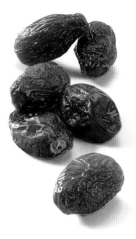

index, such as some varieties of dates, is better for your body and for your skin.

It is important to emphasize, however, that the glycemic index of dates varies greatly by variety or type—scientists have found values ranging from as low as 31 to as high as 103—so choose your dates with care. According to a 2002 United Arab Emirates University study, three particular varieties of dates—khalas, barhi, and bo ma'an—were found to have low glycemic index values of 35.5, 49.7, and 30.5, respectively. Such values make these three types healthy choices for your skin regime.

Toss some dates together with your favorite skin-healthy nuts and some oats and you've got the start of a powerful, skin-beautifying breakfast. Or use dates in our Apple, Pear, and Dried Fruit Strudel (on p. 280) for a healthy dessert.

Eggs

Crack, boil, or scramble eggs into your diet and enjoy tight, toned, and sag-free skin. Eggs are a good source of selenium, which is a natural nip and tuck nutrient for your skin. You can also find choline, protein, and other skin-beautifying nutrients in eggs.

No Choline, No Collagen

Another health benefit of eggs is their choline content. Choline is a B vitamin essential in the normal functioning of all cells, including those involved with brain and nerve function and the transportation of nutrients throughout the body. It is also a key component of the fat-containing structures in cell membranes.

Without choline, your skin cells can become less flexible, which can lead to wrinkles. Although our bodies can produce some choline, we need to supplement it with what we eat as well. Insufficient choline in your diet can lead to a choline deficiency, which makes it difficult for your body to maintain proper levels of other B vitamins, including those required to produce energy in your skin. No energy means no way to make collagen, elastin, and other components of the skin that act like natural face lifts. Luckily, we can obtain choline easily by eating eggs—just two contain 280 mg of choline, or half the recommended daily supply.

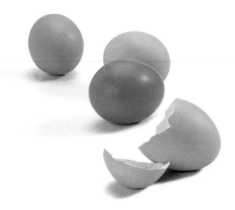

It's All in the Yolk

According to recent research, there may be more bioavailable lutein in eggs than in green vegetables such as spinach, which has typically been considered the major dietary source of the cartenoid. In a study published in a 2004 issue of the *Journal of Nutrition,* researchers found that lutein is best absorbed from egg yolk, rather than from lutein supplements and spinach, because of components in the egg's yolk such as lecithin (another nutrient important to cell health). Antioxidants like lutein can neutralize free radicals, preventing damage to your skin—and just one egg a day can increase your body's levels of it by 26 percent.

Lutein can also make your skin more elastic—a naturally great way to look like you had a face lift. In an Italian study conducted on women between the ages of 25 and 50, researchers found that 10 mg of lutein taken daily for twelve weeks increased the skin's elasticity by 8 percent. The study also confirmed that lutein is a necessary antioxidant for healthy skin, protecting it from damage that can lead to sagging. If you make a point of eating eggs and using lutein topically, research studies suggest that you can increase your skin's elasticity by 20 percent.

Get Cracking

It's easy to add eggs to your diet: Keep hard-boiled eggs in the refrigerator for a quick and nutritious snack, dice cooked eggs onto salads, or mash them up with celery and onions for a great-skin tightening combination. Just one egg a day is all you need to get a healthy dose of choline and other skin-saving nutrients.

Powerful Protein

An excellent source of high-quality protein, just one egg gives you 5.5 g of protein (and only 68 calories). Protein helps build the muscles and tissue below your skin that support your skin's outward appearance, and healthy muscles can help your skin look tight and youthful.

Green Peas

There is a fairy tale about a beautiful princess who was so delicate and sensitive that she could feel a pea buried under twelve mattresses. That princess may have been bruised by one tiny pea, but your skin will glow with health if you welcome these powerful pods into your diet.

Saves Collagen and Elastin

Peas are commonly used to describe the small, round seeds of the legume. Typically considered a vegetable, peas are actually a fruit in the botanical sense. They have long been an important part of our history and diet. Today, they are the latest way to get a nonsurgical face lift.

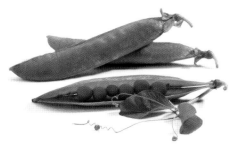

Peas contain a full range of nutrients that support, tone, tighten, and beautify skin. Green peas are a very good source of vitamin C, vitamin K, manganese, dietary fiber, folate, and thiamin (vitamin B1). They are also a good source of vitamin A, phosphorus, vitamin B6, protein, niacin, magnesium, riboflavin (vitamin B2), copper, iron, zinc, and potassium. Many of these nutrients are particularly effective at promoting tight, toned skin.

Folate (folic acid) and vitamin B6 are perhaps the stars of this natural face-lifting food. These two nutrients help reduce the buildup of homocysteine, a byproduct of fat metabolism in your body that can prevent collagen cross-linking. Collagen cross-linking makes your skin strong, firm, and toned, and when it is blocked—by homocysteine, for example—sagging results. Folate and vitamin B6 can convert homocysteine into a less damaging substance, freeing your skin to make collagen and retain its firm, tight, and toned appearance.

Vitamin C, also found in peas, protects your skin's structure from damage. This antioxidant fights off free radicals that like to damage collagen and elastin, the two compounds that play a part in your skin's tone and firmness. Vitamin C is a relentless free radical scavenger, protecting your collagen and elastin, and leaving you looking youthful and radiant.

Pea-For-All

The French king Louis XIV popularized peas in the seventeenth century by including them on his palace's party menus. Give your skin the royal treatment by using fresh peas to brighten up any soup or salad, or sauté them with mushrooms for an elegant side dish. When fresh peas aren't readily available, try one of the other varieties (canned or dried). Make a batch of split-pea soup or try our recipe for Smokey Black-Eyed Peas on page 252.

Mango

Mangoes are a tropical treat that contribute to beautiful, tight, young-looking skin. They are typically green and red on the outside, with a nutrient-rich orange flesh on the inside that can do wonders for your skin.

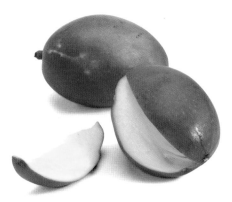

Captures Water and Fights Free Radicals

Mangoes originated from Asia but are grown in warm climates throughout the world today. Loved by many for their sweet taste, mangoes are uniquely refreshing to eat because of their high water content. Water helps nourish the skin cells and gives them a plump, toned appearance—it may be the simplest way to give your skin a lift.

There is more than water to these delectable fruits, however. Mangoes contain vitamins, minerals, antioxidants, and enzymes (magneferin and lactase), which help you absorb other nutrients needed for beautiful skin.

Mangoes contain vitamins A and C, two great protectors of your skin's tight, toned appearance. These antioxidants can stop free radicals from causing damage, thereby preventing droopy skin and keeping your skin fit and beautiful. And since vitamin A is fat-soluble and vitamin C is water-soluble, mangoes protect your skin in a two-fold way.

Fruit Implants

The most potent nip and tuck nutrient in this fruit is silica, a mineral that gives structural support to your hair, muscles, bones, teeth, and skin (and to artificial implants as well). Silica can also hold 300 times its weight in water, and thereby gives your skin a plump, hydrated appearance. It also plays a role in keeping the skin tight and smooth by supporting both bone and collagen formation. When there is not enough silica in your diet, your skin turns weak and loses elasticity.

Unfortunately, only about 40 percent of the silica in your diet gets absorbed. With age, your ability to absorb silica further decreases, making it even more imperative that you seek out silica-rich foods like mangoes.

Mangoes, Mangoes, Everywhere

Mangoes have one of the most beautiful flavors of any fruit. How can you get them into your diet? Most people eat them peeled and sliced for breakfast or as a snack. In addition, mangoes are a common ingredient in chutneys and salsas. Try adding diced mango to your salad—see page 228 for Mango, Spinach, Sorrel, and Pistachio Salad—or chop dried mango into your oatmeal for a rich, sweet zing and sag-free skin.

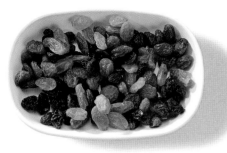

Raisins

Drying grapes into raisins has been practiced since ancient times. Raisins were produced in Persia and Egypt as early as 2,000 B.C. Raisins were also highly prized by the ancient Romans, and should also be prized by you. These dried fruits are a handy, high-energy, low-fat snack, packed with fiber and nutrients that help keep your skin looking beautiful.

Fight Wrinkles with Wrinkles

There are many types of this wrinkly treat to choose from, including Sultana, Malaga, Monukka, Muscat, and Thompson. Which is best? In 2007, the *Journal of Agricultural and Food Chemistry* published a study that compared the amount of antioxidants from fresh green seedless Thompson grapes (the most commonly consumed grape in North America), sun-dried Thompson raisins, and Thompson golden raisins. In the study, fifteen people ate one of these three types daily for four weeks. The researchers discovered that those who ate the Thompson golden raisins had highest amounts of antioxidants in their body.

So are raisins better than grapes? In the cited study, it appears that they are; however, most researchers suggest that fresh grapes are still better for you. In either case, the raisin appears to be a very healthy food to include in your diet.

Raisins contain high amounts of phenols, a potent antioxidant. Antioxidants can prevent oxygen-based (free radical) damage to skin cells, collagen, and other components that keep the skin firm, tight, and free of sags. Raisins are also a source of the trace mineral boron, which is important for the health of your bones.

Like all dried fruits, raisins are easy to add to your healthy-skin regime. Toss them into oatmeal, baked goods, salads, and more. We've included them in both our Pumpkin and Chickpea Stew with Couscous (p. 268) and our Tamari-Flavored Snack Mix (p. 204).

Rosemary

Rosemary is a fragrant herb used to enhance a wide array of dishes. However, antioxidant-rich rosemary is much more than a culinary accent. It contains essential oils that offer your body many healthy benefits, including improving the skin's elasticity and giving you a natural face lift.

A Collagen Protector

Studies have shown that rosemary has a strong antioxidant ability, which enables it to neutralize free radicals and prevent them from causing damage to the skin. Left unchecked, free radicals can damage the parts of your skin that keep it tight, toned, and youthful looking, leaving your skin to sag.

Rosemary, in the dried form, is a good source of iron, calcium, and vitamin B6. Vitamin B6 is one of the vitamins required to keep your body's levels of homocysteine—a byproduct of fat metabolism in your body that can prevent collagen cross-linking—in check. Vitamin B6 can help keep homocysteine levels low and thus help keep your skin from sagging due to weak collagen.

Both fresh and dried rosemary are used liberally in traditional Mediterranean cuisine. Fresh rosemary has 25 percent more manganese than the dried form, but dried rosemary has 40 percent more calcium and iron, so both have their advantages (and disadvantages). Manganese is involved in the body's energy production and helps fight free radicals, which damage the skin, trigger inflammation, and cause wrinkles. Calcium supports the proper functioning of nerves and muscles, and iron helps your body produce energy and keeps your immune system healthy.

Have a Dinner Date with Rosemary

The herb's aromatic, slightly astringent taste is a lovely complement to foods such as fish, lamb, and chicken (see p. 258 for our Rosemary Ginger Chicken with Orange-Honey Glaze). Sprinkle crushed rosemary leaves on your vegetables before roasting them for added flavor, or try combining rosemary with garlic and asparagus for a tasty dish that combats sagging skin.

A Rosy-Colored Picture
Rosemary oil also contains cineole, borneol, camphor, and pinenes, which are helpful for soothing the muscles in your intestinal tract. The oil can also be used topically to improve blood circulation and wound healing.

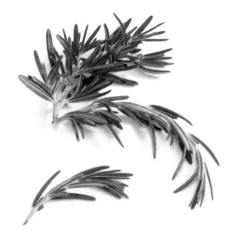

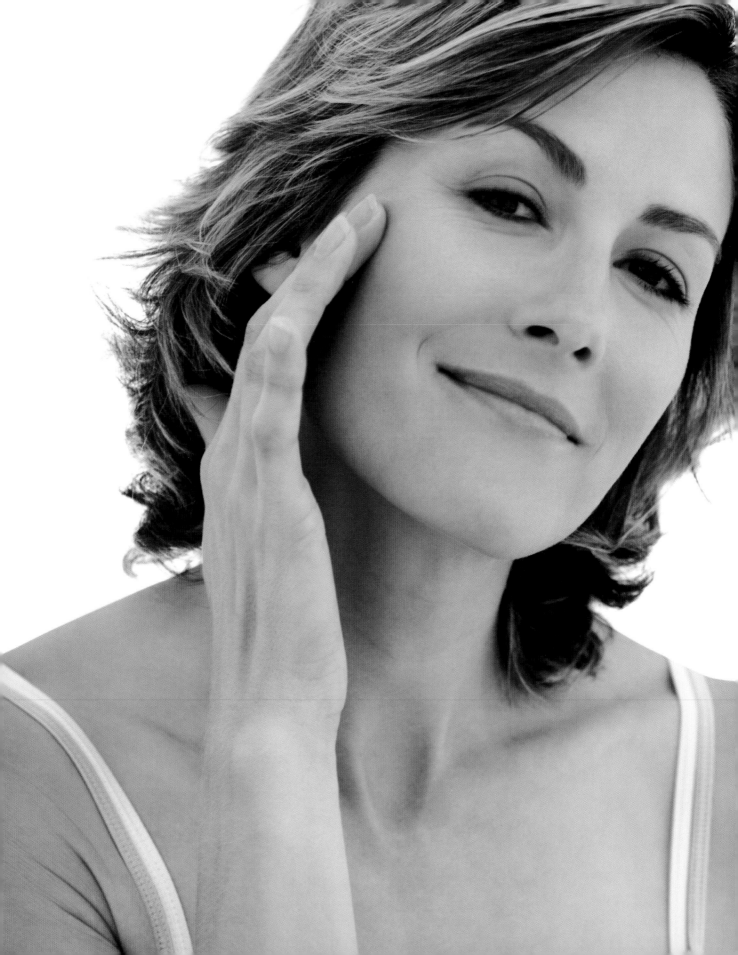

Foods That Brighten Your Complexion

THERE ARE A NUMBER of reasons why your complexion can appear dull, spotted, or blotchy. Inflammation, sun damage, and poor skin cell turnover, for example, are all factors that might prompt you to reach for concealer and blush. But with a diet rich in nutrients such as folate, chromium, copper, and vitamins A, B12, and C, you can banish the need for makeup and transform your complexion from dull to radiant in no time.

What Is Rosacea?

Rosacea is a skin disorder that causes redness on the cheeks, nose, chin, and forehead. People with rosacea can also have small visible blood vessels and bumps or pimples on their face. They sometimes have watery, irritated eyes as well. According to the National Rosacea Society, 70 percent of people with rosacea say it negatively affects their self esteem and social life.

Sun exposure, wind, emotional stress, alcohol consumption, spicy foods, medication, and dairy foods are some of the common triggers of rosacea. Treating your skin gently and eating foods that fight inflammation can help reduce the symptoms. Antibiotics can also be used to treat rosacea, due to their anti-inflammatory properties.

Defeat Dullness

Is your complexion looking a little sallow? It could be because you have too many dead skin cells on the top layer of your skin, or it could be that not enough blood is being circulated to your skin. The look and health of your skin depends on your skin's two main layers: the dermis and the epidermis. (The third skin layer is the hypodermis, but its role in your skin's complexion is very limited.)

The dermis is the inner layer of the skin that contains nerves, fat cells, blood vessels, sweat and oil glands, collagen, and elastin. If your dermis fails to produce enough moisture (oil and sweat), your complexion can appear dry, flaky, and pale. Your complexion also can look pale if your blood vessels are not providing your skin with adequate nutrients and oxygen. Having a healthy vascular system means that more blood can get to the farthest parts of your body, like your skin. Keeping your vascular system healthy requires good fats like omega-3s (found in fish), fiber (found in fruits, vegetables, nuts, seeds, and grains), and antioxidants (also found in fruits, vegetables, nuts, seeds, and grains). The dermis is key to having—and keeping—a complexion that glows.

The outer layer of your skin, or epidermis, plays an equally important role in your complexion. It contains melanocytes, or pigmented cells, that, when exposed to the sun, can cause spotting on your skin. The epidermis is otherwise made up of dead cells that slough off over time. (Did you know that 90 percent of household dust is dead skin cells?) New cells generated by the dermis continually replace your epidermis.

If the epidermis becomes too thick, it can give your skin a flaky, white, or even yellow appearance. Certain foods encourage your skin to slough off dead cells, promote healthy skin cell growth, and allow the natural beauty of your dermis to shine through. Exfoliating and using abrasive cleansers on your skin can also help, but you need to be careful: Removing too much of your epidermis can expose your very sensitive dermis. If you've ever scraped or burned your skin, you know what this can feel like.

To keep that natural, youthful glow to your skin, your dermis needs to continually grow new, healthy skin cells, a process which requires the help of specific nutrients found in foods. Vitamin A, for example, stimulates skin cells to divide (mitotic cell division) and increases the rate at which your skin creates new cells, giving you a more radiant complexion. Folate and vitamin B12 are also needed for cell division. Such vitamins can be found in foods like brewer's yeast, mushrooms, and wheat germ—just to name a few—and can give your skin a glowing complexion.

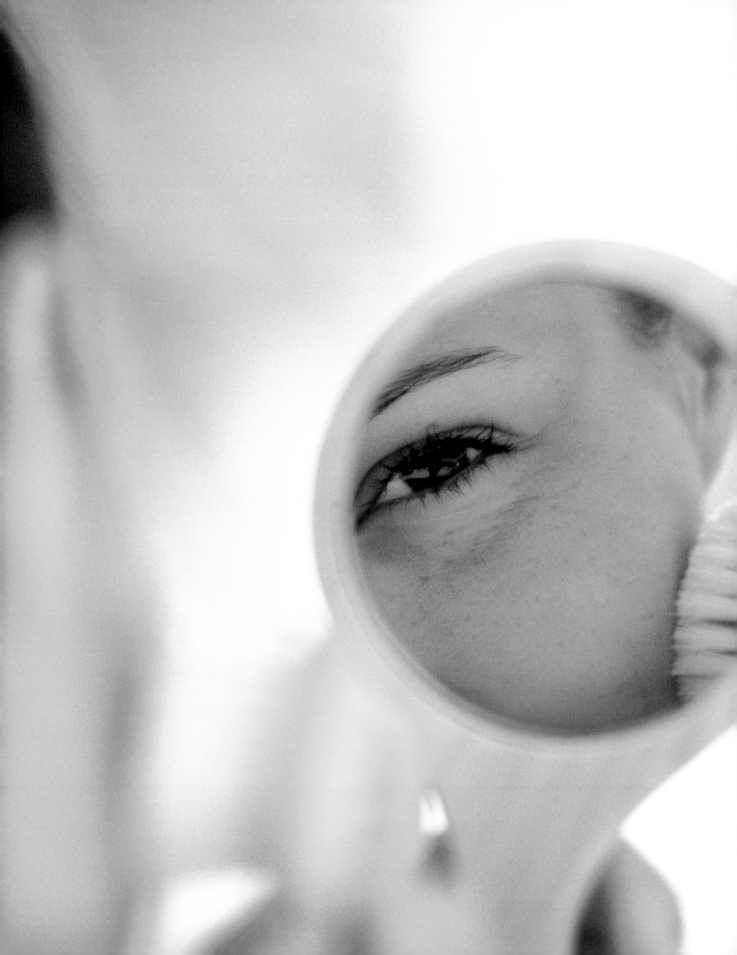

Dump the Concealer

In addition to eating foods that encourage cell growth, you can also improve your complexion by adding foods that fight inflammation to your diet. Inflammation, which often appears in the form of red or blotchy skin, is caused by trauma (rubbing of the skin, ultraviolet light, or chemical damage), allergic reaction, or rosacea. Consuming foods rich in essential fatty acids and antioxidants, such as sardines, oranges, strawberries, and mangosteen (all of which are featured in this chapter), is one of the best ways to fight this inflammation.

Spot It

Is your complexion spotted? Age spots, freckles, and moles can make your complexion appear uneven. While some consider these spots a problem, others see them as a unique dimension of their beauty. Either way, it is important to know that two of these types of spots—freckles and age spots—are caused by sun damage and can actually be prevented with antioxidants found in many foods.

Age Spots

Age spots are collections of melanin, the skin pigment, on the top layer of the skin (epidermis). Like freckles, they are a sign of photoaging (skin damage due to the sun). Age spots can be prevented and potentially reduced with the help of antioxidants; selenium and vitamins A, C, and E are all thought to be particularly helpful.

Freckles

When the skin is exposed to the sun, the body attempts to defend the dermis from damage by increasing production of a dark pigment called melanin. Freckles are concentrated spots of color that result.

The medical terms for the three main types of freckles are ephelids, lentigoes, and lentigines. Common in people with fair skin, freckles are usually round, flat spots that can be yellow-brown, tan, brown, or black. They tend to appear on areas of the skin that see the most sun and become more prominent with age.

Be Careful What Remedies You Use

For centuries, people have tried to diminish the appearance of freckles and age spots. Ancient Egyptians used fenugreek oils to fade them. More recently, lemon juice has been used as a favorite lightening remedy, along with modern cosmetics and bleaching agents. Note that none of these methods is terribly effective. More advanced techniques, such as freezing, chemical peels, dermabrasion, and laser resurfacing, may get rid of freckles and age spots, but these treatments can be painful and may damage healthy skin or cause scarring.

Moles

Moles are clusters of colored skin cells called melanocytes, and are typically benign. Though usually small and dark brown, they can be a wide range of colors and sizes, and they can be raised or flat. You can have moles anywhere on your body. Unlike freckles, which are made by sunlight, moles can be present at birth. They may also appear later in life; most people have between 10 and 40 moles by adulthood.

Seventeen Foods That Brighten Your Complexion

Nutrients in foods can help your skin have a glowing, radiant complexion. Foods that fight inflammation, promote skin cell growth, and keep your vascular system healthy can make your skin shine with its full beauty. The following foods are helpful aids to brighten your complexion.

Dullness Busters

- Brewer's Yeast
- Lima Beans
- Multigrain Bread
- Mushrooms
- Oysters
- Peppermint
- Psyllium
- Pumpkin Seeds
- Sweet Potatoes
- Wheat Germ

Natural Concealers

- Mackerel
- Mangosteen
- Sardines

Spot Preventers

- Chicken
- Oranges
- Sesame Seeds
- Strawberries

DULLNESS BUSTERS

Are you faced with a dull complexion when you wake up in the morning? Perhaps you turn to blush or even pinch your cheeks to try and perk up your look? Luckily, there is a better way to get your bright complexion back—and it's tasty too! Try adding the following ten foods to your diet and you'll not only jazz up your skin, but spice up your diet as well. From beans and bread to peppermint and pumpkin seeds, dullness will have no place to hide!

Brewer's Yeast

Also known as nutritional yeast, brewer's yeast is one of the healthiest foods on earth, and it offers your skin many healthy benefits. It is the yeast that is left behind after making beer or alcohol and is considered a health food because it is easily digested and has a high nutrient content.

Be Beautiful with Bs

Not many people know about brewer's yeast, however, and even fewer people include it in their diet, which is a shame since it's a rich source of B vitamins, all essential amino acids, and fifteen minerals. Many of these nutrients offer your skin the tools it needs to have a glowing, radiant complexion.

B vitamins give your skin the energy it needs to generate new cells. A youthful complexion has lots of new skin cells created by the dermis, the second layer of your skin, and B vitamins ensure that these cells divide and grow.

In addition, these cells are involved in every type of energy metabolism in your skin—and skin cells that produce enough energy to work properly (thanks to B vitamins) have a beautiful appearance.

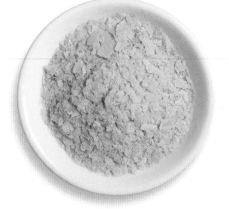

Energizing Skin Cells

Brewer's yeast also contains high quantities of chromium. A high quality brewer's yeast provides as much as 60 mcg per tablespoon (15 ml)—half the recommended daily allowance. This mineral is involved in the metabolism of all forms of energy: carbohydrates, protein, and fats. Your rapidly growing skin cells need chromium to extract energy from these sources.

Chromium also helps insulin move sugar into cells. If your blood sugar levels stay too high because insulin is not working, it can damage your nerves and blood vessels, particularly the delicate ones in your fingers and eyes (a particular problem for diabetics).

When blood properly feeds your skin oxygen and sugars, on the other hand, the skin looks healthy and can divide and grow properly. And healthy blood vessels mean a bright complexion.

Yeast Infections?

Some may believe that eating yeast causes yeast infections. Quite the opposite, in fact: The species of yeast that brewer's yeast belongs to is known to offer many healthy benefits to the body. Side effects have not been reported from using brewer's yeast, although some people are allergic to it. It can be found in the health section of your local grocery store in powder or flake form.

Brewer's yeast is terrifically nutritious and certainly worth adding to your diet. If you like popcorn, top it off with a dusting of brewer's yeast. Mix some into your yogurt or oatmeal or bake it into low-fat bran muffins. Enjoy brewer's yeast however you can, and you'll notice a brighter complexion.

Lima Beans

Lima beans contain molybdenum, a lesser-known mineral that plays a very important role in the body. They also contain folate, iron, and manganese, all of which promote healthy skin. Toss these beans into your recipes and let your skin glow—it doesn't get much easier than that!

Beans of Energy

Every new cell requires molybdenum to help synthesize DNA, the cell's genetic material. In the parts of your body—such as the skin—that create new cells at a rapid rate, molybdenum is indispensable. Not only that, but molybdenum is an important part of sulfite oxidase, an enzyme responsible for detoxifying (removing) damaging toxins called sulfites. Lucky for us, just one ½-cup (85 g) serving of lima beans provides nearly 95 percent of the recommended daily value of molybdenum.

Nutrients like B vitamins and iron also help skin cells make energy. Lima beans are a good source of the B vitamins folate and thiamin—one cup of cooked beans (170 g) provides 39 percent of the suggested daily value for folate and 20 percent of the suggested daily value for thiamin. Their iron content (25 percent in one cup) is involved in transferring oxygen from your lungs to your skin cells, which helps brighten your complexion.

Insulin—Not Just for Diabetics

Chromium plays a critical role in our bodies because without it, the hormone insulin fails to work. Insulin is like the master hormone of metabolism. It not only controls blood sugar levels, as well as many other aspects of carbohydrate breakdown and storage, but it also directs much of the metabolism involving fat, protein, and energy. Insulin helps skin obtain the energy it needs to repair damage, making chromium an essential nutrient for healthy skin.

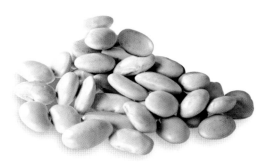

Buttery Beauties

Lima beans are a source of the trace mineral manganese. Manganese is an essential cofactor in several enzymes involved in energy production. Moreover, manganese helps fight free radicals, which damage the skin, trigger inflammation, and can negatively affect your complexion.

Sometimes called butter beans because of their creamy texture, lima beans have a subtle flavor that complements a whole variety of dishes, from soups (like the Corn, Squash, and Lima Bean Soup on p. 216) to salads to sides. My grandmother used to steam lima beans with a bit of oil as a delicious accompaniment to roast chicken.

Multigrain Bread

No more white bread. Multigrain bread is here, and store shelves are packed with it. What prompted this revolution in the bread aisle? The many healthy benefits of fiber. Fiber has been proven to lower your risk of heart disease, fight breast cancer and gallstones, improve digestion, help detoxify the body, and improve your complexion.

White Bread, Palid Complexion

In its natural form, wheat has a host of skin-beautifying nutrients, but refining it to make white bread strips it of most of its natural goodness. For example, most breads, pastas, and cookies in the United States are made with 60 percent extraction wheat, which means that 40 percent of the original wheat was removed during the refining process. The most nutritious parts of the wheat—the germ and bran—are removed during this process, and more than half of the B vitamins, vitamin E, calcium, phosphorus, zinc, copper, iron, and fiber are lost.

It is important not just to choose whole wheat bread, but to opt for multigrain as often as possible. Multigrain bread contains more than just the nutrients from wheat; it also provides nutrients from other grains.

New Beauty with B Vitamins and Iron

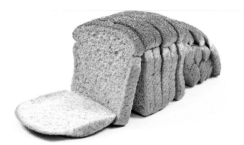

Multigrain breads are fortified with B vitamins and iron. B vitamins are required for every aspect of metabolism in your skin. The dermis, the second layer of your skin, also relies on these vitamins to keep healthy, new cells growing. Your skin is a very active tissue that is constantly growing and dividing, and if it does not have enough B vitamins, it cannot grow quickly. This can give your complexion a dull appearance.

Iron is another important nutrient for your complexion. It is part of the hemoglobin in your red blood cells, which is responsible for carrying oxygen from your lungs to your skin cells. When you have steady blood flow to your skin, your skin looks rosy and radiant. Without oxygen, however, your cells cannot function properly.

Fiber Is Your Friend

The most important complexion compound in multigrain bread is fiber, which helps your digestive tract work well. Fiber traps fat in your intestines and prevents it from being absorbed. This is great as bad fats like cholesterol can cause damage to your blood vessels, including those in your skin, and therefore dull your complexion.

Fiber also improves the rate at which your body eliminates toxins. Your liver clears toxins from your blood and sends them to your digestive tract in bile to be eliminated. Fiber can trap these toxins and carry them out of the body when you go to the bathroom. Without fiber, toxins can accumulate in the fat cells in your dermis and damage your skin.

There's no reason to settle for white bread when high-fiber bread, pasta, and cereal all taste better—and are better for you. Once you start scanning the shelves for multigrain products, you'll be amazed at what's available. Have you tried multigrain nacho chips? How about multigrain waffles? You'll love the richer texture and taste, and you'll love what the nutrients do for your skin.

What Is Multigrain?

A food labeled "multigrain" contains more than one type of grain. Whole wheat products contain only wheat, but they contain more of the wheat than "white" food products. Spelt, kamut, wheat, and barley are examples of grains found in multigrain products.

Mushrooms

Earthy and delicious, mushrooms are packed with nutrients, making them a great addition to your skin-beautifying diet. They're also available in a wide range of varieties, so you can slice, dice, and sauté these fungi in all sorts of ways.

Choose Your Shrooms Carefully

While the white button variety is the most popular in the United States, coffee-colored crimini mushrooms have a richer flavor and more nutrients than their white button cousins. Shiitake, oyster, king oyster, and maitake mushrooms also deliver skin-healthy nutrients, but are larger and have more distinct flavors. Portabello mushrooms are another tasty choice—their large, flat shape and steak-like flavor make them a hit with vegetarians and meat-eaters alike.

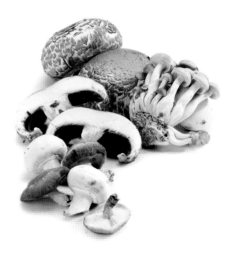

Gets Skin Growing

Mushrooms are best known for their content of B vitamins, which are required for metabolism in your skin and assist with new skin cell growth. The cells of the dermis that produce new skin cells are some of the hardest working cells in your body, which means that they have a high metabolism rate and require lots of B vitamins to perform their job properly.

Mushrooms are packed with vitamins B1 (thiamin), B2 (riboflavin), B3 (niacin), B5, and B6. Together, these vitamins form an all-star team in your body, making you feel energized and boosting your immune system.

Protection Against Dullness

Just five ounces (142 g) of crimini mushrooms offers you more than 52 percent of the suggested daily amount of selenium. Why is selenium so important to your skin? Because it acts as an antioxidant, protecting the skin from damaging free radicals that form as a result of inflammation and exposure to chemicals and ultraviolet radiation (sunlight).

New skin cells are created in the dermis, the second layer of your skin. They give the skin a youthful, glowing appearance. Selenium can stop free radicals from damaging these cells, keeping you looking radiant.

Which Mushroom Is Best?

When it comes to selenium content, the crimini mushroom gets top billing, as it contains more of this mineral than its white button or portabello counterparts. Compared to other known food sources of selenium, however, all three of these mushrooms are at the head of the class:

Food Source	Quantity	Daily Value of Selenium
Turkey, light meat	3 oz	45 percent
Crimini mushrooms	5 medium	31 percent
White button mushrooms	5 medium	22 percent
Portabello mushrooms	1 medium	21 percent
Egg, whole	1 medium	20 percent
Brown rice	½ cup (95 g)	15 percent

New Source of Powerful Antioxidant

Mushrooms contain the powerful antioxidant L-ergothioneine, which was once thought to be available only in chicken liver and wheat germ. According to researchers at the Pennsylvania State Mushroom Research Laboratory, mushrooms contain significant levels of this antioxidant, which acts as a scavenger of free radicals. Better yet, the presence of selenium in mushrooms enhances this antioxidant activity.

Maitake, oyster, king oyster, and shiitake mushrooms have the highest amounts of L-ergothioneine—up to forty times as much as wheat germ—followed by portabello, crimini, and white button. And because this antioxidant is heat-stable, it is not destroyed if mushrooms are cooked.

So grab your shopping bag and fill up. You can eat mushrooms raw in salads, with hummus, cooked into sauces, or as a pizza topping. For a wonderfully earthy entrée, try the Mushrooms Stuffed with Barley, Kale, and Feta (p. 248), or pair grilled fish with the Braised Lentils with Eggplant and Mushrooms (p. 250).

Button, crimini, and shiitake mushrooms are available in most grocery stores. If your local store does not carry fresh reishi or maitake mushrooms, look for them at an Asian market in your area. Select mushrooms that are firm, plump, and clean. Stored in your fridge in a loosely closed paper bag, mushrooms can last about a week.

Oysters

Oysters are not only delicious, they are also among the most nutritionally balanced foods. Containing protein, carbohydrates, and lipids, oysters are considered so healthy that the National Heart and Lung Institute suggests they be added to low-cholesterol diets. They also contain vitamins A, C, and D, plus many B vitamins, and a high amount of zinc—all of which can make your complexion shine as beautifully as a pearl.

Brightening In Multiple Ways

Oysters contain B vitamins, which help your skin produce energy and new skin cells. They also contain vitamins A and C, which are great antioxidants, as well as selenium, a potent antioxidant that helps your skin fight inflammation and prevent wrinkles.

On top of all that, one serving of oysters (four or five medium) supplies the recommended daily allowance of iron, copper, iodine, magnesium, calcium, zinc, manganese, and phosphorus.

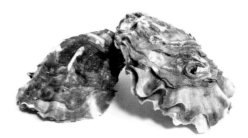

Pearly Complexion

Let oysters be the pearl of your complexion. Oysters are the richest source of the trace mineral zinc, with one serving giving you more than 100 percent of the recommended daily intake.

Zinc acts as an antioxidant in your body and is involved in more than three thousand reactions. In your skin, it helps fight the signs of aging, in part by neutralizing free radicals that form due to inflammation and sun exposure. In this way, zinc helps maintain collagen and elastin fibers that give skin its firmness and help prevent sagging and wrinkles.

On the Half-Shell

Folklore says that oysters should be eaten only in months that contain the letter R, meaning that you would eat them from September to April. This may have been true in the past when hotter temperatures would spoil oysters as they traveled from the ocean to the market, but thanks to modern refrigeration, we can now treat ourselves to oysters each and every month of the year.

If you like raw oysters, you're in luck, as they are actually more nutritious than cooked oysters. Keep in mind, however, that raw shellfish carry a risk of contamination, so be sure to purchase your oysters at their very freshest from a reputable market.

Peppermint

Peppermint could be regarded as one of the world's earliest medicines, with archaeological evidence tracing its use as far back as ten thousand years ago. The leaves of the peppermint have long been known to soothe upset stomachs and freshen breath, but few people know the health benefits that peppermint offers your skin.

Fight Red with Green

A cross between watermint and spearmint, peppermint is thought to restore elasticity, tone to your skin, minimize pores, and reduce swelling and redness. While peppermint is used topically because it cools, refreshes, stimulates, and revitalizes, it's just as beneficial when taken internally, where its many nutrients energize your skin from the inside out.

Peppermint contains manganese, vitamin A, and vitamin C in high quantities. The two antioxidants, vitamins A and C, fight the damaging effects of inflammation that you notice in the skin as redness. For this reason, peppermint reduces swelling and thereby improves the skin's com-

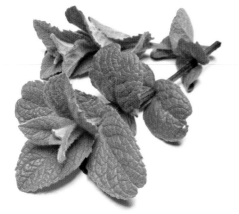

plexion. It's also worth noting that peppermint contains small amounts of iron, as well the B vitamins folate and riboflavin. These nutrients are known to help brighten your complexion.

Peppermint is native to western, central, and southern Europe. Today, it is grown throughout the world and can be found in a variety of products, including peppermint teas, bottled drinks, chocolates, candies, and gum. Try to avoid peppermint products that are high in sugar, which can adversely affect your skin. Instead, add fresh peppermint leaves to sparkling water or mix up a pitcher of Iced Minted Green Tea (p. 272). For a real minty treat, use peppermint oil to create homemade ice cream and peppermint candies.

Psyllium

Psyllium comes from the seeds and seed husks of the *Plantago ovata* plant, an herb native to parts of Asia, the Mediterranean, and North Africa. Used in herbal remedies and considered one of the most popular laxatives in North America, psyllium is increasingly finding its way into breakfast cereals and other products, mainly due to its high fiber content.

Detox to Avoid Dullness

Psyllium and the fiber it contains bulks up in the intestines, taking on water, which helps you feel full and encourages proper bowel excretion. Fiber also eliminates the nasty toxins in your body and helps your skin look more clear and beautiful.

There are more than eighty thousand toxic chemicals manufactured in the United States. These toxins can be in our water and food supplies and in our cosmetics. When toxins enter your body, the liver filters them out of your blood and sends them, along with bile, into your intestines, where fiber can trap them and send them out of your body. Without fiber, however, these toxins can become reabsorbed and build up in your system, eventually damaging your skin and resulting in a dull complexion.

Fiber, such as that in psyllium, can help lower your body's toxins levels. Psyllium seed husks are nature's most concentrated source of toxin-trapping, cholesterol-lowering soluble fiber, with their husks containing about 60 percent fiber (oats, on the other hand, are only about 5 percent fiber). Just one tablespoon of whole husk provides about 9 grams of soluble fiber, more than one-third of the recommended daily intake.

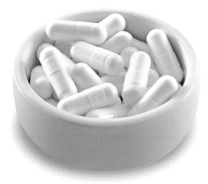

Strong Skin with Psyllium

Researchers in Germany have found that the carbohydrates in psyllium can help your skin. These carbohydrates improve the way cells attach to each other. For your skin, this means better cell-to-cell adhesion, which contributes to firmer, more elastic skin. Additionally, psyllium can play a role in your skin's fibroblast cells, which produce the compounds that keep your skin strong, firm, smooth, and elastic.

You can find psyllium husk seeds or psyllium as a dried powder at any health food store. You can also find psyllium marketed as treatments for constipation at your local pharmacy. Sprinkle the powder on your cereal, add it to your favorite baking recipe, or blend it into yogurt. The powder has little or no taste and can be added to just about anything.

Pumpkin Seeds

Worlds better than candy, pumpkin seeds, also known as "pepitas," are a good source of many nutrients that keep your complexion bright, including iron, zinc, vitamins, and essential fatty acids. They also contain phytosterols that help lower cholesterol levels and may also promote prostate health in men.

Iron Out Dullness

Iron can help your skin regain a rosy, healthy glow. Involved in energy metabolism, iron acts as an oxygen carrier in hemoglobin, which carries oxygen in your red blood cells from the lungs to every cell in your body. Because the cells in your skin are far away from your lungs and need lots of oxygen due to their high rate of metabolism, your skin needs a steady supply of iron to get the job done. In just ¼ cup (16 g) of pumpkin seeds, you'll find nearly 29 percent of the daily value for iron.

The trace mineral zinc is also on your side in pumpkin seeds, with ¼ cup (16 g) providing 17 percent of the daily value. Zinc acts as an antioxidant, neutralizing free radicals before they cause the damage that stimulates inflammation. The result is beautiful, redness-free skin.

Pumpkin seeds are a healthy snack for your entire body. To make your own, start by cutting off the top of a pumpkin and removing the seeds from the orange flesh. Toss the seeds lightly with vegetable oil and toast them in the oven at 375°F (190°C, or gas mark 5) until they turn light brown. Sprinkled with sea salt, roasted pumpkin seeds are one of my favorite skin-healthy snacks (and they're wonderful paired with dried fruit and nuts in the Tamari-Flavored Snack Mix on p. 204).

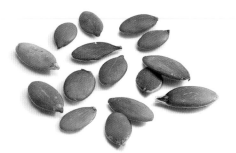

Sweet Potatoes

Although sweet potatoes typically grace the dinner table during colder seasons, it is of great benefit to your skin to prepare these wonderful, naturally sweet vegetables throughout the year. Sweet potatoes are a great source of vitamin A, vitamin C, and fiber, all of which add radiance to your complexion.

Hot Potato

Vitamin A supports the growth of beautiful new skin cells and stimulates skin cells to divide. It also increases the rate at which your skin creates new cells, giving you a more glowing complexion. In just one baked sweet potato, you'll find more than 200 percent of the recommended daily value of vitamin A.

Vitamin C acts as a powerful antioxidant that neutralizes damaging free radicals that form in your skin from inflammation or sunlight exposure. One potato provides nearly 30 percent of your daily value.

Finally, the 3 g of fiber you'll find in one potato help your digestive tract work properly, reducing the number of toxins in your body, which can cause damage to your skin and dull its appearance.

No Zinc, No Vitamin A

Researchers have determined that without zinc your skin cannot properly use vitamin A to fight wrinkles and maintain a healthy complexion. This is because zinc is required to make retinol-binding protein, which transports vitamin A to the skin. Therefore, if you do not have sufficient zinc in your diet, your body struggles to move vitamin A from its stores in the liver to the skin. To make the best use of vitamin A from sweet potatoes, try to eat them along with zinc-rich foods, such as beans, nuts, and whole grains.

Orange Is the New Black

The sweet potato has yellow or orange flesh, and its thin skin appears either white, yellow, orange, red, or purple. Sweet potatoes can be shaped like a white potato (short and blocky, with rounded ends) or can be longer, with tapered ends. Bake, peel, and mash them for an autumn-hued, skin-healthy version of regular mashed potatoes, or, for a healthier version of French fries, slice sweet potatoes into wedges, toss lightly with oil and salt, and bake in the oven at 375°F until the desired crispness is reached. Sweet potatoes can go anywhere that regular white potatoes do: soups, stews, side dishes, you name it!

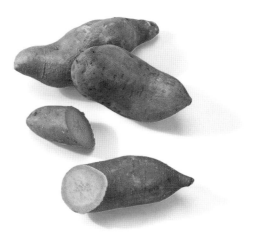

Wheat Germ

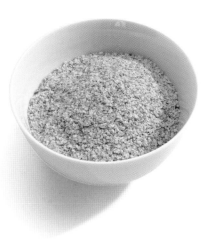

Wheat germ is a star when it comes to delivering health benefits for your skin. This vitamin- and mineral-rich heart of the wheat kernel, which gets removed when wheat is refined to make white flour (another reason why you should always choose whole grain products), is a highly concentrated source of nutrients like zinc, magnesium, manganese, vitamin E, and B vitamins.

A Bundle of Nutrients

Wheat germ contains folate, thiamin, and B6—three B vitamins that can support the high rate of cell division taking place in your skin cells. These vitamins are also needed for energy and digestion; for the health of your nerves, muscles, skin, hair, and organs; and for the growth and repair of tissues.

Wheat germ is also a great source of vitamin E, a fat-soluble antioxidant that helps protect the fatty parts of your skin, including cell membranes, from damage by free radicals. Fats and cholesterol are very susceptible to free radical damage caused by toxins, chemicals, sunlight and inflammation. A steady supply of vitamin E is vital for keeping this damage at bay.

Wheat germ can easily be incorporated into muffins, casseroles, and pancakes or sprinkled over hot or cold cereal. Add wheat germ to smoothies or yogurt for a little bit of texture and a lot of nutrition.

NATURAL CONCEALERS

Red spots, blotches, and pimples are always problems we wish we could conceal. But instead of reaching for your latest cosmetic solution, why not try preventing the appearance of unwanted blemishes by eating the right foods? Healthy foods such as the fish and fruit discussed next can help your skin stay healthy and keep your complexion in perfect shape.

Mackerel

"Mackerel" commonly refers to the Atlantic mackerel fish, also known as the Boston mackerel, which lives in the northern parts of the Atlantic Ocean. A serving (3.5 oz, or 100 g) of cooked Atlantic mackerel contains about 1300 mg of omega-3 fatty acids, which are among the most potent anti-inflammatory nutrients available.

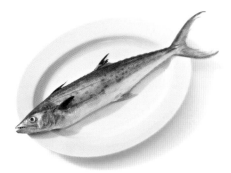

Reduce Redness with Fish

The American Heart Association recommends that everyone eat at least two servings of fish per week, and that people who are at risk for heart disease consume 1000 mg of omega-3 fatty acids each day. Fatty fish like mackerel, lake trout, herring, sardines, albacore tuna, and salmon are all high in omega-3 fatty acids. (Note: King mackerel has about one-third the amount of omega-3 fatty acids that Atlantic mackerel contains, so shop for Atlantic mackerel whenever possible.)

Omega-3 fatty acids from fish have anti-inflammatory effects. By competing with arachidonic acid, which triggers bad inflammation, omega-3s help you reduce the amount of negative inflammation and damage in your skin. Fish oil is so good at reducing inflammation that it has been tested as a treatment for many diseases, including heart disease, psoriasis, inflammatory bowel disease, and arthritis.

More Than Omega-3s

Mackerel also contains selenium, a mineral that supports the body's natural antioxidant abilities and, like omega-3s, helps neutralize the free radicals produced by inflammation.

Finally, mackerel is a good source of vitamins B6 and B12, which are required for the production of new skin cells that rejuvenate the look of your complexion and keep you looking beautiful.

Mangosteen

Ever heard of mangosteen? Probably not. This fruit is a newcomer to most people in North America, and has nothing to do with the more familiar mango. The mangosteen is actually a tropical evergreen tree that bears fragrant fruit with a sweet, creamy, citrus-like flavor. Considered a super-food because of its antioxidant power, nutrient richness, and delicious taste, the mangosteen is gaining popularity as a fruit to include in any healthy diet—including diets designed to improve your complexion.

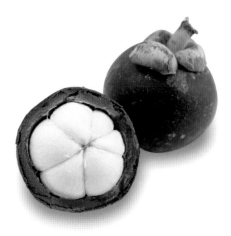

On the Hunt for Mangosteens

Most mangosteen is grown and harvested in the Far East, mainly in Thailand, Vietnam, China, and Taiwan. It takes about 15 years before the mangosteen tree bears fruit, and when the fruit is ripe, the rind turns a deep, red-purple color. At the center is a soft, opaque white fruit that can be pulled apart in sections.

Mangosteen fruit does not ripen well after harvesting. It is usually eaten fresh, but it can be stored for a few weeks or juiced for longer shelf life. While the fresh variety may be difficult to find in the United States, canned and frozen options can typically be found in well-stocked grocery stores.

Inflammation No More

The antioxidants in mangosteen fight inflammation, the cause of redness and blotchiness that can adversely affect your skin's complexion. In a study published in 2002, an antioxidant component from mangosteen called xanthone gamma-mangoestin was found to reduce the activity of a chemical (cyclooxygenase) involved in inflammation and pain.

In that same year, Japanese researchers also found that mangosteen reduces histamine and prostaglandin E2, two markers of inflammation.

In addition to mangosteen's benefits for your skin, new research is investigating its ability to help prevent breast cancer and leukemia. With all that this fruit has going for it, it'd be silly not to add it to your fruit bowl.

Sardines

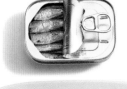

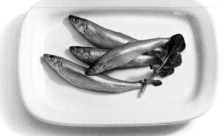

If your skin seems red or blotchy, you may be suffering from inflammation. Low levels of damage and irritation to your skin can cause inflammation of this sort. But there's good news: Omega-3 fatty acids, like those found in sardines, can resolve these skin issues and get you back on the healthy skin track.

Omega-3s for You and Me

You may have read in the newspaper that fish oil is being used to fight diseases such as arthritis and heart disease. This is because the omega-3 fatty acids found in fish are excellent at reducing inflammation, a major cause of such diseases.

Sardines, relatives of herrings, are a tremendous source of omega-3 fatty acids. One 4-ounce (113 g) serving of sardines canned in oil delivers between 0.8 g and 1.8 g of omega-3s (a daily intake of 1.1 g of omega-3 fatty acids for women and 1.6 g for men is recommended).

Sardines are also low in mercury, PCBs, and other contaminants found in larger fish. Mercury levels are higher in bigger fish because they feed on smaller fish, causing them to accumulate this toxin. This process is called bioaccumulation. Because sardines are at the start of the food chain in this scenario, their contamination levels are much lower. This works to our benefit in terms of healthy eating (but certainly not to theirs!).

Pop Open a Can of Health

Sardines are usually packed in small, flat tin cans. If you like anchovies on your pizza, experiment with sardines. In Russia, they serve pizza covered with mockba, a combination of sardines, tuna, mackerel, salmon, and onions. Sardines are also great in sandwiches and stews. Some people like to mash sardines into a paste to spread on crackers. However you include this inflammation-fighting nutrient into your diet, you'll enjoy a beautiful, bright complexion.

Green Fishing

Sardines are a great fish to eat for environmental reasons. Unlike tuna, salmon, and cod, sardines are very resilient to fishing. Because they reach sexual maturity quickly and spawn several times a year, they can quickly replenish their numbers.

SPOT PREVENTERS

Murphy's Law says that if a big social event is coming up, you will most definitely develop unwanted spots in your complexion. Prevent spots on those special days, and every day, by including these four antioxidant-rich foods in your diet—in fact, you may have some of them in your fridge or fruit basket already. Eating right has never been so easy!

Chicken

Lean poultry like chicken is a great source of selenium, vitamin B3 (niacin), and the compound CoQ10, all of which can brighten your complexion. Poultry also contains plenty of protein, which helps keep your muscles in gear and your skin tight. With all these elements working for you, you'd be a chicken not to add some to your plate.

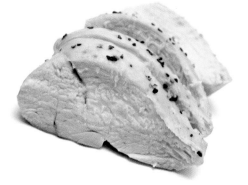

Rare Source of Beauty

Selenium, a mineral found in animal meats and plants that have been grown in selenium-rich soil, is used to make compounds that act as antioxidants, which can neutralize free radicals, and thus reduce damage that can lead to wrinkles, dryness, and age spots. In four ounces (113 g) of roasted chicken breast, you'll find 40 percent of the recommended daily value for selenium.

Your skin cells divide rapidly and have a high metabolism which requires B vitamins, making it imperative that you seek out B-vitamin–rich foods. Niacin, or vitamin B3, is one such vitamin you'll find in chicken that supports the health of your skin by helping it grow and repair quickly. One 4-ounce (113 g) serving of roasted chicken breast contains approximately 72 percent of the recommended daily value of this valuable nutrient.

CoQ10, or coenzyme Q10, is a vitamin-like compound that you can find in almost every cell of your body. It plays a key role in producing energy in the mitochondria and acts as a powerful antioxidant, helping to protect your DNA and the energy-producing parts of your skin cells.

CoQ10 levels are highest during the first twenty years of life and decline with age, making it increasingly important to include in your diet as you get older. Though tough to find in most foods, CoQ10 is present in small amounts in poultry, as well as in oily fish, organ meats, and whole grains.

The Power of Protein

Chicken is a great source of amino acids, which are the building blocks of proteins. Everyone knows that our muscles are made of protein, but enzymes and hormones are proteins as well.

You need amino acids for many actions in your skin. Enzymes cause the skin to grow, divide, repair—and appear beautiful. Two particular amino acids are helpful for your skin: methioine and cysteine. Methionine is involved in many processes in the body, including acting as an antioxidant to help protect the skin from free-radical damage. Cysteine can be made in the body from methionine, and after one more metabolic step, it is converted into the potent antioxidant glutathione. Cysteine also promotes skin cell growth and repair, helping your complexion look healthy, youthful, and free of damage.

These antioxidants protect the skin from free radical damage and prevent the formation of free radicals by toxins. However, this tag-team of amino acids is present in lower levels as you age, making it vital that you seek out foods like chicken and other poultry as your birthday candles multiply. To feed your body right and fight the signs of aging, give our Rosemary Ginger Chicken with Orange-Honey Glaze on page 258 a try.

Niacin Fights Spots

Niacin, when applied topically, can reduce the appearance of spots and blotchiness, improve the appearance of skin wrinkles and yellowing, and improve elasticity.

Oranges

Kiss your age spots good-bye with the help of vitamin C from oranges. These juicy, sweet fruits are grown in the southern United States, Brazil, Mexico, Spain, China, and Israel. Before the twentieth century, oranges were expensive, and some cultures gave them as a treat in Christmas stockings. Today, oranges are widely available and easily affordable—and they are a great way to fight the signs of aging.

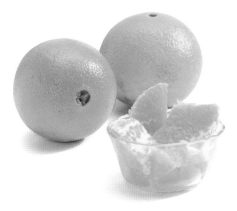

Clear Up Your Complexion with Vitamin C

Just one orange provides your body with about 115 percent of your daily requirement of vitamin C. This potent antioxidant prevents free radical damage from sunlight, which can cause age spots and inflammation. Age spots, a sign of photoaging (skin damage due to sunlight), are collections of the skin pigment melanin on the top layer of the skin (epidermis).

Supplements with high dosages of vitamin C are popular today as there is evidence that vitamin C boosts your immune system. However, your body absorbs vitamin C from food sources much more easily than from supplements. In fact, a study conducted at the University of Milan in Italy tested the effect of consuming a vitamin C supplement drink versus drinking pure orange juice. Free radical damage was lowered when orange juice was consumed, but no change was seen with the supplemented drink. This is likely due to the fact that oranges (and orange juice) contain bioflavonoids, which are required for vitamin C absorption.

To Squeeze or Not to Squeeze?

Oranges are the perfect snack and add a special tang to many recipes. They are generally available from winter through summer, with some seasonal variations. Toss some orange segments into your salad, or serve some slices alongside your morning oatmeal.

Drinking orange juice is not as nutritious for your skin as eating a fresh orange, but it is certainly a better choice than coffee or soda. If you don't have time to squeeze your own, look for a juice that is pure, without added flavors or sugars. Stay away from concentrated juices, as concentrating a juice involves removing the water from the juice before shipping it, and the removed water contains many water-soluble vitamins and minerals. If possible, go organic; you'll benefit from more nutrients and fewer contaminants.

An Orange a Day Keeps the Doctor Away

There's more to oranges than vitamin C. An important flavanone in oranges called herperidin has been shown to reduce high blood pressure and cholesterol in animals. Herperidin also has strong anti-inflammatory properties, which makes oranges a powerful tool in fighting the three risk factors associated with heart disease.

Sesame Seeds

Sesame seeds date back more than 5,000 years and are believed to be one of the oldest condiments known to man. Ancient Egyptian tomb paintings even depict the seeds being added to bread dough—a practice still popular today. And it's no wonder that these seeds have withstood the test of time—they're versatile, full of flavor, and packed with nutrients that help your skin have a radiant, bright complexion.

Open Sesame!

Let's unlock the secrets of this beautifying food. First, you will find vitamin E in sesame seeds. This fat-soluble antioxidant is a great friend to your skin because it prevents the formation of free radicals, which cause damage to the fatty parts of your skin. Free radicals develop when your skin is exposed to toxins and sunlight.

There is also an amazing amount of copper in sesame seeds: One-quarter cup (36 g) provides your body with 74 percent of your daily need. How can copper help your complexion? It is a cofactor needed by your skin to make superoxide dismutase, a powerful antioxidant. This antioxidant disarms free radicals formed when your skin is exposed to sunlight and prevents photoaging (skin damage due to sunlight). In other words, copper can help your skin prevent age spots. It also helps your complexion stay bright, as superoxide dismutase is very good at protecting the mitochondria from free radicals. This means that your skin cells can generate much-needed energy without any interference, keeping your skin looking youthful, healthy, and radiant.

Finally, sesame seeds contain a considerable amount of zinc, an antioxidant involved in more than three thousand reactions in your body. In your skin, it helps fight the signs of aging, in part by neutralizing free radicals that form due to inflammation and sun exposure. In this way, zinc helps maintain collagen and elastin fibers that give skin its firmness. One-quarter cup (36 g) of sesame seeds provides you with approximately 18 percent of the recommended daily value for zinc.

Sprinkle Away

Sesame seeds add a nutty taste and crunch to many dishes, from stir fries to salads. They also make a light and delicious coating for poultry and fish (try the Sesame-Crusted Salmon Bake on p. 262). In paste form, sesame seeds turn into tahini, a key ingredient in many Middle Eastern dishes, including hummus. The seeds are available throughout the year, so sprinkle them into your diet anytime to enjoy all their skin-beautifying benefits.

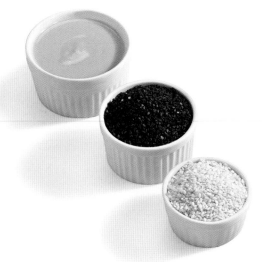

Strawberries

It might surprise you to discover that there are more than six hundred varieties of this sweet, juicy berry. If they aren't already your favorite fruit, strawberries may soon be when you discover how they can improve your complexion.

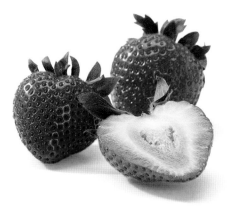

Berry Youthful Skin

Strawberries are a great source of vitamin C: One cup (145 g) supplies about 130 percent of your daily need—more vitamin C than you will find in an orange! This great antioxidant helps your skin fight free radicals that can cause damage to your skin, including age spots—an obvious sign of photoaging (skin damage due to sunlight).

There are even more powerful antioxidants hiding in this delicious berry. Strawberries contain phenols like anthocyanins and ellagitannins. These super powerful compounds are great antioxidants that can protect your skin cells' structures and prevent free-radical damage. In fact, these antioxidants are so good at protecting your cells from harm that strawberries are considered heart-protective, cancer-fighting, and anti-inflammatory.

Slice and Dice Your Way to Clear Skin

Add strawberries to salads, slice them over oatmeal, and blend them into smoothies made from yogurt or other skin-beautifying foods. Choose fresh, firm strawberries, as skin complexion-improving nutrients are lost when strawberries are old, canned, or processed.

Also keep in mind that strawberries are among the fruits most contaminated by pesticides. They tend to be heavily sprayed to prevent bugs from eating them. With that in mind, wash your berries thoroughly before eating and purchase organic strawberries whenever possible.

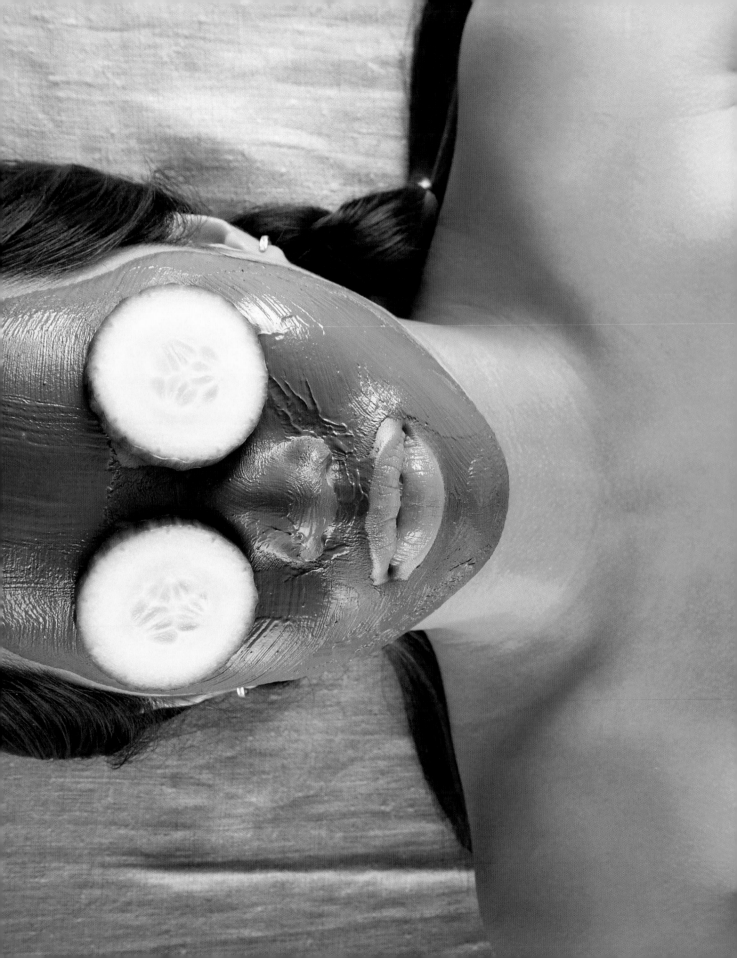

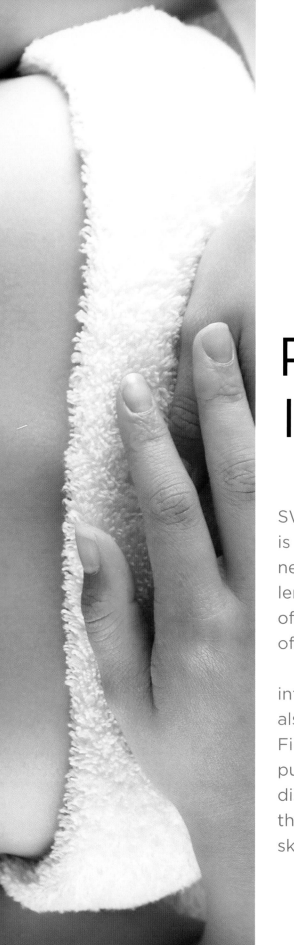

Foods That Fight Puffiness and Inflammation

SWOLLEN, RED, and unattractive skin is a nightmare we all want to avoid. Puffiness and inflammation can cause problems for your complexion, increase aging of the skin, and promote the appearance of wrinkles.

There are many foods that can trigger inflammation in your skin, but there are also many foods that fight inflammation. First, we'll take a look at what causes puffiness and inflammation. Then we'll discuss the foods you should skip, and those you should seek out to help your skin look beautiful.

Puffiness: The How and Why

When you glance in the mirror in the morning, is the skin below your eyes puffy? Puffy eyes are a common problem and are caused by fluid building up between your skin cells. In medical terms, the accumulation of fluid between cells is called edema. It occurs when fluid from your blood vessels is forced into your tissues.

Inflammation and burns to the skin can cause puffiness. Changes in your blood, such as low levels of protein or too much sodium, can also force fluid into your tissues. To battle puffiness with a proper diet, it's necessary to design meals that have all of the essential amino acids so your blood can make the proteins it needs to work properly.

You also need to make sure to eat a diet rich in natural foods so that your sodium intake is not elevated. Diets high in sodium greatly affect the water balance in your body, causing puffiness in your skin, as well as high blood pressure and kidney problems. Processed foods—particularly soups, salad dressings, and chips— are very high in sodium. Avoid these foods and drink plenty of water to help flush out sodium.

What Is Inflammation?

The immune system is responsible for protecting you from foreign invaders like bacteria and viruses. White blood cells are the army of the immune system. They travel to an infected area of your body and guard it against infection. To do so, they destroy infected cells and engulf viruses and bacteria. White blood cells act like a clean-up crew, vacuuming up broken components of the skin. In the process of protecting and cleaning, however, white blood cells can leak chemicals that harm healthy cells. This release of chemicals increases blood flow to the affected area, resulting in redness and swelling (inflammation).

Inflammation involves an influx of fluid (puffiness) and results in the creation of free radicals that can damage the skin in many ways. Free radical damage to the structural components of your skin means wrinkle formation. If free radicals damage the moisture barrier, your skin can become dry and scaly.

What Triggers Inflammation?

Inflammation in the skin can be triggered by any source of damage, including sunlight, chemicals in your environment, cosmetics, and soaps. Sunlight is you skin's number one enemy. It is the main reason that skin looks red, puffy, wrinkled, and rough and can have dark spots. Sunlight damages the skin with its ultraviolet radiation.

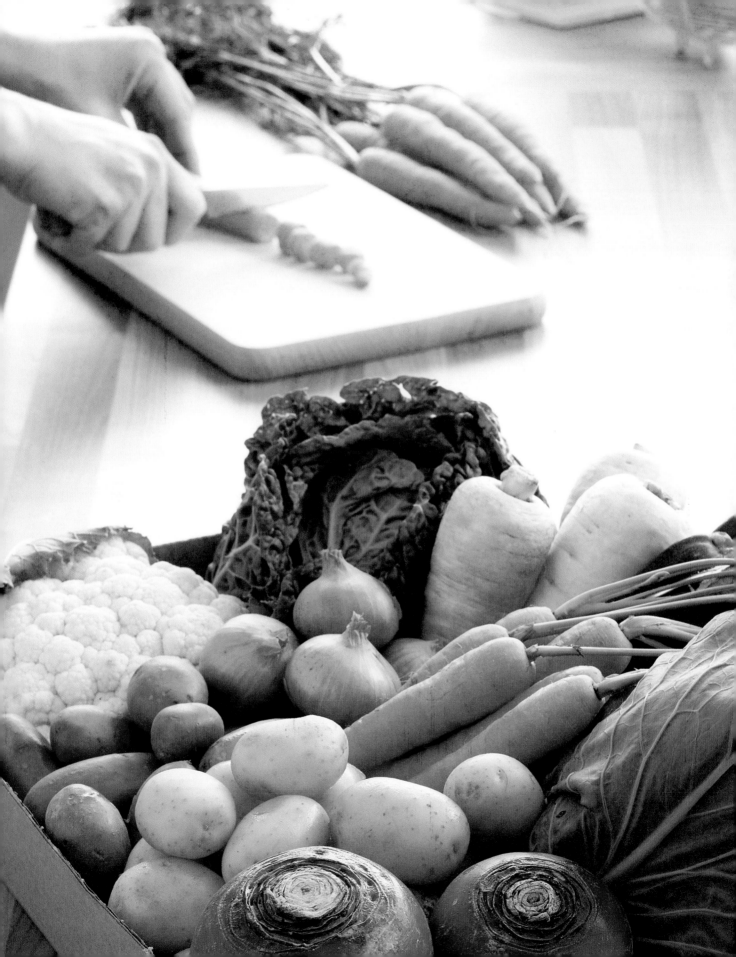

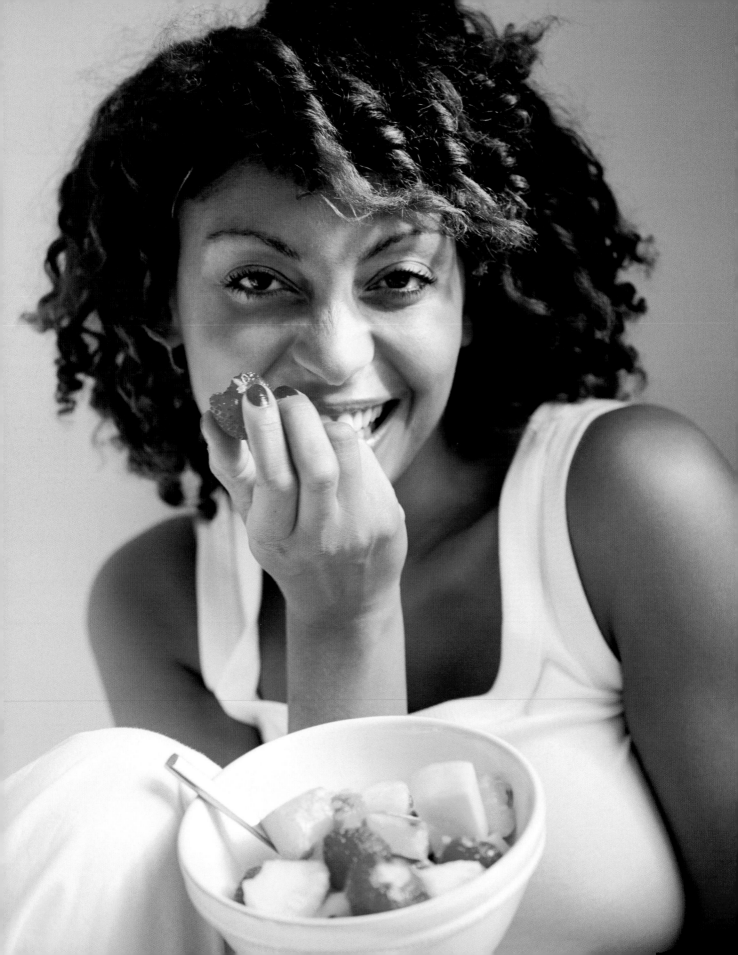

Don't believe sun damage is real? Compare the skin on the outside of your arm with the skin on the underside. Which looks younger? Skin that is exposed to sun shows far more signs of aging than unexposed skin.

Sun Exposure Triggers Inflammation and Aging

Damage to the skin through sun exposure is called photoaging. Photoaging can lead to skin inflammation, cancer, wrinkles, and age spots. Sun exposure reduces the number of blood vessels in your skin. Blood vessels provide your skin with the oxygen and nutrients that it needs to repair and rebuild and look beautiful. When sun exposure reduces the number of blood vessels, the skin becomes malnourished and is unable to repair itself. This damaged skin is unhealthy and tends to get inflamed.

Sunburns are probably the most painful result of too much sun exposure, and cause a great deal of inflammation. Sunburns also cause elastic fibers to clump in the skin, leading to leathery (rough and wrinkled) skin.

To protect itself from sun damage, the skin produces the pigment melanin when exposed to sunlight. In many people, melanin production results in a tan and protects the DNA in your skin from the damaging effects of the sun's ultraviolet radiation. However, no matter how much melanin you have, sunlight can still damage the skin.

Your Diet Can Trigger Inflammation

The sun is an external cause of inflammation, but making poor food choices can lead to inflammation as well. Junk food and foods that are high in sugar are associated with puffy, zapped-looking skin, so it's important to avoid foods such as chocolate bars, candy, soda, fried foods, and processed foods for these reasons.

Unhealthy fats such as saturated and trans fats also make inflammation worse. Trans fats are the so-called "bad fats" added to processed foods to extend their shelf life. These fats build up and cause problems in your circulatory system. The bigger problem, however, is saturated fat, which contains arachidonic acid. Too much arachidonic acid in your diet can make inflammation worse.

When a cell is damaged, fats from its cell membrane trigger inflammation messengers to initiate the clean-up process. However, bad fats such as arachidonic acid trigger inflammation that is more intense, and therefore more damaging. In other words, eating bad fats means increased puffiness, redness, and damage to the area. For your skin, this type of inflammation can cause an uneven complexion, puffy eyes, and wrinkles. To avoid this, pass up the butter and fried foods, and reach instead for foods like fish and vegetables that supply your skin with good fats that keep it looking its best.

Some Rays Are Worse Than Others

Ultraviolet rays are categorized by wavelengths: UVA, UVB, and UVC. The ozone layer filters out most of the UVC and many of the UVB rays, but it has little effect on UVA rays, which make up 90 percent or more of the radiation that reaches the earth's surface. Exposure to UVA causes most of the photoaging damage to the skin, including premature wrinkles, loss of elasticity, sun spots (hyperpigmentation), and a dry, dull, leathery appearance.

Fewer UVB rays reach your skin, but they too are very damaging. These rays can cause sunburns and basal-cell cancers of the skin, and they can increase your risk of melanoma, the most serious type of skin cancer. UVB rays are most intense between the hours of 10 a.m. and 2 p.m.

Antioxidants and Sunscreen: A Healthy Cocktail

Beta-carotene, lycopene, flavanols, selenium, vitamin E, and vitamin C are all thought to shield your skin from sun damage. In a double-blind, controlled trial, healthy young women took a supplement containing these nutrients and also used topical sunscreens. The researchers concluded that these nutrients offer the skin added protection against sunlight. To prevent sunburns and subsequent skin damage, include such antioxidants in your diet or as a supplement, in addition to applying plenty of sunscreen.

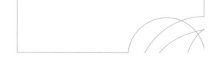

Making the Right Food Choices

Good fats can counteract the effects inflammation. Essential fatty acids like omega-3s are known to play an anti-inflammatory role in the skin. Foods rich in antioxidants can also help your skin in its fight against puffiness. Antioxidants are capable of neutralizing the free radicals made by white blood cells during inflammation. By neutralizing these free radicals, antioxidants protect the skin's structures (collagen and elastin) and reduce the formation of wrinkles. Antioxidants also prevent free radicals from damaging the skin's moisture barrier, keeping the skin beautiful, moist, and glowing.

Eighteen Foods That Fight Puffiness and Inflammation

A diet rich in a variety of colorful foods delivers the antioxidants and good fats your skin needs to fight the free radicals caused by inflammation. Puffiness can be further averted with a low sodium diet rich in amino acids and other nutrients. Feed your skin and starve inflammation and puffiness with the following skin-beautifying foods:

Puffiness Protectors
- Cauliflower
- Cucumber
- Turkey

Inflammation Fighters
- Barley
- Beets
- Hemp Seeds
- Maple Syrup
- Olives
- Pears
- Pomegranate
- Salmon
- Yogurt

Damage Controllers
- Broccoli
- Cherries
- Grapes
- Honey
- Nectarines
- Potatoes

PUFFINESS PROTECTORS

Inflammation is a natural reaction in your body that occurs every day. When it happens under your eyes, your skin can develop a puffy appearance. Fight back with the help of the following three foods, which contain key vitamins and nutrients to prevent inflammation and puffiness.

Cauliflower

This neutral-hued vegetable is packed with nutrients that can help you detoxify, fight cancer, and safeguard your skin against puffiness. A great source of vitamin C, most of the B vitamins, and all of the minerals your skin needs to stay healthy, cauliflower is one of the only white-colored foods that will do your body good.

Detoxifying Florets

Cauliflower contains phytonutrients that encourage the production of enzymes in your body that detoxify, clean, and eliminate harmful compounds. These enzymes also clear free radicals and cancer-causing chemicals from your skin.

Research proves that the detox-promoting phytonutrients in cauliflower are very protective. In a Dutch study on diet and cancer, researchers followed 100,000 people for six years and found that those who ate the most cruciferous vegetables (cauliflower included) had almost twice as low a risk for developing colorectal cancer. Similarly, a study in Singapore found that smokers who ate cruciferous vegetables had a 69 percent reduction in their risk of lung cancer.

How much cauliflower do you need to eat to help reduce puffiness and inflammation in your skin? One daily serving of vegetables from the cruciferous family (which includes cauliflower, broccoli, kale, Brussels sprouts, and collard greens) has been shown to lower your risk of cancer, so eating just one cup (100 g) each day is surely enough to help your skin.

Cauliflower is low in fat and rich in fiber, water, and vitamin C. It also has a very high nutritional density (the ratio of nutrient content to the total energy content, or calories) and is a very versatile ingredient in the kitchen. You can smash it up for a healthier alternative to mashed potatoes, roast it (see our recipe on p. 242), add it to a stir-fry, or even munch on it raw. With so many options, this is one white food you'll have a hard time getting bored with!

More than Just White

Did you know that cauliflower comes in other colors too? The common white variety is packed with nutrients, but there are even more skin beautifying nutrients in orange, green, and purple cauliflower. Orange cauliflower has 25 times the level of vitamin A as white cauliflower. Green cauliflower, sometimes called broccoflower, combines the physical features of cauliflower with the chlorophyll of broccoli. Purple cauliflower contains anthocyanins, a group of antioxidants (also found in red cabbage and red wine) with anti-inflammatory properties.

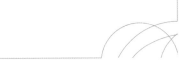

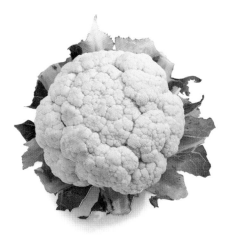

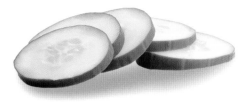

Cucumber

Placing cucumber slices over your eyes has long been heralded as a method to fight puffiness, but eating them can also help you look your best. This is because a cucumber is mostly water, so eating it hydrates your skin, flushes out toxins, and relieves the inflammation that can cause your skin to appear puffy.

Soothes and Reduces Swelling

Cucumbers belong to the same family as watermelon, zucchini, pumpkin, and other types of squash. In the flesh of cucumbers, you will find ascorbic acid (vitamin C) and caffeic acid. These two nutrients soothe skin irritations and prevent water retention. Their presence may also explain why cucumbers, when applied topically, can help swollen eyes, burns, and dermatitis (skin inflammation).

Leave the Peel On

The outer green skin of cucumbers is a rich source of fiber, potassium, and magnesium. These three nutrients are core requirements in diets designed to help people lower high blood pressure. High blood pressure is closely linked to inflammation, as it forces fluids out of your blood and into your tissues, including your skin, which can cause puffiness.

Cucumber skin also contains silica, an essential component of healthy connective tissue, which includes the skin. Silica helps improve the skin's structure, keeping it tight. When puffy skin swells, it gets stretched; when the puffiness disappears, the skin hangs loose. The silica in cucumbers can help the skin regain its firmness again and improve complexion.

Whether you use sliced cucumber to lay over your eyes or munch on it as a snack, this cooling vegetable is a great way to help your skin reduce puffiness. For a colorful dish that tosses cucumber together with a whole rainbow of ingredients, from scallions to plum tomatoes, try making our Gazpacho Salad on page 232 .

Do Pickles Count?

Pickles are cucumbers that have been cured in brine, so technically they are vegetables. Nutritionally speaking, pickles are lightweights, but they make for a tasty, fat-free, low-calorie condiment or snack. Keep in mind, however, that one large dill pickle provides approximately 1200 mg of sodium, or 50 percent of an adult's suggested daily supply, and too much sodium can cause puffiness in your skin.

Turkey

Eating turkey is good for your skin because, unlike red meat, it is low in the saturated fat that can promote inflammation in your skin. It's also a great source of protein—with one 4-ounce (113 g) serving providing 65 percent of your daily value—and other nutrients.

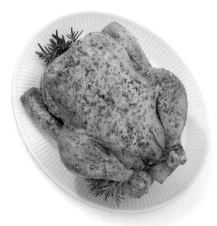

Protein and Minerals to Keep You Looking Supple

Protein is important to your skin because it forms the building blocks of the enzymes that keep your skin going. It also plays a role in reducing puffiness in the skin. Edema, the movement of fluids from the blood vessels in your skin to the area between your skin cells, can be caused by a lack of protein.

Another cause of puffiness is inflammation, which increases the permeability of blood vessels, allowing fluids to enter your skin and make it appear swollen. You can reduce puffiness by preventing inflammation, and two nutrients in turkey, cysteine and selenium, do exactly that.

Cysteine fosters healthy skin. It belongs to the group of cells (melanocytes) that give your skin its color, and it promotes the production of melanin by these cells, which helps protect your skin from the most common source of inflammation: sun damage.

Turkey also contains selenium, which is needed to make one of the body's most potent antioxidants, glutathione peroxidase. This antioxidant neutralizes free radicals that form from exposure to sunlight or toxins in the skin, thus stopping inflammation. The result is healthier, more beautiful skin. In just four ounces (113 g) of roasted turkey breast, you'll find 47 percent of your daily recommended value of selenium.

Be Thankful for Turkey

Holiday feasts may be peak times for turkey consumption, but don't wait for the holidays to take advantage of its wonderful taste and nutritional offerings. Sliced turkey is a perfect sandwich meat, and cooked, cubed turkey is a great substitute for beef in stews and chili. In place of chicken, make a turkey pot pie or turkey salad with walnuts, chunks of apple, and dried apricots. For double the protein, cook up a batch of Bean Soup with Turkey Sausage (p. 214).

Say No to Lunch Meat

Many deli meats contain added fat, which triggers inflammation, and added sodium, which causes puffiness in your skin. For a healthier sandwich, prepare a turkey breast at home and slice it into your own deli-style cold cuts. It will taste much better and be kinder to your skin.

INFLAMMATION FIGHTERS

Every day, it's your skin against the world. Sometimes the world wins and your skin gets damaged, leading to inflammation and puffiness. But it's possible to fight back against damage by including the following nine foods in your eating regimen. While you'll surely recognize a few, some of the foods may be new to you, so have fun experimenting! Your skin, and your taste buds, will be forever grateful you did.

Barley

The fourth most popular grain harvested today is barley, although it is mostly used as feed for animals and to make beer and whiskey. Our skin would greatly benefit if we spent more time eating it ourselves, however, because one cup (157 g) of cooked barley provides 52 percent of your daily value for selenium, a potent inflammation fighter, as well as other valuable nutrients.

Stops the Cause of Inflammation

Selenium is an important part of a protein in your skin known as glutathione peroxidase, which acts as a potent antioxidant, destroying the free radicals that form as a result of exposure to sunlight and toxins. Because these unstable compounds (free radicals) are missing an electron, they will scavenge around your skin to find another compound from which to steal an electron. Whichever part of your skin gets robbed becomes damaged.

When this damage affects your skin's structural parts, it can lead to wrinkles and sagging. When the damage is to your skin's moisture barrier, it can give your skin a dry, scaly texture. No matter where the damage is, however, inflammation is triggered and redness, puffiness, and unhealthy-looking skin result. In addition, inflammation produces even more free radicals that can damage your skin. Thankfully, with enough selenium in your diet, you can stop inflammation at its source and never suffer from red, puffy, inflamed skin again.

Lignans Turn Back the Clock

A major factor in the skin's aging is hormones. Hormonal shifts that occur naturally as we age alter the metabolism of collagen and elastin, the main components that keep skin strong and youthful. For example, the drop in estrogen levels that accompanies menopause is thought to cause aging of

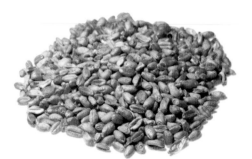

the skin. Animal studies suggest that lower estrogen levels correspond to a drop in the skin's collagen levels.

Lignans, the fats in many grains—including barley—can promote your skin's health by mimicking estrogen. These phytoestrogens (lignans) may offer a way to help stimulate collagen formation in menopausal skin and, consequently, prevent the collagen loss associated with lower estrogen levels.

Barley and other whole grains are a tasty way to get lignans into your skin. In a Danish study published in the *Journal of Nutrition,* blood levels were measured in more than 800 postmenopausal women. The study found that women who ate the most whole grains were found to have significantly higher levels of lignans in their blood. The presence of these lignans translates into a more youthful appearance and is also associated with a lower risk of breast cancer.

Barley is a wonderfully versatile cereal grain with a rich, nut-like flavor, and its quick cooking time makes it easy to include in a number of dishes. Add the grain to any casserole or soup, or use it as the basis for a nourishing, hearty salad. For a filling vegetarian entrée, try our Mushrooms Stuffed with Barley, Kale, and Feta (p. 248).

Fiber Free-for-All
One cup (157 g) of cooked barley provides a whopping 13 g of fiber—more than half of the recommended daily value.

Beets

Did your mother used to tell you to eat your beets or there would be no dessert? Your mother may have stopped saying it, but scientists will still tell you to eat your beets, or your skin will not look as beautiful as it could. Beets have a deep, ruby red color thanks to their high content of anthocyanins—potent antioxidants that are fabulous inflammation fighters.

Red Beets Eliminate Red Skin
A red, puffy complexion is caused by inflammation, a natural process triggered by many types of damage, including free-radical damage. Antioxidants are your best weapon against this damage, and anthocyanins, found in beets and other red- or purple-colored produce like berries and purple cabbage, are great antioxidants.

Anthocyanins protect in a two-fold way. First, they neutralize enzymes that destroy connective tissue, thereby preventing further damage, and then they repair proteins in blood-vessel walls. According to a study published in the journal *Pharmacological Research,* animal experiments have shown that supplementation with anthocyanins effectively prevents inflammation and subsequent blood-vessel damage.

B Beautiful

Beets also contain folate, a B vitamin that is required for normal tissue growth. Just one cup (170 g) of boiled beets contains 136 micrograms of folate—more than one-third of the daily requirement.

Once cooked, beets take on a soft, buttery sweet flavor. Never cooked them before? Start with our quick and beautiful Roasted Beet Soup (p. 218) for an introduction. Once you get started, you'll be surprised at how easy it is to include them in your diet. Steamed, roasted, or boiled, beets are a lovely addition to any salad. You can even turn them into a dip by pureeing them with chickpeas and almonds. If you want to keep things simple while maximizing your antioxidant intake, pull out your juicer and make a tall glass of beet juice. Nothing beats beets!

Hemp Seeds

Hemp is a versatile crop that is used to produce rope, clothing, paper, and many other products. When the hemp seed is shelled, you've got one of the most nutritious foods on earth. The seeds, which are commonly made into oil, butter, and flour, are a source of fiber, protein, and many healthy fats that prevent inflammation in your skin and give you a more radiant complexion.

Full of Rejuvenating Fatty Acids

The two essential fatty acids found in hemp, linoleic acid (LA) and alpha-linolenic acid (ALA), help mitigate damage to your skin. Just one to two tablespoons (15 to 30 ml) of hemp oil is sufficient to meet the daily nutritional requirement for essential fatty acids completely.

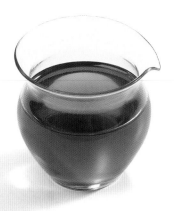

Both LA and ALA cannot be made by the human body and must be obtained through the diet. In your body, they are responsible for the luster in your skin, hair, eyes, and even your thought processes.

Hemp seeds also contain gamma-linolenic acid. This omega-6 fatty acid is known to support skin health by reducing inflammation and promoting healthy moisture levels in the skin. As a result, it has been used in the treatment of acne and psoriasis.

Packed with the Protein Your Skin Desires

Hemp seeds are considered to have the most complete edible and usable protein of any member of the plant family. They contain all twenty-one known amino acids, including the eight essential acids are bodies cannot produce and therefore must obtain from nature.

An important aspect of hemp seed protein is its high content of the sulfur-containing amino acids methionine and cysteine, which are needed to form key antioxidant enzymes. These antioxidant enzymes shield your skin from the free-radical damage that triggers inflammation.

Hemp is one of the best skin-beautifying foods on earth and should be included in every skin-healthy diet. Hemp seed butter, oil, flour, and protein powder are available in health food stores and some grocery stores. Hemp seed butter is a terrific alternative to peanut butter. Try using hemp-based products instead of other grains, flours, seeds, butters, and oils in your favorite recipes. Hemp pancakes are one of my particular favorites. And since hemp powder is loaded with protein and fiber, it is the perfect power boost to add to smoothies.

Maple Syrup

First recognized by the Native Americans as a good source of energy and nutrition, maple syrup has become a favorite treat the world over. Unlike white sugar, which can actually cause problems for your skin and has also been linked to inflammation, maple syrup contains several nutrients that can benefit your outer beauty. Time to get those pancakes started!

More than a Treat

Maple syrup has roughly the same number of calories (50 calories/ tablespoon) as white cane sugar and brown sugar. It is, however, a much better bet nutritionally as it contains malic acid, calcium, potassium, and trace amounts of vitamins.

Potassium helps with puffy skin by keeping sodium levels in check and maintaining the body's water balance. Because there are about 35 mg of potassium per tablespoon (15 ml) of maple syrup and only 2 mg of sodium per tablespoon, it is a great puff-fighting food choice.

Maple syrup is also a source of the essential elements iron and thiamin. Iron helps carry oxygen in your blood to your skin, which helps skin cells grow and give off a radiant glow. Thiamin is a B vitamin involved in many energy processes in the skin that help it stay beautiful.

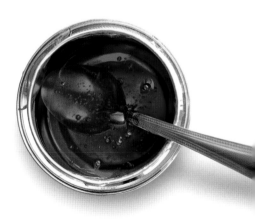

Put Syrup on Tap

Maple syrup is collected in the early spring when maple trees are in their dormant state. Native Americans made the syrup by boiling 40 gallons (152 L) of sap over an open fire until it reduced to a single gallon (3.8 L) of syrup, and although the process is less labor intensive today, it follows many of the same principles.

Maple syrup is the obvious accompaniment to wholegrain or cornmeal pancakes; we've included it in our recipe for Cottage Cheese Pancakes with Blueberry Maple Syrup on page 198. Also try drizzling it over plain yogurt, fruit, or ice cream. You can also use it to glaze fish or poultry, or to give baked squash a sweet touch. For a special dessert, broil plums or peaches and top them with syrup and a sprinkling of cinnamon.

Olives

Olives are as rich in nutrients as they are in cultural history. The leafy branches of the olive tree are symbols of abundance, glory, and peace—and for our purposes, you can think of the olives themselves as symbols of beauty and radiance for your skin.

Vitamin, Minerals, and Monounsaturated Fats Galore

Olives are a source of iron, copper, and vitamin E, all of which support the health of your skin. Iron helps carry oxygen to your skin cells so that they can create energy and grow. It also helps keep your immune system healthy. In one cup (100 g) of olives, you'll find nearly one-quarter of the recommended daily intake of iron.

Copper is a trace mineral that keeps your skin radiant and healthy in many ways. It helps your body use iron, reduces tissue damage caused by free radicals, helps maintain the health of your bones and connective tissues, and aids your body in the production of melanin, the pigment that helps protect your skin from sun damage. One cup (100 g) of olives contains 17 percent of your daily value of copper.

Vitamin E is a fat-soluble antioxidant, which means that it can penetrate the fatty parts of your skin and protect them from damage by free radicals. Such damage can cause wrinkles, sagging, and dryness. Vitamin E is thought to improve skin moisture, softness, and smoothness and to provide mild protection from sun damage. You'll find 20 percent of your daily value of vitamin E in one cup (100 g) of olives.

Finally, olives are a rich source of monounsaturated fats. These fats are not easily damaged, and are therefore good to have in your skin cells. The stability of monounsaturated fats means your skin cells are less likely to get damaged, and less damage means less inflammation and more beautiful skin. Better still, when combined with the antioxidant pow-

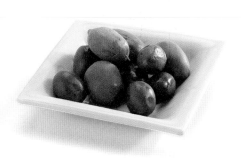

ers of vitamin E, these fats can actually lower your risk of damage and inflammation.

The Tree of Youth

Olives make a zesty addition to salads, pizzas, and poultry dishes. You can also turn them into a lively sandwich spread or appetizer dip by making tapenade.

Most gourmet shops carry a dazzling array of olives to suit your fancy. Some are picked when they are unripe (green), while others are allowed to fully ripen on the tree (black). Olives can be cured in oil, water, brine, or salt. Sample them all, and enjoy beautiful skin.

Pears

Pears originated in Asia and are related to the apple, another skin-healthy fruit. Available in the summer and fall, pears come in many different varieties, each offering your skin nutrients to help prevent inflammation.

Super Inflammation Prevention

Pears are a good source of the trace mineral copper. One pear supplies you with 10 percent of your daily copper requirement. Copper plays a very important role in your ability to block inflammation. It is required by superoxide dismutase, one of the skin's most important antioxidant enzymes, in its work to protect your skin from damage and eliminate the need for inflammation. Copper also helps maintain the health of your bones and connective tissues, and aids your body in the production of melanin, the pigment that helps protect your skin from sun damage.

One of your skin's favorite antioxidants, vitamin C, can be found in this fruit (11 percent of your daily requirement in one pear). This vitamin neutralizes free radicals and prevents damage to your skin that would otherwise stimulate inflammation.

Detoxification for Your Skin

Pears are a fabulous source of fiber, which helps your body trap toxins in your digestive tract and excrete them. Left alone, these toxins can be absorbed by the body and travel in the blood to your skin, where they cause free radicals to form and trigger inflammation. Luckily, pears help prevent this from happening, as just one of these fruits arms you with 4 g of dietary fiber (15 percent of the recommended daily value).

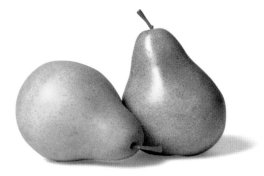

Ripe pears are perfect to eat on their own, but there are lots of ways to cook with them as well. Their natural sweetness makes pears perfect for including in desserts like our Apple, Pear, and Dried Fruit Strudel (p. 280) and our Polenta Soufflé with Caramel and Pear (p. 284). Pears are super in salads; combine them with arugula, pecans, and dried cranberries, or with goat cheese, pistachios, and grapes. Sliced and quickly sautéed, pears are wonderful as a topping for frozen yogurt.

Pomegranate

Considered a superfood, pomegranates have an exceedingly high ORAC (oxygen radical absorbance capacity) value, which is a measure of the antioxidant power of a food. According to this rating, they have the ability to neutralize twice as many free radicals as red wine and seven times as many free radicals as green tea. Your complexion will surely thank you for including this fruit in your diet.

Antioxidant Power Like No Other

One of the main causes of skin damage is free radicals. Luckily, antioxidants can neutralize and destroy free radicals, stopping damage and inflammation before they occur. Like blueberries, grapes, cranberries, and other deep-colored fruits, pomegranates contain anthocyanins, a powerful class of antioxidants that bolster your skin in the fight against inflammation. The ORAC value for the pomegranate ranks highest in this lineup at 105 ORAC units/gram, followed by cranberries at 93 ORAC units/gram, blueberries at 77 ORAC units/gram, and blackberries and raspberries at 55 ORAC units/gram.

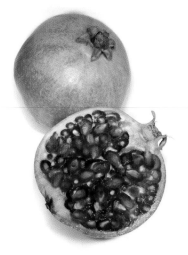

Prevents Sun Spots

Ellagic acid is a skin-beautifying compound in pomegranates proven to help your skin protect itself from sun damage. Sunlight can cause the skin to change color, producing sun spots, which are a sign of photoaging (skin damage due to the sun).

Such damage may be prevented by eating pomegranates, scientists say. According to a study in Tokyo, researchers found that when an ellagic-rich pomegranate extract was orally administered to subjects, it helped protect the skin from the sun's ultraviolet radiation.

Sip or Snack on It

Native to the Middle East and the Himalayas, pomegranates have recently become popular in North America, in part due to their superfood status, which has brought them to the forefront of consumers' minds. Juices, snack bars, cocktails, and even cereals now contain pomegranate. The fresh fruit is available from October through December in North America, but advances in agriculture have extended its season, allowing you to find pomegranates for more than three months of the year—leaving you with no excuse not to pick one up on your next shopping trip.

Salmon

Salmon is a delicious way to healthy, inflammation-free skin. It is packed with antioxidants, vitamins, minerals, and good fats like omega-3s that promote your skin's health.

Omega-3s for You and Me

The chief reason to eat salmon is because it is an excellent source of omega-3 fatty acids, which have anti-inflammatory effects in the skin. These fats interact with the immune system and discourage damaging inflammation that can lead to red, puffy, wrinkled skin. One 4-ounce (113 g) serving of baked or broiled salmon provides roughly 87 percent of the recommended daily amount of omega-3s.

In 2005, the *Journal of Investigative Dermatology* published a study in which researchers from the University of Manchester in the UK suggested that eating fish rich in omega-3 fats (like salmon) can also reduce the inflammation caused by sunlight (UVB radiation). The omega-3 fatty acids, they explained, prevent sunlight from triggering a pro-inflammatory chemical called tumor necrosis factor-alpha. This means that omega-3 fatty acids inhibit the ability of damaging chemicals to wreak havoc in the body.

Raw, smoked, or baked, salmon is a delicious, skin-beautifying food to include in your next meal. Note, however, that farmed fish is linked with higher levels of toxins. For nutritional and environmental reasons, therefore, choose to buy and consume wild salmon instead.

Vitamin D Times Three

Pick sockeye salmon and enjoy another skin healthy benefit. Sockeye salmon is an exceptionally rich source of vitamin D: one 4-ounce (113 g) serving of baked or broiled sockeye salmon provides 739.37 IU of

Easy Kitchen Trick
Most people bypass pomegranates because it can be difficult and messy to extract the seeds from them. Here is an easy way to get the skin-beautifying benefits of pomegranate without mess or frustration: Cut off the crown of the pomegranate and slice the fruit into sections. Place the sections in a bowl of water and gently roll out the seeds with your fingers. The seeds will sink to the bottom and the membrane will float to the top.

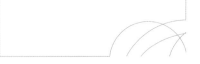

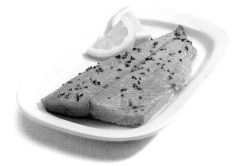

vitamin D—more than three times the total recommended daily value! The same 4-ounce (113 g) serving of chinook salmon supplies 411 IU (still a winner at 102 percent of the daily value).

Vitamin D is manufactured in your skin when it is exposed to sunlight; however, most people avoid the sun to prevent aging of their skin. This presents us with a catch-22, as research has found that a lack of vitamin D increases the risk of osteoporosis, type 1 diabetes, rheumatoid arthritis, tuberculosis, multiple sclerosis, and other conditions.

Thankfully, we can obtain vitamin D through food instead of the sun. The *American Journal of Clinical Nutrition* found that taking a vitamin D supplement reduces the risk of cancer (colorectal and breast) in post-menopausal women. Vitamin D may also reduce the risk of prostate cancer in men.

Serve up some salmon and eat to your skin's health. If you need some inspiration, give our Sesame-Crusted Salmon Bake on page 262 a try.

Yogurt

Yogurt is back in fashion, and for good reason. Research suggests that it can help your skin fight inflammation and wrinkles due to the probiotics it contains. These helpful microbes promote healthy inflammation throughout the body, including the skin. Along with riboflavin, a B vitamin involved in energy production, yogurt packs a one–two skin punch.

Probiotic Rescue for Your Skin

Probiotics are the good microbes that live in your intestines. Researchers believe that this healthy bacteria may improve overall health by helping to keep inflammation in check, thereby preventing inflammatory disorders from intensifying. While there is no proof that eating yogurt can reduce inflammation in the skin itself, probiotics are known to promote healthy inflammation in other parts of the body, including the intestinal tract and lungs.

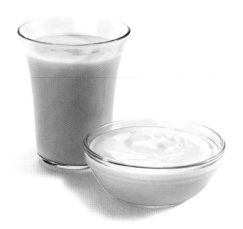

Yogurt is a good source of riboflavin, with one cup (230 g) providing you with 30 percent of your recommended daily value. This B vitamin helps protect cells from oxygen damage and supports cellular energy production. When you are deficient in riboflavin, inflammation can occur (and cause deep ridges to form by your mouth). Eating yogurt can help prevent this type of inflammation from occurring.

Delicious, Beautifying, and Helps You Live Longer

Considered the original health food, yogurt has been enjoyed for centuries. Even Caesar believed in eating yogurt to improve health. Yogurt is easy to include in your diet as a light snack, a base for a smoothie, a substitute for sour cream, or as dessert. For the ultimately skin healthy snack, try stewed rhubarb with yogurt, and you'll be battling inflammation and wrinkles in the same bowl.

DAMAGE CONTROLLERS

No matter how much you try to avoid it, your skin can suffer from damage. Your cosmetics may include chemicals that are harmful to your skin, you may forget to apply sunscreen before meeting a friend for lunch on the patio, or you may over-indulge (just a little!) with that plate of fries—no matter the culprit, it's so easy for your skin to become damaged. But you can take control of that damage with the help of the nutrients in the following foods, which can reduce inflammation, help speed skin recovery, and keep your skin looking beautiful. With six delicious foods to choose from, you'll have no problem launching an all-out assault against skin damage!

Guide to the Supermarket

There are so many yogurts on the market. Which one is best? All natural, plain yogurts are always a good choice. Try to stick with organic versions that do not contain added sugar or artificial sweeteners, as these additives can have toxic effects on your skin. Some new yogurts have added probiotics that may offer your skin more benefits, especially those with Bifidobacteria species.

Broccoli

Kiss an Italian and say thank you for broccoli, an amazing vegetable for your skin. In ancient Rome, broccoli was developed from wild cabbage, and it has remained a popular vegetable ever since. When it comes to your skin, broccoli can help prevent and fight inflammation, detoxify, and more.

More Vitamin C Than an Orange

One cup (156 g) of steamed broccoli is bursting with nutrients to help your skin fight free radicals, which form in your skin when it is exposed to sunlight or toxins. These unstable molecules wreak havoc in all parts of your skin, leading to wrinkles, dryness, blemishes, and inflammation. If you can stop free radicals from causing damage, you can prevent inflammation. To do this, you need antioxidants.

Broccoli delivers two great antioxidants: vitamin C and vitamin A. In fact, one cup (156 g) of steamed broccoli has more than double the amount of your daily needs of vitamin C—that's more vitamin C than an orange provides! Broccoli is also packed with vitamin A, a carotenoid that is a great antioxidant and skin beautifier. You'll find 45 percent of your daily vitamin A needs in one cup (156 g) of this steamed veggie.

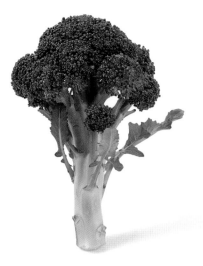

Firms, Protects, and Improves Elasticity

Another carotenoid in broccoli, lutein, offers your skin a tag team of benefits. First, this antioxidant helps your skin maintain its youthful appearance by protecting it from inflammation and damage caused by sunlight. Second, it increases skin elasticity, helping stretched skin spring back to place and not form wrinkles. The more elastic the skin, the more effectively it can rebound from damage and puffiness.

In addition, broccoli contains sulforaphane, an anticancer and antimicrobial compound. This antioxidant stimulates the production of enzymes in your body that help remove the toxins that damage skin and trigger inflammation.

Best Cooked

Broccoli contains another anticancer nutrient known as indole-3-carbinol. This compound is particularly good at protecting the DNA of your skin cells, which may explain why broccoli is thought to reduce the risk of cancer. To date, broccoli has been found to reduce the risk of prostate, ovarian, and bladder cancer.

Indole-3-carbinol is more bioavailable in cooked broccoli than raw, so be sure to lightly steam your broccoli to get the most benefit. (Be careful not to overcook, however, as this can deplete nutrients.) Of all methods of preparation, steaming broccoli is best as it causes the least loss of nutrients.

Broccoli is an easy vegetable to add to your table. Toss it into a salad or pasta sauce, on pizza, or in any baked dish. Try sprinkling steamed broccoli with feta cheese for a yummy, skin-beautifying side dish.

Cherries

People suffering from arthritis are quick to reach for a bowl of cherries, and you should take a tip from them. These sweet, juicy fruits have awesome anti-inflammatory properties and should be included in your diet to avoid inflamed, puffy skin.

Well-Known by Arthritis Sufferers

The two varieties of cherries eaten most often are wild or sweet cherries and sour cherries (principally used in cooking). No matter which variety you choose, your skin will enjoy anti-inflammatory effects. This is because all cherries contain anthocyanins, potent antioxidants that give the fruit its stunning red color. Anthocyanins have been shown to reduce pain and inflammation—hence their popularity among arthritis sufferers. Other foods rich in anthocyanins include berries, beets, and grapes (all featured in this book).

Protection from Radiation and Aging

Another anti-inflammatory nutrient found in cherries is melatonin, an antioxidant hormone that protects the skin against the sun's ultraviolet radiation. Scientists have found that tart cherries contain more of this powerful antioxidant than what is normally produced by the body. Melatonin stimulates cell growth, which can help the skin repair more effectively after damage, and may also have a role in repairing burned skin.

According to a study conducted at the University of Granada in Spain, melatonin may also slow the aging process. Researchers there found that melatonin neutralizes the oxidative and inflammation process caused by aging, leading them to suggest that daily melatonin intake from the age of 30 or 40 could potentially help delay the development of age-related illnesses.

Red, Delicious, and Antiwrinkling

Here's the bad news: Fresh cherries are available only in the summer. Dried cherries are a suitable choice but are not as healthy for you because they have lost some of their nutritional value, and they tend to be sprinkled with preservatives and sugar. Frozen cherries, however, have a nutritional value fairly close to that of fresh cherries, so buy a bag and keep it in your freezer for adding to smoothies or yogurt.

Cherry juice is a great source of inflammation-fighting nutrients as well. Look for organic, 100 percent pure cherry juice that is not from concentrate, as concentrated juice loses most of its water-soluble nutrients during processing.

Grapes

The health benefits of grapes may be most readily associated with red wine, but are there other health benefits in these small, juicy fruits? There certainly are. Grapes are actually the better choice if you want healthy skin because they contain proanthocyanidins, nutrients that help reduce inflammation.

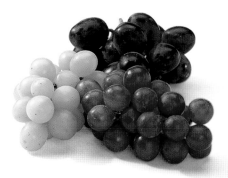

The New Treatment for Inflammation

Inflammation in the skin results in an increased level of free radicals, the unstable compounds that steal electrons from your skin and leave damage in their wake. This damage can affect both the collagen that is responsible for keeping your skin firm and stable, and the DNA of your skin cells, and both kinds of damage can then result in wrinkle formation.

The class of flavonoids known as proanthocyanidins come to the rescue in this scenario. Proanthocyanidins act as antioxidants and play a role in the stabilization of collagen and maintenance of elastin, two critical proteins in connective tissue that support organs, joints, blood vessels, and muscle. By fighting the damaging forces at work in your body, the proanthocyanidins in grapes add luster, instead of wrinkles, to your skin.

Fresh, Frozen, or Fermented

Grapes are great additions to salads and cheese trays, and make for a healthy dessert alternative (try our Glacéed Grapes on p. 286). Of course, you can also toast your health with a glass of red wine, which contains the proanthocyanidins we know are so healthy for our hearts and our skin. With a bunch of grapes in one hand and a glass of red wine in the other, you'll be a symbol of glowing health.

Honey

The preferred food of storybook bears, honey should also be a preferred food for anyone in search of beautiful, glowing, healthy skin. Since the times of ancient Greece, when Olympians used honey to enhance their sports performance, honey has been a sweet choice for health.

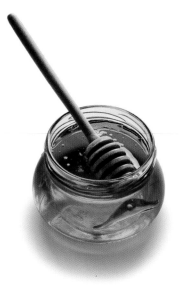

Sweet Antioxidants

According to research conducted at the University of California, Davis, daily consumption of honey raises levels of protective antioxidant compounds in humans. In the study, 25 study participants were given four tablespoons (20 g) of buckwheat honey daily for 29 days in addition to their regular diets, with their blood drawn at given intervals following consumption (to monitor antioxidant levels). Researchers concluded that honey increased the level of antioxidants in the participants' blood, thus helping manage the free radicals formed from exposure to sun and chemicals.

In another study, published in the *Journal of Agricultural and Food Chemistry*, honey's antioxidant levels were found to equal those in many fruits and vegetables. Different types of honey, however, contain varying levels of antioxidants, with dark honey having higher levels than light.

A Spoonful a Day

Use honey in place of sugar to sweeten your tea, slather it on multigrain toast, drizzle it on oatmeal, or add it to salad dressings and marinades. We use it in both our Roasted Garlic and Mustard Vinaigrette on page 234 and our Rosemary Ginger Chicken with Orange-Honey Glaze on page 258. Experiment with the many delicious ways to include this sweet treat in your diet, and you'll be well on your way to beautiful skin.

Nectarines

Few people know that nectarines are actually peaches, just without the fuzzy skin. When it comes to your skin, it doesn't much matter which variety you choose to eat since both offer your skin the same beautifying nutrients.

Peachy Keen Skin

Nectarines contain lycopene, lutein, niacin, copper, and vitamins A, C, and E. Eating nutrients like these is believed to help protect your skin from sun damage because the nutrients act as antioxidants, preventing inflammation and minimizing damage to the skin. Scientists even recommend including these nutrients in your diet (or as a supplement) to prevent sunburns and the ensuing skin damage they cause.

Vitamin C is one of the most important antioxidants in your skin because it is water-soluble and can therefore neutralize free radicals in the watery parts of your skin. Vitamins A and E, on the other hand, are fat-soluble antioxidants, so they can patrol the fatty parts of your skin and skin cells to make sure that free radicals do not cause damage and trigger inflammation there. Together, these vitamins provide you with full coverage in the fight against wrinkles.

One nectarine provides you with 9 percent of your daily value of vitamin A, 12 percent of your vitamin C, and 3 percent of your vitamin E. Peaches provide only half that amount of vitamin A, and slightly less vitamin C, making nectarines the better choice.

For the Love of Lutein
Foods rich in lutein, like nectarines, protect your skin from the damaging effects of free radicals (think inflammation) and promote elasticity. Elastic skin is better at bouncing back after inflammation has caused it to swell and stretch.

Research suggests that carotenoids like lutein may also promote eye health through their antioxidant ability to protect the eyes from light-induced oxidative damage and filter out UV light.

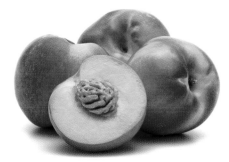

Perfect for Any Meal

Grown around the world and available year round, nectarines (and peaches) are ideal foods to include in your skin diet. Packed with nutrients that fight inflammation, they guard the skin from damage, encourage elasticity, and prevent the formation of wrinkles. Add diced nectarine to chicken salad or make a pretty, low-fat dessert by filling a glass with layers of diced nectarine, fresh berries, and yogurt (topped with maple syrup and a mint leaf). Nectarines are also perfect in muffins, salsas, sauces, and glazes.

Potatoes

You needn't assume that the baked potato on your plate is a nutritional dud; this tuber is packed with nutrients that can help your skin prevent damage. Damage to your skin can trigger inflammation, which can cause your skin to appear puffy and red. But with the help of plain old potatoes, you can bust out a beautiful complexion in no time.

Better than Broccoli—and Brussels Sprouts

You might be surprised to learn that potatoes contain levels of flavonoids that rival those found in broccoli, spinach, and Brussels sprouts. Flavonoids protect cells from oxygen damage and prevent inflammation.

According to a 2007 study published in the journal *Agricultural Research,* scientists found that in addition to their high flavonoid levels, potatoes are rich in vitamin C, folic acid, and kukoamines. Kukoamines, in particular, are a rare compound, found only in one other food—goji berries—and may have blood pressure lowering potential.

Hot Potatoes for Health

In particular, potatoes contain three nutrients that help control damage in your skin: vitamin C, copper, and vitamin B6.

Potatoes may not offer the same amount of vitamin C as kiwi, oranges, or other vitamin C powerhouses, but a single potato contains about 25 percent of your daily recommended intake. This antioxidant can help prevent free radicals in your skin from causing damage that leads to puffiness.

The trace mineral copper is another antioxidant that can help your body prevent damage. Copper works with vitamin C to help make elastin, a component of your skin's connective tissue that keeps your skin looking strong, smooth, and youthful. One cup (122 g) of baked potato provides 18.5 percent of your daily copper needs.

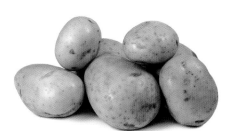

You will also find vitamin B6 in potatoes—one cup (122 g) provides 21 percent of your daily value. Involved in more than one hundred reactions in your body, vitamin B6—like all B vitamins—is essential to your health. B6 is particularly important if your skin tends to get red or puffy, a sign that you are fighting inflammation. This is because the immune system, which is responsible for inflammation, requires vitamins like B6 to work properly. Skin that is red and puffy is evidence that your immune system is hard at work. You can bolster your immune system and help keep your skin healthy with a dose of vitamin B6 from potatoes.

Skip the Fries

Baked, mashed, or roasted—anything but fried—potatoes are a delicious vegetable to include in your next skin-healthy meal. Skip the fries and potato chips, as they contain trans and saturated fat that can harm your skin. Moreover, the processing that goes with making those foods destroys all of the potato's skin-healthy nutrients.

Potato Peels

Did you know that potato peels are better than gauze for dressing burns? According to research conducted in India, potato peels—in place of a plain cotton gauze dressing—applied to burns can reduce infection and accelerate skin cell regeneration. Why? Because potato peels have antibacterial properties that actively help wounds heal. Potato peels are an easy, low-cost dressing for burn wounds when you're in a pinch (or perhaps on your next camping trip).

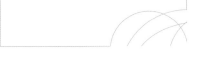

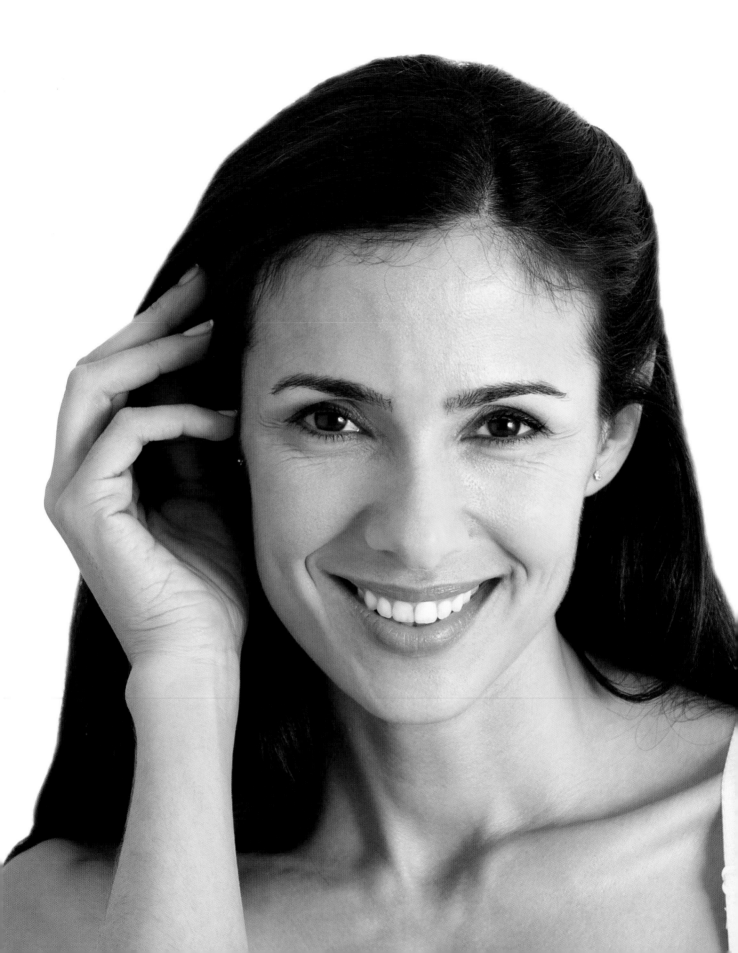

Foods That Fight Acne and Psoriasis

ACNE AND PSORIASIS are not merely skin conditions; they can be crippling diseases that leave sufferers feeling depressed and self-conscious, and can make social interaction difficult and embarrassing. While there are medical treatments available to reduce the severity of acne and psoriasis, nourishing your skin from the inside out is an additional remedy that can help correct the underlying problems causing or aggravating the condition. A diet rich in key foods (like those highlighted in this book) can help your skin rebuild, repair, and regain its natural, beautiful complexion.

Acne: On the Rise

The *British Journal of Dermatology* reported in 2005 that the rate of acne is on the rise. In fact, the journal noted that in addition to an increased number of patients suffering from the condition, the average age of patients in acne clinics is increasing. In 1984, the average age of acne patients was twenty years old; by 1994, that age had risen to twenty-six years. Today, more patients are suffering from acne and for long after their teenage years.

One of the main culprits behind this increase in the prevalence of acne is diet. Over the last century, we have shifted further and further away from diets rich in fresh foods to eating regimes that favor prepackaged and processed foods. Such foods are nutritional wastelands and lead to physical imbalances in our skin.

To better understand just how our food choices can cause (or prevent) acne, let's first take a look inside the skin and the underlying forces at work in our bodies.

The Sebaceous Glands: The Oil Moguls of Our Skin

The sebaceous glands are small oil-producing glands at the base of hair follicles in the skin. They have two functions: to moisturize the skin and to help clean away dead cells that line the hair follicle shaft. When problems arise with these glands, acne can develop.

There are four major problems that can occur in the sebaceous glands and lead to acne: too much sebum (oil) production; clogging of the hair follicle shaft; overgrowth of the bacteria *Propionibacterium acnes* in the skin; and/or rupturing of a clogged follicle into the skin, which causes inflammation. These four problems all lead to the same outcome: blackheads and whiteheads.

Hormones and the Nervous System

Hormones and the nervous system also influence the behavior of the sebaceous glands. Teenagers are most commonly afflicted with acne because their hormones are changing dramatically and adjusting to their new bodies. The result can be lead to an over-production of oil in the skin, and acne can result.

Hormone levels can also be affected by the quality of your diet. Poor food choices can create hormone imbalances, which then disrupt the sebaceous glands and lead to acne outbreaks. Similarly, the chemicals in your nervous system that are responsible for the structure and function of sebaceous glands are also affected by diet.

Acne-Fighting Foods

Populations that do not consume a high percentage of processed foods tend not to have acne. Such findings indicate a strong correlation between a natural, healthy diet that keeps blood sugar levels stable and clear skin. The lack of acne in these populations may also be linked to the high amounts of good fats (omega-3 fatty acids) and antioxidants such populations consume.

Australian researchers put this diet–acne theory to the test in a 2007 study conducted by the Royal Melbourne Institute of Technology. Researchers there took 50 men between the ages of 15 and 25 with mild-to-moderate acne, and broke them into two groups. One group followed a diet rich in lean meat, poultry, fish, fruits and vegetables, and whole grains. The other ate a typical Western diet (high in processed foods and sugar). After 12 weeks, the acne of the group following the healthier, higher-protein, low-glycemic index diet had improved by more than 50 percent—an increase not even achieved by topical acne solutions.

While more research is needed to establish a conclusive link between diet and acne, it is safe to assume that a diet high in greasy, high-fat, and sugary foods does little good for one's health and complexion. Diets high in protein, whole grains, and fresh produce, on the other hand, have proven again and again that they do a body good. For those of us in search of great skin, the choice is clear.

Does Milk Cause Acne?

For some time, a connection has been made between milk consumption and acne problems. In the 1960s, many researchers and magazines (including *Time*) reported that milk consumption was linked to acne. In 1996, researchers at Harvard studied six thousand girls aged 9 to 15 and found that those who consumed the most milk had the worst acne.

Then, in 2005, the *Journal of the American Academy of Dermatology* released the "Nurses Health Study II," which studied nearly 50,000 women and their milk drinking habits as teenagers. The results showed that those who drank milk were more likely to develop teenage acne; researchers theorized that this connection was due to the growth and reproductive hormones and bioactive molecules in milk.

More research is needed before the milk-acne relationship is fully understood. For those acne-sufferers who do decide to eliminate milk products from their diet, it is recommended that they consult their doctor first and take care to substitute other calcium-rich foods into their eating plans.

Aim Low with the Glycemic Index

The glycemic index is a measure of how quickly a food breaks down into sugar in your body. White sugar has a glycemic index value of 100, the highest possible value. Foods with high glycemic values break down quickly into sugar in your body, causing a spike in blood sugar levels and a peak in insulin. High-fiber foods, such as most vegetables and whole-grain breads, have lower glycemic index values. These foods do not cause peaks in blood sugar or insulin and are therefore considered healthier to eat. Low glycemic index foods are more filling, do not induce cravings, and are thought to help with weight loss. They are also easier on your body, as they do not stimulate the pancreas to produce large amounts of insulin or require cells to process large quantities of sugar.

Does Chocolate Cause Acne?

Chocolate has long been demonized as a primary cause of acne, but that's nothing more than a myth. Thanks to a number of research trials, we now know chocolate is actually a skin protector and not a culprit of acne. Dark chocolate in particular is an excellent source of flavonoids, which are powerful antioxidants that protect the skin from free radical damage and the inflammation acne brings on. Studies have also found that the flavonoids in cocoa drinks improve blood flow to skin cells, improve the hydration and texture of the skin, and prevent free radical damage to the fatty components of skin cells. All of that translates to healthier, less acne-prone skin.

Chocolate also appears to improve the way the body responds to blood sugar. The *American Journal of Clinical Nutrition* reported in 2005 that chocolate may help regulate sebum (oil) production, which is affected by blood sugar, thus helping with acne.

It is important to note that research supporting the use of chocolate to help fight acne did not use conventional chocolate bars. Most chocolate bars are high in refined sugar and saturated and trans fats. High-quality dark chocolate is the best kind to help in the battle against acne.

Pesky Psoriasis

Psoriasis is a noncontagious, life-long skin condition that affects more than seven million Americans. It causes scaly patches, called psoriatic plaques, to develop on the skin. These patches are areas of inflammation and excessive skin production.

While the exact cause of psoriasis is not known, researchers believe it is immune-related. In psoriasis sufferers, the immune system receives faulty signals that damage has occurred in the body, which then triggers an increase in the growth cycle of skin cells to repair the (nonexistent) damaged cells. While normal skin cells mature and are shed from the skin's surface every 28 to 30 days; skin cells in psoriasis patients mature in 3 to 6 days and quickly move to the skin surface. But instead of being shed, these skin cells pile up, causing visible lesions and patchy skin.

There are five different types of psoriasis:

1. Plaque psoriasis, the most common form, appears as raised, red patches or lesions covered with a silvery white buildup of dead skin cells, called scales.
2. Guttate psoriasis appears as small red spots on the skin.
3. Inverse psoriasis occurs in the armpits, groin, and skin folds.
4. Pustular psoriasis appears as white blisters surrounded by red skin.
5. Erythrodermic psoriasis causes intense redness over large areas of the skin.

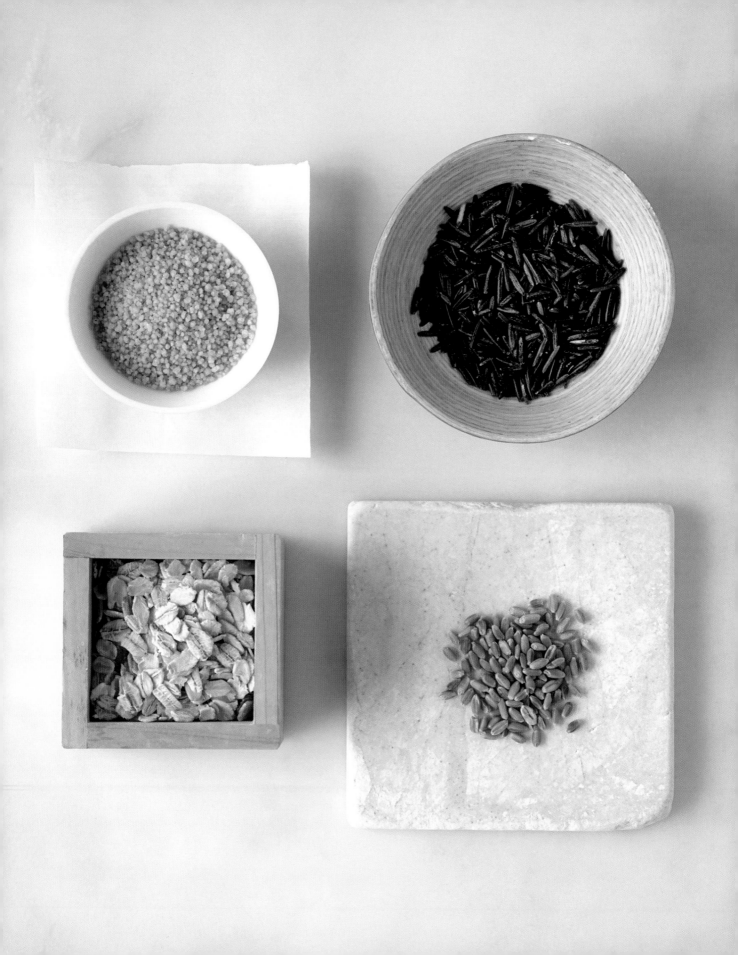

Is There a Cure?

The treatment of psoriasis depends on the extent and severity of an individual's condition. Treatment options can range from topical medications to phototherapy, or the practice of exposing a person to sunlight for a prescribed amount of time in order to improve or help clear the condition.

Even with treatment, flare-ups are common among psoriasis sufferers and can be caused by factors such as stress, skin injuries, certain medications, and diet. Eating a healthy diet, however, can help reduce some of the symptoms of psoriasis by providing the body with key nutrients that keep the immune system healthy and inflammation to a minimum.

Psoriasis-Fighting Foods

Several of the foods mentioned in earlier chapters are helpful in fighting psoriasis. Cherries, for example, may benefit skin plagued with psoriasis due to the anti-inflammatory melatonin they contain. People with psoriasis and eczema do not have normal melatonin secretion—their melatonin peaks in the day when it should not, and there is a low supply at night when it should normally be produced by the pineal gland. Eating cherries may therefore help tip melatonin levels back to a healthy balance.

Green tea can also help fight psoriasis. Research reported in 2007 found that green tea contains polyphenols that can reduce the lesions in flaky skin that typifies psoriasis. Exactly how green tea does so is yet unknown.

Finally, recent studies have indicated that consuming borage oil suppresses chronic inflammation and that dietary supplementation of borage oil for patients with skin disorders (such as psoriasis patients) can improve the condition of their skin. Borage oil also plays a role in restoring the moisture barrier of skin that is either chronically dry or has been environmentally damaged.

Ten Foods That Fight Acne and Psoriasis

Because acne and psoriasis are skin conditions that involve inflammation, they can be alleviated by eating foods that help keep such inflammation to a minimum. Fruits and vegetables that are rich sources of antioxidants, such as lemons, grapefruit, raspberries, and eggplant, can help do this by stopping free radicals from causing damage that triggers inflammation. The omega-3 fatty acids found in fish can also curtail such skin irritations.

Good fats, zinc, lycopene, selenium, and vitamins A, B6, C, and E are just some of the nutrients that are known to help your skin fight acne and psoriasis. By eating foods that deliver these skin-beautifying nutrients, you can fight back against any skin disruptions that attempt to come your way.

Many of the same foods that fight wrinkles; tighten, smooth, and fight sagging; brighten your complexion; and fight inflammation and puffiness will benefit acne- and psoriasis-prone skin. The following is a list of foods that were mentioned in earlier chapters, but are equally useful in the prevention and treatment of these immune-based skin problems:

- Açai
- Asparagus
- Avocado
- Beets
- Bell Peppers
- Blueberries
- Borage Oil
- Broccoli
- Brussels Sprouts
- Cherries
- Dried Fruit
- Fish (Salmon, Mackerel, Tuna, Sardines)
- Green Tea
- Kale
- Nuts
- Oranges
- Pears
- Peas
- Pomegranate
- Spinach
- Strawberries

In addition to the foods above, here are several additional foods we'll discuss in this chapter that can help fight both of these problems:

Acne and Psoriasis Fighters
- Couscous
- Eggplant
- Fish Oil
- Ginger
- Grapefruit
- Lemons
- Limes
- Quinoa
- Raspberries
- Sage

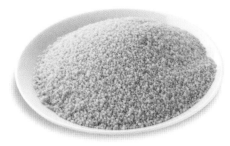

Couscous

A staple in Middle Eastern cooking, couscous is a delicious, skin-beautifying food you should try (or eat more of if you're already familiar). This versatile pasta is a great source of manganese and selenium, two nutrients that do wonders for your skin.

Manganese Stops Damage at Its Root

Manganese is a mineral and trace element that plays many essential roles in the body. It helps in the metabolism of food, functioning of the nervous system and thyroid, and production of sex hormones (which are one of the factors associated with the onset of acne).

Manganese also works as an antioxidant and thus helps prevent damage in the skin caused by free radicals. In skin suffering with acne and psoriasis, inflammation is a chronic problem, which means that free radicals are continually causing damage to the skin. You can restrict damage to your skin by adding couscous to your diet and (thereby) upping your intake of manganese; in one cup (157 g) of cooked couscous, you'll get 7 percent of your recommended daily intake of this skin-savvy mineral.

Up Your Antioxidant Levels

People with psoriasis tend to have low levels of glutathione peroxidase, a very potent antioxidant in the skin that helps protect against free-radical damage that triggers inflammation. Studies have found that when selenium and vitamin E are consumed, people with skin disorders, including psoriasis, demonstrate improved levels of glutathione peroxidase.

Couscous is a rich source of selenium; one cup (157 g) of cooked couscous provides you with 62 percent of the recommended daily value. And while there isn't much vitamin E in couscous, it can be easily—and deliciously—paired with other foods rich in vitamin E, such as spinach and almonds.

If you're not sure how to cook couscous, turn to our basic recipe on page 256. Or, if you're feeling more adventurous, give our Pumpkin and Chickpea Stew with Couscous on page 268 a try. Your taste buds—and your skin—will thank you.

The Specs

Couscous is made by rolling moistened semolina wheat (or durum wheat) into balls and coating them with finely ground wheat flour. While traditional couscous requires considerable preparation time and is usually steamed, quick-cooking or instant couscous is now widely available and takes just minutes to prepare.

Eggplant

Dark-colored vegetables are full of antioxidants, which can help your skin stay healthy even when it is plagued with acne and psoriasis. Eggplant's dark purple skin is a signal that it is packed with the reddish-blue pigments known as anthocyanins, powerful antioxidants that protect the integrity of support structures in the skin and veins.

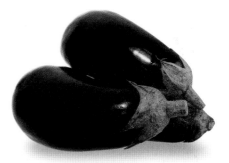

Nasunin Rescues Cells

In addition to anthocyanins, eggplant contains another antioxidant known as nasunin. This potent phytonutrient acts as a free radical scavenger, protecting cell membranes from damage and inflammation, two symptoms that can plague acne and psoriasis sufferers.

Nasunin also functions as an iron chelator, or remover. Although iron is an essential nutrient that plays a role in oxygen transport, normal immune function, and collagen synthesis, an excess of iron in the body can increase free radical production. By chelating iron, nasunin prevents the formation of free radicals, thereby stopping cellular damage that can promote acne and psoriasis.

Menstruating women lose excess iron each month during menstruation and are therefore at lower risk of over-accumulating iron. Men and postmenopausal women, however, cannot easily excrete iron and may benefit more greatly from nasunin intake.

Support the Troops

Eggplant also contains niacin, folate, and manganese—nutrients that are important to the health of your skin and body. B vitamins like niacin and folate are needed by the rapidly growing cells in your skin. B vitamins also support the skin in repairing damaged cells, making the skin healthier and stronger.

Manganese is a mineral and trace element that works as an antioxidant and thus helps prevent damage in the skin caused by free radicals. You'll find nearly 7 percent of your daily value of manganese in one cup (100 g) of cooked, cubed eggplant.

Be a Purple Produce Eater

Packed with antioxidants and other nutrients, eggplant is a great addition to your skin-healthy diet. Grilled eggplant, zucchini, and roasted red peppers make a wonderful sandwich, and eggplant is a main ingredient in ratatouille (see p. 270 for recipe), a delicious dish that can be served hot or cold. From sides to spreads, eggplant is a versatile vegetable to feed your skin.

A Mineral That Helps Vitamins

Manganese also helps activate enzymes that the skin needs in order to use vitamin C and the B vitamins biotin and thiamin. Vitamin C is a potent antioxidant that prevents damage caused by the inflammation associated with acne and psoriasis and B vitamins supply your skin with energy to repair the damage that occurs from such skin conditions.

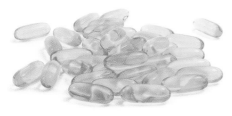

Fish Oil

Good fats are good news for skin suffering from psoriasis and acne, and fish oil is a very good fat because it contains omega-3 fatty acids. These fatty acids are an important part of your cell membranes: They make them more fluid, allow them to communicate better with other cells, and help them find nutrients and dispose of waste. For your skin, this means improved overall health and a better moisture barrier.

Promotes Good Fats, Fights Bad

The role of fish oil in preventing inflammation makes it an ideal food for a diet geared toward fighting acne or psoriasis. The omega-3 fatty acids abundant in fish oil are responsible for these anti-inflammatory powers.

Unlike the saturated fat found in most processed foods and some meats, which triggers aggressive and damaging inflammation, omega-3 fatty acids compete with bad fats in the inflammation pathway, blocking the production of chemicals that promote inflammation. Moreover, omega-3 fatty acids' anti-inflammatory abilities are thought to explain fish oil's role in reducing the risk of heart disease.

For Acne, Too

People suffering from acne sometimes avoid iodine-rich foods such as fish, shellfish, and seaweed, believing that they cause acne. However, there is no firm proof linking iodine to acne. In fact, coastal populations with diets rich in saltwater fish and seafood show a lower level of acne than inland populations.

This low prevalence rate, however, may have more to do with omega-3 fatty acids and less to do with iodine. Studies have shown that people who consume high amounts of fish have the lowest rates of acne. The omega-3 fatty acids found in fish promote an anti-inflammatory pathway that discourages acne, making fish a prime candidate for acne protection.

Mercury and PCB Concerns

When selecting which fish to eat, your best choices are sardines, anchovies, salmon, and mackerel because they are very high in the omega-3 fatty acids called EPA and DHA. These two fatty acids are very healthy as they promote health in your brain, eyes, joints, and heart.

If you are concerned about the mercury content in these fish, here's the scoop: Contrary to popular opinion, the mercury in both farmed and wild salmon is negligible. Although higher levels of mercury may be found in fresh tuna, swordfish, shark, grouper, orange roughy, and bluefish, none of these levels are thought to be of concern either.

What is concerning is that farmed salmon may be tainted with toxic environmental chemicals such as polychlorinated biphenyl compounds (PCB), making wild fish a better—albeit more expensive—option.

Eat fish more often, ideally two to three times a week, or include fish oil as a supplement in your diet to help your skin resist psoriasis and acne. Fish oil may be unpleasant to swallow, so try hiding it in a smoothie or taking it in capsule form. (If you experience fishy burps after ingesting fish oil, try an enteric-coated fish oil capsule.) Whether fresh or in pill form, making fish a centerpiece of your diet will contribute to beautiful, healthy skin.

Ginger

Ginger may best be known for its ability to relieve nausea and alleviate intestinal discomfort, but current scientific research now tells us that it also has strong antioxidant and anti-inflammatory abilities. For those dealing with psoriasis or acne, this means that enjoying the spice and flavor of ginger may also benefit their skin.

Antioxidants Helping Other Antioxidants

Psoriasis and acne are skin conditions that involve inflammation, which is triggered in response to damage. One of the leading causes of skin damage is free-radical activity, which occurs during exposure to sunlight, inflammation, and toxins in cosmetics or the foods you eat. That's right: Inflammation is both caused by free radicals and causes free radicals to form. In skin plagued by psoriasis and acne, therefore, free radicals are a significant problem due to constant inflammation. Ginger contains antioxidants that can neutralize free radicals, meaning less damage to your skin and, ultimately, less inflammation.

What in ginger makes it such a great antioxidant? A 2003 study suggests that an antioxidant called 6-gingerol makes this root highly effective at neutralizing free radicals in your body. This antioxidant also helps increase the skin's levels of glutathione, another antioxidant in your body. Glutathione is one of the natural antioxidants in your antioxidant pool, which includes such compounds as vitamin E, glutathione, superoxide dismutase, and ubiquinone (CoQ10).

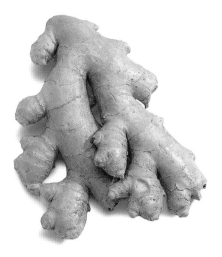

Great for Joints and Skin

Ginger has more to offer than just 6-gingerol. It contains very potent anti-inflammatory compounds called gingerols, which are believed to help fight inflammation. People with inflammation-based joint diseases such as osteoarthritis or rheumatoid arthritis notice a reduction in their pain levels when they eat ginger regularly. Additionally, in 2005, the *Journal of Alternative and Complementary Medicine* reported that ginger can suppress compounds like cytokines that promote inflammation. Perhaps ginger's anti-inflammatory abilities work to reduce the inflammation that occurs in psoriasis and acne as well. Reducing inflammation in these skin conditions prompts the skin to heal and appear smoother, tighter, and less red.

Add fresh ginger to your diet to enjoy more beautiful skin. Thinly sliced ginger makes a zesty condiment (commonly served with sushi), and grated ginger wakes up any salad dressing. You can also use grated or minced ginger wherever you use garlic, particularly in marinades, stir-fries, peanut sauces, or Thai dishes. For two recipes that deliver ginger's antioxidant benefits, check out our Rosemary Ginger Chicken with Orange-Honey Glaze (p. 258) and our Braised Lentils with Eggplant and Mushrooms (p. 250).

Grapefruit

Sweet and tangy, grapefruits are a refreshing, delicious way to relieve acne and psoriasis. Packed with lycopene and vitamin C, grapefruit is a great food for your skin. Slice one open to start your morning out right.

Powerful Vitamin C

The most valuable compound in this citrus fruit is vitamin C; in fact, you can satisfy your entire daily vitamin C requirement by eating just one grapefruit. (If you prefer just eating half, no worries—you'll still get a whopping 78 percent of your daily value.)

Those with acne and psoriasis require lots of vitamin C because it acts as an antioxidant, stopping free radicals from causing damage to the skin and triggering inflammation. Vitamin C also helps support the immune system, making it a particularly beneficial nutrient for psoriasis sufferers (as psoriasis is thought to be an immune-related condition).

Pink Is Beautiful

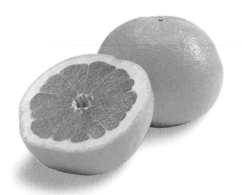

Grapefruit's blushing pink color is your signal to build it into your skin-healthy diet. The red color in fruits and vegetables comes from lycopene, a type of carotenoid. Foods high in cartenoids boost your immune system and protect your cells from the damaging effects of free radicals (compounds that can damage skin cells).

One of the Best Juices for Your Skin

Not all fruit juices are created equal in terms of what they offer your skin; their antioxidant amounts can differ greatly. Of all juices tested in a study by the University of Glasgow in the UK, Concord grape juice was found to have the highest and broadest range of antioxidants, and grapefruit juice was not far behind—it ranked at the top of the list with cloudy apple, pomegranate, and cranberry juices, beating out orange, tomato, and white grape juices.

A Versatile Citrus

Help your skin repel free radicals that aggravate acne and psoriasis by drinking grapefruit juice or enjoying some fruit segments. Create your own fresh juice blend with grapefruit and your other favorite fruits, drizzle half a grapefruit with honey and broil for a delicious dessert, or sprinkle grapefruit segments into your salad—just as we did in our Avocado, Grapefruit, Pomegranate, and Red Onion Salad on page 230.

> ### Grapefruit Interacts with Some Drugs
> Grapefruit juice is known to interact with enzymes in the liver that metabolize pharmaceuticals. If you are on medication, be sure to speak with your doctor or pharmacist about how your prescription might interact with grapefruits and grapefruit juice.

Lemons and Limes

Blimey, limey! Lemons and limes are packed with vitamin C and contain unique compounds that are great antioxidants for your skin. These compounds, called flavonoids, not only enhance the power of vitamin C, but also protect cells from oxygen damage and help prevent inflammation.

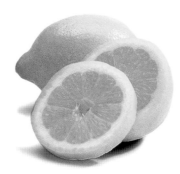

Pucker Up for Puff-Free Skin

One of nature's most effective antioxidants, vitamin C is present in good quantities in lemons and limes. In one-quarter cup (60 ml) of lemon juice, you'll find 46 percent of your daily value.

Vitamin C is very important to your immune system and to your skin, where it helps with collagen formation. For those with acne and psoriasis, vitamin C's ability to prevent free radical damage is of greatest benefit. Free radicals damage the skin and trigger inflammation, which in turn causes the formation of free radicals. Lemons and limes can help break this destructive cycle.

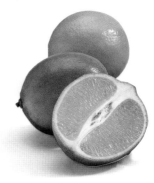

Better than Green Tea

Antioxidants known as limonins, which are found in citrus fruits, have been shown in clinical trials to fight skin and other types of cancer. These antioxidants are present in citrus fruits in the same amount as vitamin C and stay in your blood stream longer than other antioxidant compounds. In fact, in a study conducted by the U.S. Agricultural Research Service, researchers found that traces of limonin were still present in some volunteers 24 hours after consumption. The phenols in green tea and chocolate, on the other hand, remain active for only 4 to 6 hours.

Squeeze Your Way to Better Skin

Lemons and limes may not be your top choice for an afternoon snack, but they are great for your skin. Use them liberally to enhance the flavors in other foods, such as fish or fruit salad, or to turn a regular glass of water into a skin-beautifying refreshment.

You'll find various recipes that use lemons and limes in chapter 9, including Asparagus with Anchovy, Garlic, and Lemon Sauce (p. 244); Mango, Spinach, Sorrel, and Pistachio Salad (p. 228); and Watermelon Punch (p. 274).

Quinoa

Quinoa (pronounced keen-wah) is an amino acid–rich seed with a texture that is at once fluffy, creamy, and crunchy. This grain is quickly gaining in popularity due to its many health benefits and can be enjoyed cold or warm, making it well worth experimentation.

Supports a Super Antioxidant

Quinoa is a very good source of manganese, copper, and zinc, all of which help your skin battle psoriasis and acne. Manganese and copper are two minerals that are cofactors for superoxide dismutase, an enzyme that is a potent antioxidant that protects your skin from free-radical damage. In one-quarter cup (43 g) of uncooked quinoa (which yields three-quarters to one cup, or 139 to 185 g, cooked), you'll get 48 percent of your daily requirement for manganese and 17 percent of your daily requirement for copper.

Zinc is an essential mineral that is involved in more than three hundred different reactions in your body. It can be found in oysters, lean meats, beans, nuts, and whole grains like quinoa. This important antioxidant and anti-inflammatory agent assists in the battle against acne and

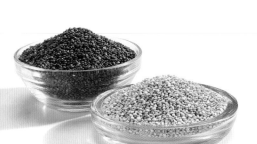

is involved in the metabolism of omega-3 fatty acids. It is also responsible for releasing and transporting vitamin A, an anti-acne nutrient, from liver storage to various parts of the body, including the skin.

Not surprisingly, population studies indicate that people who suffer from acne often have low levels of zinc in their bodies. This may be due to the fact that zinc helps clear away and break down a nerve chemical known as substance P that promotes sebum (oil) production in the skin when you are under stress. When your body does not receive adequate amounts of zinc, sebum production can get out of control, resulting in blemishes and breakouts.

Full of Fiber

When grains are processed, they lose precious vitamins and minerals, such as zinc, selenium, and vitamin B6, all of which help protect your skin from acne. Foods made from processed grains (such as white bread) are also devoid of fiber, and can cause elevations in blood sugar and insulin release. Such spikes in blood sugar and insulin levels may be significant players in the production of sebum (oil) that clogs follicles in the skin and leads to acne.

Fortunately for your skin, quinoa is a whole grain, meaning that all of its nutrients—including fiber—are intact. In fact, in just one cup (185 g) of cooked quinoa, you'll find more than 5 g of fiber, or 20 percent of your recommended daily value.

Serve up some quinoa to add zinc, fiber, and other nutrients to your acne-fighting arsenal. Vegetarians can build an entire meal around quinoa, but it also makes an easy and lovely side dish; try our Quinoa Pilaf with Roasted Tomatoes and Pine Nuts on page 254.

Vitamin A Fights Acne

Vitamin A has many functions in the body, including supporting the immune system, red blood cell production, healthy skin, and vision. Having low levels of vitamin A has been associated with inflammation and acne.

For years, dermatologists have used oral and topical vitamin A to treat acne. Vitamin A is essential in the normal shedding of cells that line follicle walls, and it also prevents cells from building up in the pores, which can cause pimples to form.

Raspberries

A member of the rose family, raspberries can make your skin as beautiful as the flower to which they are related. These amazing berries offer your skin many healthy benefits and can help you win the battle against psoriasis and acne.

Packed with Skin Protectors

A good source of manganese and vitamin C, raspberries are packed with free-radical fighting power. These antioxidant nutrients help your skin neutralize free radicals, preventing them from causing damage and

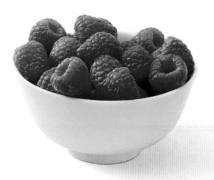

Better than Strawberries and Kiwis

The antioxidant capacity of raspberries is almost 50 percent greater than that of strawberries, three times that of kiwis, and ten times that of tomatoes.

triggering inflammation. Free radicals form in your skin from sun exposure, cosmetics, toxins in foods, and even from inflammation itself. They are a major problem for your skin as they can cause dryness, wrinkles, and complexion problems.

In one cup (125 g) of raspberries, you'll find 62 percent of your recommended daily value of manganese and 51 percent of your daily vitamin C requirement. Aside from protecting your cells from damage, these two nutrients have other beneficial qualities as well. Manganese helps keep your bones strong, your nerves healthy, and your blood sugar levels normal, and vitamin C improves iron absorption and helps in the regeneration of vitamin E, another skin-healthy nutrient.

Antioxidants Galore

Raspberries contain a host of other powerful antioxidants, from ellagic acid to anthocyanins (the latter of which give the berries their bright color). Ellagic acid belongs to the family of phytonutrients called tannins and is responsible for a good portion of the antioxidant activity of raspberries and other berries. It helps neutralize free radicals, thereby preventing unwanted damage to cell membranes and skin.

The anthocyanins in raspberries make up 25 percent of their antioxidant capacity. These antioxidants protect in two ways. First, they neutralize enzymes that destroy connective tissue, thereby preventing further damage. Then, they repair proteins in blood-vessel walls. According to a study published in the journal *Pharmacological Research,* animal experiments have shown that supplementation with anthocyanins effectively prevents inflammation and subsequent blood-vessel damage.

A Barrage of Berries

How you enjoy raspberries is limited only by your imagination. Toss them on your cereal, blend them into a smoothie, bake them into muffins, add them to salads or yogurt, or eat a bowlful of these ruby-colored berries on their own.

While fresh is always best, studies have found that freezing raspberries does not significantly affect their antioxidant levels (though their vitamin C content does diminish), so if you're in a pinch or it's the wrong season, frozen raspberries are a fine stand-in. No matter how you eat these sweet little fruits, they will bring you one step closer to healthy, vibrant skin.

Sage

Sage leaves are traditionally used for treating oily, spotty skin and wrinkled, sagging complexions. They are a common ingredient in facial cleansers as they have the ability to close pores, restore elasticity, and stimulate blood circulation. Sage is also used to treat acne because it is believed to inhibit the action of the glands in the skin. When taken internally, this savory herb is known to fight inflammation, making it a recommended food for anyone dealing with acne or psoriasis.

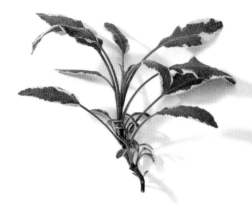

Herb on a Mission

The active compound found in the grayish-green, lance-shaped leaves of the sage plant is known as rosmarinic acid. This antioxidant—also found in rosemary (from which it gets its name), oregano, thyme, and peppermint—reduces inflammation in the skin by affecting messengers that cause inflammation.

In your body, there are a wide variety of messengers involved in inflammation, each of which stimulates a different amount and type of inflammation. The compounds in sage reduce the amount of messengers that trigger harmful inflammation and allow the skin time to heal. Less inflammation in the skin makes it appear less red and puffy, two complexion complaints from acne and psoriasis patients.

Sage can also fight the cause of inflammation because it contains superoxide dismutase and peroxidase, two antioxidant enzymes that help skin prevent free radical damage to its cells. These enzymes work alongside the flavonoids and phenolic acids in sage to stabilize oxygen-related metabolism and prevent oxygen-based damage to the cells.

Add a Dash to Your Diet

Sage, which was named the 2001 Herb of the Year by the International Herb Association, is a subtly wonderful addition that will make your dishes more delicious and your skin more beautiful. From soups to stews, roast chicken to pasta sauces, sage can be incorporated to an endless variety of dishes. To retain the most flavor, use fresh leaves if you can find them and add the herb toward the end of your cooking.

A Savory Prescription

The anti-inflammatory effects of sage are so powerful, in fact, that increased intake of sage as a seasoning is recommended for those with inflammatory conditions such as rheumatoid arthritis, asthma, and atherosclerosis.

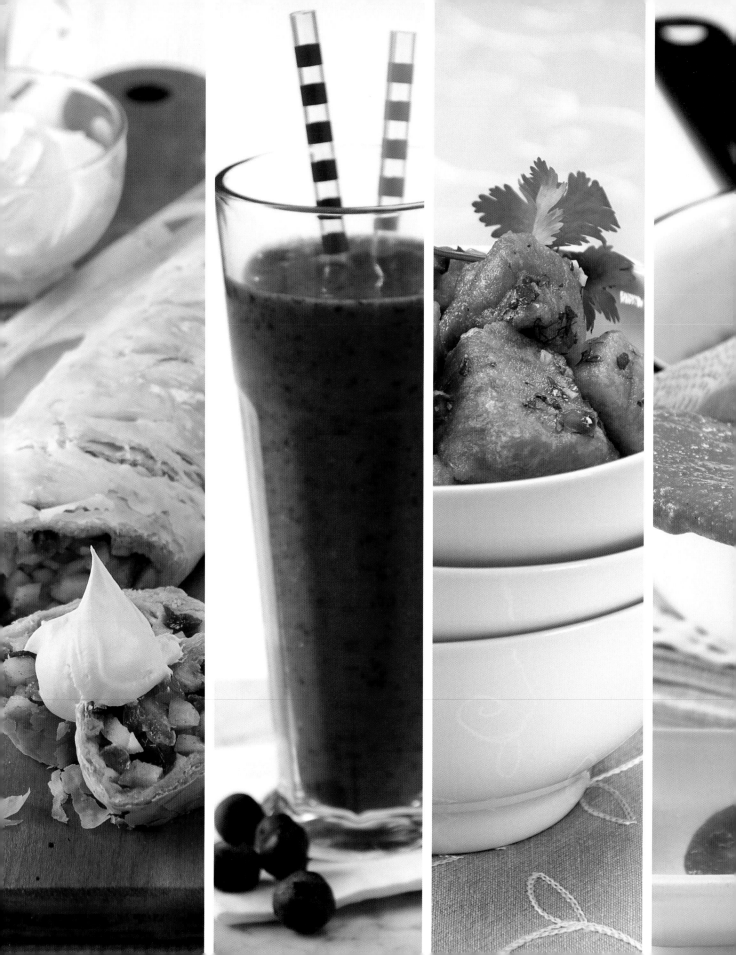

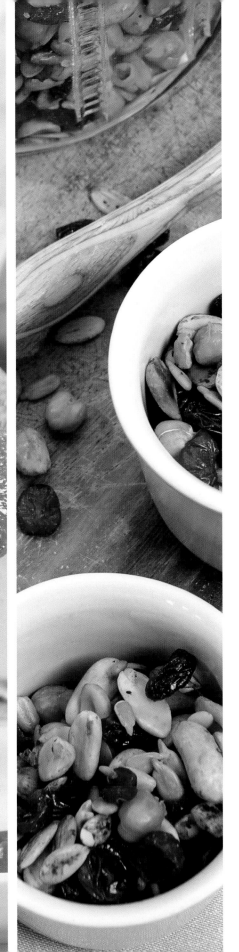

Delicious Recipes for Beautiful Skin

NOW THAT YOU'VE discovered how the skin works and which foods provide it with the greatest benefits, it's time to get your skin-healthy lifestyle started. This chapter is full of mouth-watering recipes—from soups and salads, to main courses, desserts, and more. These dishes have been formulated to brighten your complexion; moisturize, tighten, and smooth your skin; and relieve puffiness. You can look forward to having beautiful skin and delicious meals with the help of these healthy, easy-to-prepare recipes.

Creamy Fruit Smoothie

A perfect balance of good fats and antioxidants, this smoothie offers your skin the tools it needs to stay radiant, moisturized, and wrinkle-free. Add a dollop of yogurt, and you needn't worry about puffy eyes in the morning.

¼ cup (38 g) frozen berries

½ cup (120 ml) skim milk

½ banana

2 tablespoons (14 g) flaxseed meal or 1 tablespoon (15 ml) flaxseed oil

Ice cubes, optional

Yield: 1 serving

1. Combine all of the ingredients in a blender and blend until very creamy and smooth. (If you prefer a chunkier smoothie, blend for a shorter time. If you prefer a frostier smoothie, include the ice cubes.) Pour into a glass and serve immediately.

Notes

- *Alternatives to skim milk include kefir, plain low-fat yogurt, and soy milk. If these substitutions make your smoothie thicker than you'd like, thin it with fruit juice or water.*

- *You can buy flaxseed meal, or make it yourself from whole flaxseeds as follows: Measure ½ cup (84 g) seeds into a blender or food processor, and pulse until the seeds turn into a powder. Store any unused meal in a covered container in the refrigerator for up to 4 days.*

NUTRITIONAL ANALYSIS

Each serving provides: 241 calories; 14 g total fat; 1.5 g saturated fat; 5 g protein; 25.7 g carbohydrate; 3 g dietary fiber; 2 mg cholesterol.

SUPERSKIN NUTRIENTS		% DAILY VALUE*
Vitamin A	340.7 IU	7%
Vitamin B6	0.4 mg	20%
Vitamin C	7.7 mg	13%
Vitamin E	0.8 mg	4%
Magnesium	39.4 mg	10%
Manganese	0.5 mg	25%
Selenium	3.5 mcg	5%
Zinc	0.7 mg	5%

*Percent Daily Values are based on a 2,000-calorie diet. Your daily values may be higher or lower depending on your caloric needs.

INGREDIENT SPOTLIGHT

Berries

No matter which berry (or berries) you choose for your smoothie, your skin is sure to come out on top. This is because all berries contain anthocyanins, the blue- and red-colored pigments that give these fruits their beautiful color. Anthocyanins belong to the flavonoid family, a class of nutrients known for its anti-allergic, anti-inflammatory, anti-microbial, and anti-cancer properties.

Tropical Fruit Smoothie

Mornings have never tasted so good. Raise a glass filled with tropical fruits and berries and make a farewell toast to your wrinkles. Açai is among the most potent sources of wrinkle-fighting antioxidants on earth and dark-colored berries are also packed with wrinkle-fighting antioxidants (called anthocyanins). Mango contains silica, which keeps your skin tight and smooth, and flaxseed delivers fiber and omega-3 fatty acids, which help your complexion stay moist and beautiful.

¼ cup (38 g) fresh berries (raspberries, blueberries, or blackberries)

¼ cup (45 g) diced mango

¼ cup (40 g) diced melon

¼ cup (59 ml) pomegranate or cranberry juice

2 tablespoons (30 ml) açai juice or 1 tablespoon (15 ml) açai pulp (see Note)

2 tablespoons (14 g) flaxseed meal or 1 tablespoon (15 ml) flaxseed oil

Ice cubes, optional

Yield: 1 serving

1. Combine all of the ingredients in a blender and blend until very creamy and smooth. (If you prefer a chunkier smoothie, blend for a shorter time. If you prefer a frostier smoothie, include the ice cubes.) Pour into a glass and serve immediately.

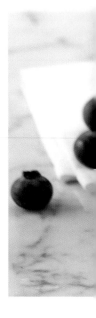

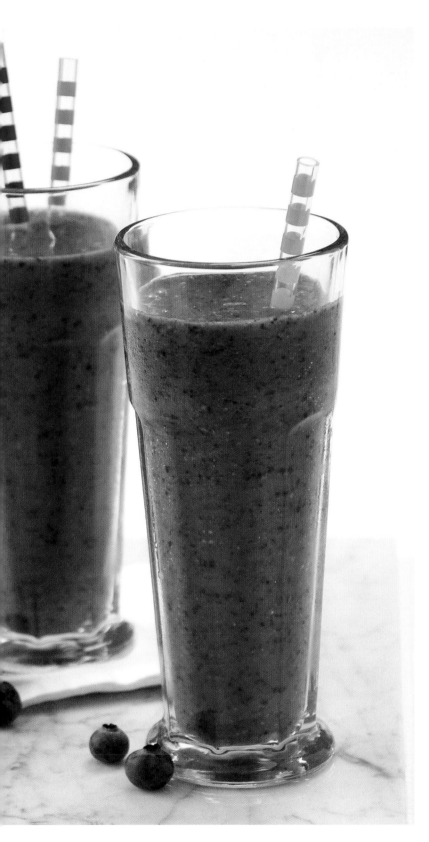

Notes

- *Açai juice and pulp are appearing more and more in the marketplace. Look for these products in specialty food or health-food stores. The pulp is typically located in the freezer section.*

- *You can buy flaxseed meal, or make it yourself from whole flaxseeds as follows: Measure ½ cup (84 g) seeds into a blender or food processor, and pulse until the seeds turn into a powder. Store any unused meal in a covered container in the refrigerator for up to 4 days.*

- *Mix and match the other fruits in this smoothie to suit your taste or the season. Whichever fruits you choose, aim for about ¾ cup (150 g) of diced fruit. Apples and pears work well with melon. Plums and blueberries have a subtly spicy flavor.*

NUTRITIONAL ANALYSIS

Each serving provides: 238 calories; 14 g total fat; 1.5 g saturated fat; 1 g protein; 30 g carbohydrate; 3 g dietary fiber; 0 mg cholesterol.

SUPERSKIN NUTRIENTS		% DAILY VALUE*
Vitamin A	2943.0 IU	59%
Vitamin B6	0.2 mg	10%
Vitamin C	55.2 mg	92%
Vitamin E	1.2 mg	6%
Magnesium	21.8 mg	5%
Manganese	0.9 mg	45%
Selenium	0.7 mcg	1%
Zinc	0.3 mg	2%

*Percent Daily Values are based on a 2,000-calorie diet. Your daily values may be higher or lower depending on your caloric needs.

Muesli

Start your day with this energizing muesli packed with antiwrinkle nutrients from oats, blueberries, and apricots. You'll keep your blood-sugar levels low with the help of cinnamon, and protect your skin from puffiness, redness, and wrinkles with almonds, which contain vitamin E and flavonols that fight free radicals.

½ cup (50 g) rolled oats

⅓ cup (28 g) oat bran

2 tablespoons (18 g) dried blueberries

5 dried apricots, chopped

1 pinch ground cinnamon

1 cup (230 g) plain yogurt

½ cup (120 ml) skim milk

1 tablespoon (7 g) slivered almonds

Yield: 2 servings

1. In a medium bowl, mix together the oats, oat bran, blueberries, apricots, and cinnamon. Stir in yogurt.

2. Cover and refrigerate overnight.

3. In the morning, pour the milk over the muesli, and sprinkle with almonds. (For extra flavor and skin-health benefits, sprinkle with fresh berries before serving.)

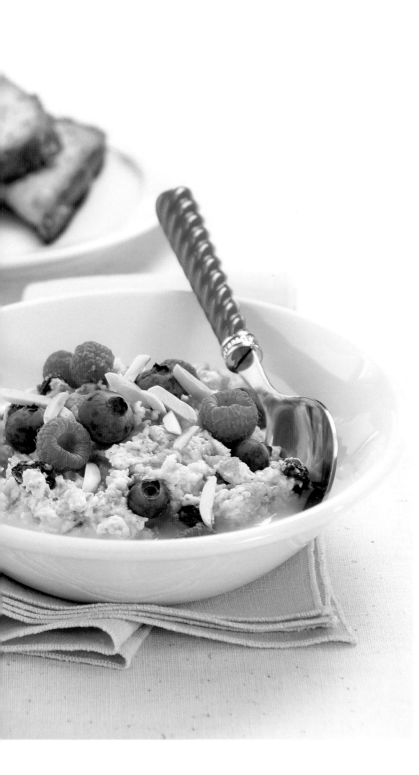

Notes

- *Use this as a sweet and crunchy filling, as a topping for papaya or mango slices, or layer it with fresh berries to make a light parfait.*

- *Instead of skim milk, try plain or vanilla-flavored soy milk, or almond milk.*

NUTRITIONAL ANALYSIS

Each serving provides: 319 calories; 6.5 g total fat; 2 g saturated fat; 16 g protein; 55 g carbo-hydrate; 7 g dietary fiber; 9 mg cholesterol.

SUPERSKIN NUTRIENTS		% DAILY VALUE*
Vitamin A	439.9 IU	9%
Vitamin B6	0.2 mg	10%
Vitamin C	8.1 mg	14%
Vitamin E	1.7 mg	9%
Magnesium	109.2 mg	27%
Manganese	1.8 mg	90%
Selenium	19.4 mcg	28%
Zinc	2.6 mg	17%

*Percent Daily Values are based on a 2,000-calorie diet. Your daily values may be higher or lower depending on your caloric needs.

Breakfast Bulgur with Dried Cherries, Apples, and Apricots

Fight puffy morning eyes with the help of melatonin from the cherries in this delicious recipe. Bursting with vitamin C, riboflavin, anthocyanins (nutrients that fight wrinkles), iron, and vitamin A, this dish is sure to improve your complexion and your health.

2 cups (475 ml) broth or water

¾ cup (105 g) bulgur wheat

½ teaspoon salt, or to taste

2 tablespoons (15 g) dried cherries

2 dried apple rings, coarsely chopped

2 dried apricots, chopped

Yield: 4 servings

1. Place the broth or water in a saucepan and bring to a boil over high heat.

2. Add the bulgur wheat and stir well with a fork to remove any lumps. Reduce the heat to low and simmer for about 3 to 4 minutes. Remove the pan from the heat.

3. Add salt, cherries, apples, and apricots to the pan, and gently fold in with a fork. Cover the pan, and allow mixture to rest for about 10 minutes before serving, allowing the cereal to absorb the flavors of the fruit.

Notes

• *Substitute dried cranberries or blueberries for the cherries, if desired.*

• *For added taste, sprinkle each serving with cinnamon sugar and add a splash of warm milk.*

• *Bulgur is often sold in three varieties, or grinds— coarse, medium, and fine. Coarse is preferred in pilaf and stuffing recipes, while fine works best in the popular Middle Eastern salad known as tabbouleh. For this recipe, medium or coarse bulgur works best.*

• *All bulgur triples in volume once cooked, so be sure your saucepan is large enough to hold everything.*

NUTRITIONAL ANALYSIS

Each serving provides: 126 calories; 0.5 g total fat; 0 g saturated fat; 4 g protein; 28 g carbohydrate; 6 g dietary fiber; 0 mg cholesterol.

SUPERSKIN NUTRIENTS		% DAILY VALUE*
Vitamin A	53.3 IU	1%
Vitamin B6	0.1 mg	5%
Vitamin C	0.9 mg	2%
Vitamin E	0.5 mg	3%
Magnesium	44.8 mg	11%
Manganese	0.8 mg	40%
Selenium	0.7 mg	1%
Zinc	0.6 mg	4%

*Percent Daily Values are based on a 2,000-calorie diet. Your daily values may be higher or lower depending on your caloric needs.

INGREDIENT SPOTLIGHT

Dried Fruit

Dried fruits are rich in the dietary minerals calcium, magnesium, phosphorus, potassium, sodium, copper, and manganese, and in vitamins A and B.

They are also a terrific source of iron, which plays a vital role in the formation of the collagen scaffolding that keeps your skin tight, strong, and smooth. Apricots and figs have the most iron per ounce of all dried fruits, each providing roughly 7 percent of the daily recommended iron intake per serving. (One serving of dried apricots is eight; one serving of dried figs is four.)

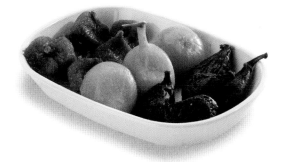

Cottage Cheese Pancakes with Blueberry Maple Syrup

Welcome your skin to a beautiful morning with these delicious pancakes. The anthocyanins in the blueberries fight wrinkles, the maple syrup is terrific for your complexion, and the eggs contain lecithin to moisturize your skin.

1 cup (145 g) fresh blueberries, rinsed and dried

½ cup (120 ml) maple syrup

4 whole eggs, separated

1 cup (225 g) small curd cottage cheese

¼ cup (59 ml) melted butter

¼ cup (31 g) sifted whole-wheat flour

½ teaspoon (3 g) grated lemon zest

¼ teaspoon salt

Canola oil

Yield: 4 servings

1. Make blueberry syrup by combining the berries and syrup in a heavy-bottomed pan. Bring the mixture to a simmer, keeping it there for about 10 minutes. Keep the syrup warm by covering the pan while preparing the pancakes.

2. Combine the egg yolks, cottage cheese, butter, flour, lemon zest, and salt in a large bowl. Stir until batter is smooth and thick (the cottage cheese will make it look a little lumpy).

3. In another bowl, using an electric mixer or a whisk, beat the egg whites into a thick foam, until soft peaks appear.

4. Gently fold the egg whites into the batter.

5. Heat a griddle or a large skillet over medium high heat. When a drop of water "skips" over the surface of the pan, it is ready. Lightly brush the pan with oil and drop the batter by large spoonfuls onto the griddle or skillet. The pancakes will spread as they cook, so leave about 2 to 3 inches (5 to 7.5 cm) between each one. Cook until the edges of the pancake are set, about 2 minutes. Flip over and cook another 2 minutes.

6. Serve the pancakes topped with blueberry syrup.

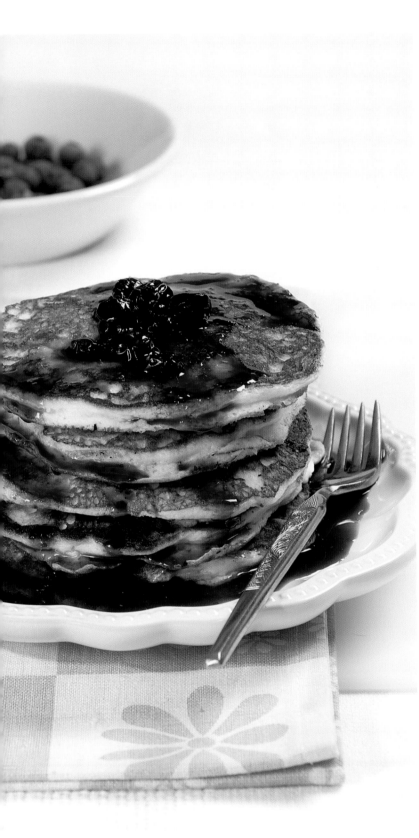

Notes

- The pancakes are very light and fluffy as they come out of the pan, but they will start to deflate as they sit. If necessary, keep them warm in an oven heated to 200°F (93°C, or gas mark ¼); they'll still taste delicious.

- The syrup can be made from other berries or fruits. Prepare it ahead of time and store in the refrigerator for up to 2 days. Reheat gently over low heat or in the microwave before serving.

NUTRITIONAL ANALYSIS

Each serving provides: 504 calories; 33 g total fat; 11 g saturated fat; 14 g protein; 40 g carbohydrate; 1 g dietary fiber; 251 mg cholesterol.

SUPERSKIN NUTRIENTS		% DAILY VALUE*
Vitamin A	873.3 IU	17%
Vitamin B6	0.1 mg	5%
Vitamin C	5.0 mg	8%
Vitamin E	4.0 mg	20%
Magnesium	4.7 mg	1%
Manganese	1.5 mg	75%
Selenium	23.4 mcg	33%
Zinc	2.5 mg	17%

*Percent Daily Values are based on a 2,000-calorie diet. Your daily values may be higher or lower depending on your caloric needs.

Spicy Maple Pecans

Fight puffy eyes and prevent inflammation with the maple syrup and pecans in this quick and easy recipe. Pecans are delicious on their own, but they taste even better when they're combined with potassium-rich maple syrup.

2 teaspoons (9 g) butter

1 cup (110 g) roughly chopped pecans

2 tablespoons (30 ml) maple syrup

Salt to taste

Pinch of ground cayenne pepper

Yield: 4 servings (1 cup, or 110 g, total)

1. Melt the butter in a small skillet over low heat. Add the pecans, maple syrup, salt, and cayenne and continue to heat, stirring until the pecans are well coated. Continue to cook until the maple syrup has reduced to a thick consistency, about 2 minutes.

2. Continue to stir the pecans over low heat until they develop a rich aroma, another 2 or 3 minutes. Stir the nuts constantly as they toast.

3. Immediately remove the pecans from the pan to cool on a baking sheet.

Notes

- *Serve the pecans on their own, or combine them with other nuts and dried fruits for a delicious trail mix (use them in either of our snack mix recipes on pp. 204 and 206).*

- *These pecans also pair perfectly with our Brussels sprouts side dish on page 240.*

NUTRITIONAL ANALYSIS

Each serving provides: 242 calories; 22 g total fat; 3 g saturated fat; 2 g protein; 12 g carbohydrate; 2 g dietary fiber; 5 mg cholesterol.

SUPERSKIN NUTRIENTS		% DAILY VALUE*
Vitamin A	133.4 IU	3%
Vitamin B6	0.1 mg	5%
Vitamin C	0.6 mg	1%
Vitamin E	1.0 mg	5%
Magnesium	39.6 mg	10%
Manganese	1.7 mg	85%
Selenium	1.6 mcg	2%
Zinc	2.1 mg	14%

*Percent Daily Values are based on a 2,000-calorie diet. Your daily values may be higher or lower depending on your caloric needs.

INGREDIENT SPOTLIGHT

Maple Syrup

Potassium helps with puffy skin by keeping sodium levels in check and maintaining the body's water balance. In maple syrup, you'll find about 35 mg of potassium per tablespoon (15 ml) and only 2 mg per tablespoon of sodium, making it a great puff-fighting food choice.

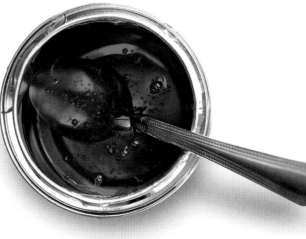

Roasted Chickpeas

Protect the collagen that gives your skin its tight, youthful appearance with the help of this delicious spin on peas. It's a perfect skin-healthy snack to have on hand and goes great with our snack mix on page 204.

One 14-ounce (400-g) can of chickpeas

2 tablespoons (30 ml) extra-virgin olive or canola oil

¼ teaspoon salt, or to taste

Yield: 3 servings (1½ cups, or 483 g, total)

1. Preheat the oven to 375°F (190°C, or gas mark 5).

2. Rinse and drain the chickpeas. Pour them from the colander onto several layers of paper towel to dry thoroughly.

3. Brush a baking sheet with oil. Spread the chickpeas onto the sheet, rolling or stirring them until they are lightly coated with the oil, and season with salt.

4. Roast the chickpeas for about 1 hour, or until they turn a deep golden brown and taste toasty and crunchy. Stir the chickpeas occasionally to ensure they toast evenly.

5. Serve warm or cold.

Notes

- *Make your own variation of this recipe by adding your favorite herbs and seasonings.*

- *To make Lemon, Garlic, and Herb Roasted Chickpeas, before roasting the chickpeas, sprinkle them with about 1 ½ teaspoons (7.25 ml) of lemon juice, ½ teaspoon of chopped fresh or dried rosemary or thyme leaves, and 1 teaspoon (3 g) minced garlic or garlic powder.*

NUTRITIONAL ANALYSIS

Each serving provides: 215 calories; 10 g total fat; 1 g saturated fat; 6 g protein; 25 g carbohydrate; 5 g dietary fiber; 0 mg cholesterol.

SUPERSKIN NUTRIENTS		% DAILY VALUE*
Vitamin A	0.0 IU	0%
Vitamin B6	0.3 mg	15%
Vitamin C	4 mg	5%
Vitamin E	1.1 mg	6%
Magnesium	70.0 mg	17%
Manganese	1.4 mg	72%
Selenium	6.5 mcg	10%
Zinc	0.0 mg	0%

*Percent Daily Values are based on a 2,000-calorie diet. Your daily values may be higher or lower depending on your caloric needs.

INGREDIENT SPOTLIGHT

Chickpeas

We all know how beneficial fiber is in controlling our cholesterol and blood sugar levels, but did you know these benefits are also good for your skin? This is because healthy cholesterol and blood sugar levels keep your blood vessels working optimally, thus ensuring that your skin receives a good supply of nutrients to keep on glowing. Lucky for us, fiber is not hard to come by, especially in chickpeas. Just one-half cup (120 g) serving provides one-quarter of your daily fiber requirement.

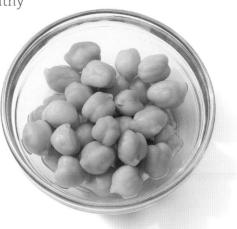

Tamari-Flavored Snack Mix

Pack this skin-beautifying mix on your next outing. It contains nutrients like fiber, magnesium, vitamin E, and manganese that tighten and smooth your skin, fight wrinkles, and improve your complexion. Consuming the phytoestrogens in sunflower seeds is an especially effective and delicious way to help your skin fight wrinkles.

¾ cup (110 g) raw shelled peanuts

¾ cup (242 g) Roasted Chickpeas (p. 202)

¼ cup (33 g) raw sunflower seeds

¼ cup (35 g) raw pumpkin seeds

2 tablespoons (30 ml) low-sodium tamari sauce

1 teaspoon (5 ml) dark sesame oil

Pinch of red pepper flakes

¼ cup (35 g) raisins

¼ cup (30 g) dried cranberries

Yield: 7 to 8 servings (about 2½ cups, or 480 g, total)

1. Heat a cast-iron skillet over medium high heat. Add the peanuts and toast them, swirling the pan to keep them in motion, until they have a rich, toasty aroma and a very light brown color. Add the chickpeas, sunflower seeds, and pumpkin seeds and continue to swirl the pan over the heat to lightly toast the seeds for about 1 minute.

2. Add the tamari sauce, sesame oil, and red pepper flakes, and continue to toast the nuts, stirring to distribute the flavoring ingredients, about 2 minutes. Immediately pour the nuts into a bowl to cool.

3. When mixture has cooled, add the raisins and cranberries and stir to combine.

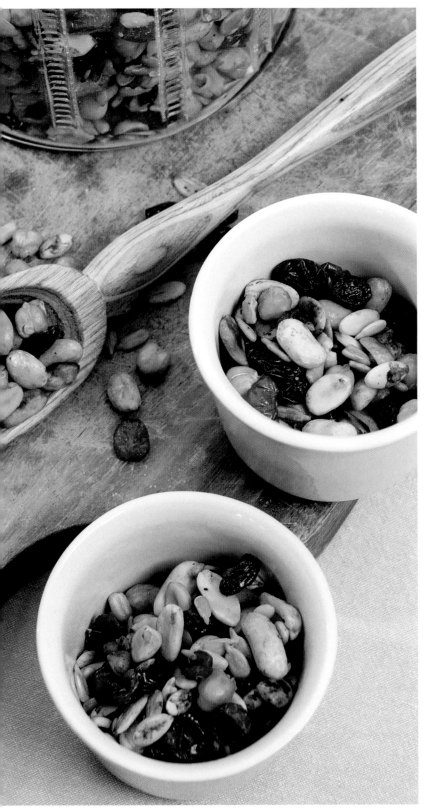

Note

This snack mix will last for up to 3 weeks in a tightly sealed storage container.

NUTRITIONAL ANALYSIS

Each serving provides: 202 calories; 13 g total fat; 2 g saturated fat; 7 g protein; 17 g carbohydrate; 3 g dietary fiber; 0 mg cholesterol.

SUPERSKIN NUTRIENTS		% DAILY VALUE*
Vitamin A	25.4 IU	1%
Vitamin B6	0.2 mg	10%
Vitamin C	1.3 mg	2%
Vitamin E	4.4 mg	22%
Magnesium	71.7 mg	18%
Manganese	0.7 mg	35%
Selenium	4.7 mcg	7%
Zinc	1.1 mg	7%

*Percent Daily Values are based on a 2,000-calorie diet. Your daily values may be higher or lower depending on your caloric needs.

Tropical Flavors Snack Mix

This tropical snack mix is a tasty blend of nutrients that help your skin repair damage while fighting wrinkles and preventing inflammation. Nuts are packed with fiber, which is good for your skin and your bowel. Mango and papaya contain silica, which keeps your skin firm, and chocolate is packed with antioxidants to fight the damage that results in puffiness and wrinkles.

Peanut or canola oil

½ cup (50 g) whole shelled pecans

½ cup (70 g) whole shelled raw Brazil nuts

½ cup (50 g) raw walnut halves

½ teaspoon salt, or to taste

⅓ cup (40 g) diced dried mango

⅓ cup (40 g) diced dried papaya

⅓ cup (33 g) banana chips

½ cup (88 g) dark chocolate chips

Yield: 9 servings (3 cups, or 630 g, total)

1. Preheat the oven to 375°F (190°C, or gas mark 5).

2. Brush a baking sheet with oil. Add the nuts in an even layer , rolling or stirring them until they are lightly coated with the oil. Season lightly with salt.

3. Roast until the nuts turn a deep golden brown, about 8 minutes. Stir the nuts occasionally as they roast to prevent those on the outer edges from burning.

4. Immediately transfer the nuts to a bowl, and let them cool completely before adding the remaining ingredients (otherwise, the chocolate chips will melt). Stir to combine.

Notes

- This snack mix will last for up to 3 weeks in a tightly sealed storage container.

- Feel free to vary your nut and dried fruit choices to suit your tastes. Pistachios and almonds would work well, as well as dried dates and pineapple.

NUTRITIONAL ANALYSIS

Each serving provides: 292 calories; 17.5 g total fat; 4.5 g saturated fat; 4 g protein; 36 g carbohydrate; 5 g dietary fiber; 0 mg cholesterol.

SUPERSKIN NUTRIENTS		% DAILY VALUE*
Vitamin A	532.9 IU	11%
Vitamin B6	0.1 mg	5%
Vitamin C	21.3 mg	36%
Vitamin E	4.5 mg	23%
Magnesium	64.9 mg	16%
Manganese	0.6 mg	30%
Selenium	228.8 mcg	327%
Zinc	1.2 mg	8%

*Percent Daily Values are based on a 2,000-calorie diet. Your daily values may be higher or lower depending on your caloric needs.

INGREDIENT SPOTLIGHT

Brazil Nuts

Brazil nuts are enriched with selenium, a mineral that your body and skin need for optimal health. This antioxidant stops free radicals—the unstable compounds that steal electrons from your skin's structures—from causing damage to your skin. Not only that, but selenium is also responsible for maintaining the elasticity of your skin. Just 3 to 4 Brazil nuts a day can provide you with enough selenium to help fight sagging skin.

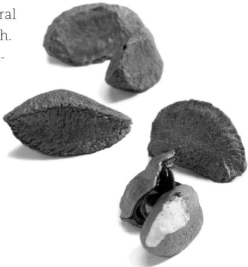

Roasted Garlic

Rebuild collagen in your skin and prevent inflammation that can make your skin look red and puffy with the help of this sweet, creamy preparation. Spread the garlic over warm whole-grain bread, mix it into baked sweet potatoes or other vegetables, or add the pureé to your whole-grain pasta—the possibilities are endless!

Kosher salt
1 head of garlic

Yield: 3 servings (about 10 cloves or ½ cup [120 g] purée total)

1. Preheat oven to 375°F (190°C, or gas mark 5).

2. In a small baking dish or skillet with an oven-proof handle, pour enough salt to make a bed for the garlic. (You don't have to cover the whole pan; just add enough to raise the garlic from direct contact with the pan.)

3. Place the garlic on top of the salt.

4. Roast the garlic for 15 to 20 minutes, or until the juices that escape from the top develop a rich, brown color and the flesh becomes soft enough to squeeze easily. Remove the garlic from the oven and allow to cool.

5. Separate the head into individual cloves and remove their peels. Leave the cloves whole, or cut the top from the entire head and squeeze the flesh into a bowl. Use a fork to mash the garlic into a smooth purée.

Notes

- *Placing the garlic on a salt bed helps it roast evenly and develop a more intense flavor.*

- *Any unused roasted garlic can be stored. Place the whole peeled cloves or purée in a small dish, and add enough oil to keep the air from coming in contact with the garlic. Store the roasted garlic in the refrigerator for up to 3 days.*

NUTRITIONAL ANALYSIS

Each serving provides: 13 calories; 0 g total fat; 0 g saturated fat; 1 g protein;
3 g carbohydrate; 0 g dietary fiber; 0 mg cholesterol.

SUPERSKIN NUTRIENTS		% DAILY VALUE*
Vitamin A	0 IU	0%
Vitamin B6	0.1 mg	6%
Vitamin C	2.8 mg	5%
Vitamin E	0 mg	0%
Magnesium	2.2 mg	1%
Manganese	0.2 mg	8%
Selenium	1.3 mcg	2%
Zinc	0.1 mg	1%

*Percent Daily Values are based on a 2,000-calorie diet. Your daily values may
be higher or lower depending on your caloric needs.

INGREDIENT SPOTLIGHT

Garlic

Manganese, a trace mineral found in garlic, functions
as a powerful antioxidant for your skin by protecting your cells from free radical damage
and helping to maintain the health
of your nerves. Studies indicate that
manganese may also play a role in
lowering cholesterol and keeping
blood sugar levels in check.

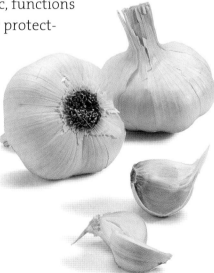

Herb-Roasted Tomatoes

Use these wrinkle-fighting tomatoes in salads and sandwiches, or as bruschetta-like topping for whole-grain bread. You can also use them to replace some or all of the fresh or canned tomatoes in your favorite sauce recipe. We've included them in our Roasted Tomato Soup (p. 224).

2 pints (960 g) plum or cherry
    tomatoes
Extra-virgin olive oil as needed
2 teaspoons (6 g) chopped
    garlic
2 teaspoons (2 g) dried orega-
    no, basil, marjoram, or parsley
    (or a combination)
Salt and pepper to taste

Yield: 6 servings (about
    3 cups, or 618 g, total)

1. Preheat the oven to 450°F (230°C, or gas mark 8).
2. Core and cut plum tomatoes into ¼-inch (0.6 cm) slices, or cut cherry tomatoes in half.
3. Pour enough oil onto a baking sheet to make a thin layer. Scatter with garlic, dried herbs, salt, and pepper to taste. Add the tomatoes, turning or rolling them until they are coated with the oil and seasoning.
4. Roast until the tomatoes are lightly browned around the edges and slightly dried, about 15 to 20 minutes (or longer, depending upon how much moisture there is in the tomatoes).

Notes

- *The tomatoes can be refrigerated for up to 6 days or frozen for up to 4 weeks.*

- *When peeling your garlic cloves for chopping, try this tip: Place the cloves in a large bowl of cold water and peel off the skins while the cloves are submerged in the water. They should easily slip right off.*

NUTRITIONAL ANALYSIS

Each serving provides: 45 calories; 2.5 g total fat; 0.5 g saturated fat; 1 g protein; 5 g carbohydrate; 1 g dietary fiber; 0 mg cholesterol.

SUPERSKIN NUTRIENTS		% DAILY VALUE*
Vitamin A	653.4 IU	13%
Vitamin B6	0.1 mg	5%
Vitamin C	19.5 mg	33%
Vitamin E	1.2 mg	6%
Magnesium	12.5 mg	3%
Manganese	0.1 mg	5%
Selenium	0.6 mg	1%
Zinc	0.1 mg	1%

*Percent Daily Values are based on a 2,000-calorie diet. Your daily values may be higher or lower depending on your caloric needs.

INGREDIENT SPOTLIGHT

Tomatoes

Tomatoes contain a powerful plant chemical called lycopene, which is one of the best scavengers of skin-damaging free radicals. Lycopene also improves some functions of cell metabolism and helps cells work more effectively. More efficient metabolism means better collagen repair and fewer wrinkles. And because lycopene appears to be more available in cooked tomatoes than in raw ones, you can feel free to roast away!

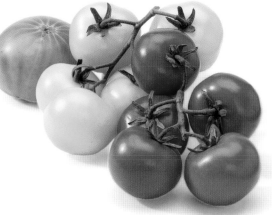

Romesco Dipping Sauce

This mouth-watering, wrinkle-fighting sauce can be served with anything from roasted vegetables to salads to fish and poultry. Its ingredients—olive oil, tomatoes, almonds, and garlic—are bursting with nutrients like vitamin C, ajoene, and lycopene that help your skin fight signs of aging and other damage. Try preparing the sauce with multigrain bread instead for an even brighter complexion.

2 dried ancho chiles

Boiling water, approximately ½ cup (118 ml)

¼ cup (59 ml) extra-virgin olive oil, divided

4 cloves garlic, peeled and halved

1 slice French or Italian bread, cut into small cubes

3 plum tomatoes, peeled, seeded, chopped (fresh or canned)

½ cup (54 g) slivered toasted almonds

¼ cup (56 ml) red wine vinegar

½ teaspoon (1 g) ground cumin

Cayenne pepper to taste

Salt and pepper to taste

Yield: 4 servings

1. Place the ancho chiles in a small bowl, and add enough boiling water to cover them. Allow the chiles to steep until they are very tender, at least 45 minutes and up to 2 hours. Remove the stem and seeds, and reserve the flesh.

2. Heat 1 tablespoon (15 ml) of the olive oil in a small skillet over low heat. Add the garlic and sauté, stirring frequently to prevent scorching, for about 3 to 4 minutes, or until the garlic cloves become golden brown and have a rich aroma. Remove from heat and set aside in a small bowl.

3. In the same oil, sauté the cubed bread until evenly toasted. Remove from heat.

4. In a blender, combine the reserved ancho chiles, garlic, cubed bread, tomatoes, almonds, vinegar, cumin, and cayenne pepper. Purée until smooth. With the blender running (if possible), add the remaining 3 tablespoons (45 ml) olive oil.

5. Taste the sauce, and add salt and pepper if needed.

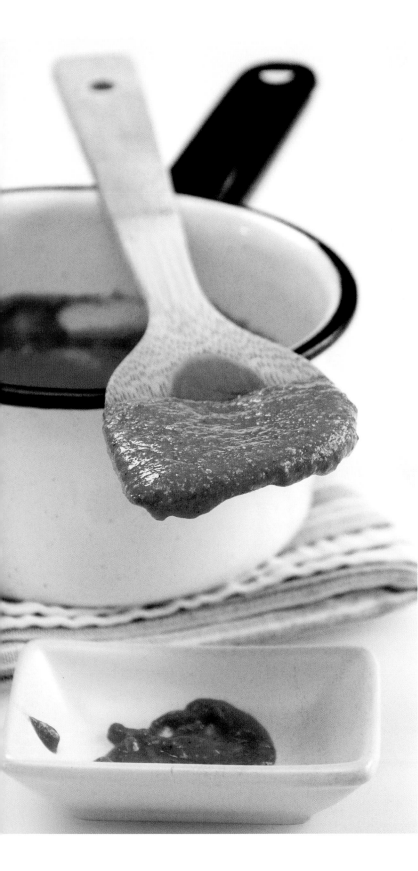

Note

The sauce can be refrigerated for up to 3 days or frozen for longer storage. Double or triple the recipe so that you can enjoy some right away and reserve some for later.

NUTRITIONAL ANALYSIS

Each serving provides: 285 calories; 23.5 g total fat; 2.5 g saturated fat; 6 g protein; 14 g carbohydrate; 4 g dietary fiber; 0 mg cholesterol.

SUPERSKIN NUTRIENTS		% DAILY VALUE*
Vitamin A	2053.1 IU	41%
Vitamin B6	0.4 mg	20%
Vitamin C	10.1 mg	17%
Vitamin E	6.0 mg	30%
Magnesium	69.4 mg	17%
Manganese	0.3 mg	15%
Selenium	2.9 mcg	4%
Zinc	0.9 mg	6%

*Percent Daily Values are based on a 2,000-calorie diet. Your daily values may be higher or lower depending on your caloric needs.

Bean Soup with Turkey Sausage

Serve this skin-beautifying meal on a cold night. Turkey helps your skin fight the inflammation that can make your complexion look red and puffy. Be sure to use lean turkey sausage to avoid the saturated fat that can have negative effects on your skin.

1 tablespoon (15 ml) canola oil

½ onion, diced

¾ cup (98 g) diced carrots

2 stalks celery, diced

1 garlic clove, finely minced

6 ounces (170 g) lean turkey sausage

Three 15-ounce (425 g) cans navy or cannellini beans, rinsed and drained

4 cups (950 ml) chicken or vegetable stock

1 white potato, cubed

3 to 4 whole black peppercorns

1 whole clove

Salt, pepper, and Tabasco sauce to taste

Yield: 8 servings

1. Heat the oil in a large soup pot over moderate heat. Add the onions, carrots, celery, and garlic. Sauté over low to medium heat for about 5 minutes, or until the garlic has a sweet aroma and the onions are a light golden brown.

2. Crumble the sausage into the mixture and cook, stirring to break up any clumps, until the meat loses its pink color.

3. Add the beans and stock to the pot. If the beans are not completely covered by the stock, add enough water to cover them by about 1 inch (2.5 cm) if necessary. Simmer for about 30 minutes.

4. Add the potato, peppercorns, and clove. Continue to simmer the soup over low heat for another 30 minutes, or until the beans and potatoes are tender enough to mash easily.

5. Use the back of a wooden spoon to mash some of the beans into the soup. Remove and discard the peppercorns and cloves if desired. Add salt, pepper, and Tabasco sauce to taste. Serve the soup very hot, in heated bowls or cups.

Notes

- *If you already have cooked beans on hand, use 3 cups (546 g) in place of the canned beans.*

- *This soup can be prepared in advance. Once the soup has cooled, it can be refrigerated for up to 3 days or frozen for up to 2 months. When reheating the soup, be sure to return it to a full boil. Bean soups tend to thicken as they are stored, so if necessary, thin the soup with additional stock or water. It also may be necessary to add more salt and pepper.*

- *Garlic-flavored croutons traditionally accompany this soup.*

NUTRITIONAL ANALYSIS

Each serving provides: 181 calories; 5 g total fat; 1 g saturated fat; 12 g protein; 22 g carbohydrate; 5 g dietary fiber; 18 mg cholesterol.

SUPERSKIN NUTRIENTS		% DAILY VALUE*
Vitamin A	3444.6 IU	69%
Vitamin B6	0.2 mg	10%
Vitamin C	3.2 mg	5%
Vitamin E	0.8 mg	4%
Magnesium	51.8 mg	13%
Manganese	0.6 mg	30%
Selenium	4.3 mcg	6%
Zinc	1.5 mg	10%

*Percent Daily Values are based on a 2,000-calorie diet. Your daily values may be higher or lower depending on your caloric needs.

INGREDIENT SPOTLIGHT

Turkey

Turkey is an excellent source of protein, providing 65 percent of your daily value in one 4-ounce (113 g) serving. Protein is important to your skin because it provides the building blocks enzymes need to keep active tissue (like your muscles) healthy and strong.

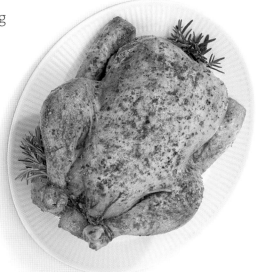

Corn, Squash, and Lima Bean Soup

Brighten your complexion with this hearty soup. Lima beans are full of nutrients that energize and beautify your skin, celery is packed with skin-smoothing silica, and the vitamin C and zinc in onions help you fight wrinkles.

1 tablespoon (15 ml) corn oil

¾ cup (120 g) coarsely chopped onion

½ cup (65 g) coarsely chopped carrots

½ cup (50 g) coarsely chopped celery

Small pinch of saffron threads, crushed, if desired

3 tablespoons (50 g) tomato paste

4 cups (960 ml) chicken broth

¾ cup (123 g) corn kernels (fresh, or frozen and thawed)

½ cup (90 g) diced tomatoes (fresh or canned)

¾ cup (181 g) lima beans (fresh, canned, or frozen and thawed)

¾ cup (105 g) diced butternut or acorn squash (fresh, or frozen and thawed)

¼ cup (15 g) chopped fresh flat-leaf parsley leaves

Salt and pepper to taste

Yield: 4 servings

1. Heat the oil in a large soup pot over medium heat. Add the onions, carrots, celery, and saffron threads, if using. Cook until the onions are tender and a light brown, stirring constantly, about 8 minutes. Add the tomato paste, and stir it into the mixture completely. Continue to cook until the tomato paste smells sweet, another 2 minutes.

2. Add the chicken broth, corn, tomatoes, lima beans, and squash.

3. Simmer the soup until all of the vegetables are cooked through and very tender, about 30 minutes. Add the parsley just before serving and season with salt and pepper.

Note

Accompany this soup with a hearty slice of whole-grain bread. Better yet, prepare a pita bread sandwich stuffed with sliced avocado, fresh tomato, and sliced red onion to go alongside. Tuck a few sprouts into the pocket for some added crunch and nutrition.

NUTRITIONAL ANALYSIS

Each serving provides: 172 calories; 5.5 g total fat; 1 g saturated fat; 9 g protein; 23 g carbohydrate; 6 g dietary fiber; 0 mg cholesterol.

SUPERSKIN NUTRIENTS		% DAILY VALUE*
Vitamin A	6756.2 IU	135%
Vitamin B6	0.2 mg	10%
Vitamin C	16.5 mg	28%
Vitamin E	3.83 mg	19%
Magnesium	42.8 mg	11%
Manganese	0.6 mg	30%
Selenium	2.9 mcg	4%
Zinc	0.8 mg	5%

*Percent Daily Values are based on a 2,000-calorie diet. Your daily values may be higher or lower depending on your caloric needs.

Roasted Beet Soup

Leave red, puffy skin behind with beets, your secret weapon against inflammation. Once you've tasted this soup's rich flavor, which comes from roasting the beets, you'll be hooked. Plus, the nutrients in the celery and onions will firm up your skin and keep wrinkles away.

5 whole beets, skin on, tops trimmed

1 tablespoon (15 ml) canola oil

1 clove garlic, finely minced

1 cup (160 g) sliced or diced onions

4 cups (950 ml) chicken, beef, or vegetable broth

⅓ cup (40 g) sliced or diced celery

½ cup (35 g) finely shredded white cabbage

2 dill sprigs, leaves removed and finely chopped

2 to 3 parsley sprigs, leaves removed and finely chopped

3 to 4 whole black peppercorns

¼ teaspoon whole fennel seeds

2 tablespoons (30 ml) red wine vinegar, or to taste

½ teaspoon (3 g) salt, or to taste

Yield: 4 servings

1. Preheat oven to 350°F (180°C, or gas mark 4). Scrub the beets well, pierce them in two or three spots with a fork or paring knife, and place them in a baking pan. Add about ¼ inch (6.25 mm) of water to the pan. Cover tightly with an oven-safe lid, and roast the beets until they are tender enough to pierce easily, about 35 to 40 minutes. (The water will cook away as the beets roast. Roasting times will vary depending upon the size and age of your beets.)

2. Let the beets cool until they can be handled, then slip off their skins and julienne or dice. Set aside.

3. Heat the oil in a large soup pot over medium heat. Reduce heat to low and add the garlic and onion. Cook gently until the onions are limp, about 5 minutes. Add the broth, reserved beets, celery, cabbage, dill, parsley, peppercorns, and fennel seeds. Simmer for an additional 5 to 6 minutes.

4. Just before serving the soup, remove and discard the peppercorns if desired. Add vinegar and salt and pepper to taste.

Notes

- *This soup can be served hot or cold, as a first course or as a one-course supper.*

- *Serve the soup topped with a dollop of yogurt and a sprinkling of chopped dill and parsley.*

- *If desired, this soup may also be puréed to a smooth consistency after having been completed through step 2.*

INGREDIENT SPOTLIGHT

Beets

Antioxidants are your best weapon against inflammation, and anthocyanins, found in beets and other red- or purple-colored produce like berries and purple cabbage, are great antioxidants.

Anthocyanins protect in a two-fold way. First, they neutralize enzymes that destroy connective tissue, thereby preventing further damage. Then, they repair already-damaged proteins in blood-vessel walls. Now beet that!

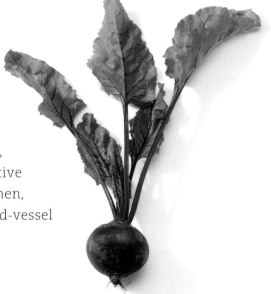

Tortilla and Avocado Soup

Travel south of the border without leaving home by preparing this satisfying soup. Avocado is a natural moisturizer for your skin, and moist skin is youthful-looking skin. This soup also has the wrinkle-fighting power of tomatoes, making it a win-win combination for your skin.

Four 6-inch (15-cm) corn
   tortillas
1 tablespoon (15 ml) canola oil
1 garlic clove, finely minced
¾ cup (120 g) finely grated or
   puréed onion
¾ cup (195 g) tomato purée
4 or 5 cilantro sprigs
1 teaspoon (2.5 g) ground
   cumin
1½ teaspoons (4 g) mild chili
   powder
6 cups (1.4 L) chicken stock
1 bay leaf
2 avocados
Lime juice to taste
Salt and pepper to taste
Cilantro, for garnish
Lime wedges, for garnish

Yield: 6 servings

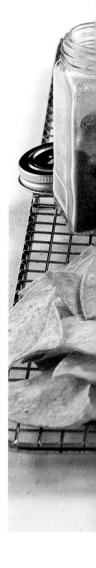

1. Preheat oven to 300°F (150°C, or gas mark 2). Cut the tortillas into wedges. You should get about 8 wedges from each tortilla, for a total of about 32 wedges. Place the wedges in an even layer on a baking sheet, and, once the oven is heated, toast in oven for about 15 minutes. Keep an eye on them to avoid burning. Set aside to cool.

2. Heat the oil in a large soup pot. Add the garlic and onion, and sauté over medium high heat until they have a sweet aroma, about 5 to 6 minutes, stirring frequently.

3. Add the tomato purée, and continue to sauté for another 3 minutes. Add the cilantro sprigs, cumin, and chili powder and sauté for another 2 minutes.

4. Add the chicken stock, 20 of the toasted tortillas wedges, and bay leaf. Stir well, and bring the soup to a simmer. Continue to simmer over low to medium heat for about 15 to 20 minutes.

5. While the soup is simmering, peel the avocados, remove the pits, and slice or cut into cubes or chunks. Sprinkle with lime juice, salt, and pepper.

6. Once the soup is done, strain through a sieve or a food mill, pushing to extract as much of the flavorful broth as possible. Make sure to discard the bay leaf.

7. Top the remaining tortilla wedges with the avocado mixture. and float on the hot soup. Sprinkle with cilantro leaves and a wedge of lime.

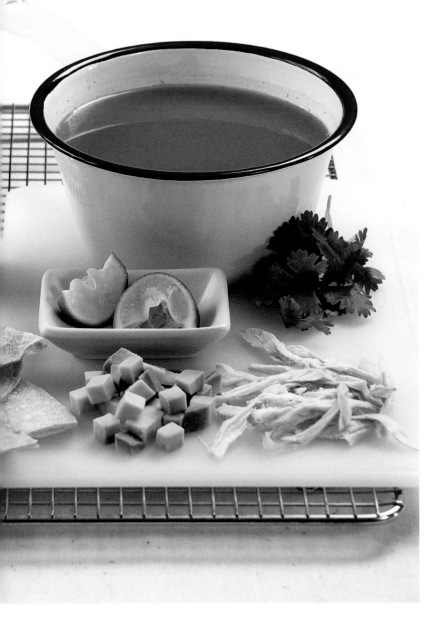

Notes

- *For a full meal, serve the soup in heated bowls and garnish with shredded chicken, cheddar cheese, tortilla, and avocado.*

- *Avocado will turn brown if it is cut too far in advance. Avoid cutting the avocado more than 1 hour before you will need it. Once it's cut, sprinkle the diced flesh with a little lemon or lime juice, tossing to coat all pieces, then cover and keep refrigerated until needed.*

- *This soup may be cooled and stored (without the toppings) in the refrigerator for about 2 to 3 days or frozen for about 2 months. To reheat the soup, bring it to a full boil and thin if necessary with additional stock.*

NUTRITIONAL ANALYSIS

Each serving provides: 252 calories; 15.5 g total fat; 2.5 g saturated fat; 9 g protein; 23 g carbohydrate; 5 g dietary fiber; 0 mg cholesterol.

SUPERSKIN NUTRIENTS		% DAILY VALUE*
Vitamin A	1046.7 IU	21%
Vitamin B6	0.3 mg	15%
Vitamin C	11.2 mg	19%
Vitamin E	2.9 mg	15%
Magnesium	24.2 mg	6%
Manganese	0.6 mg	30%
Selenium	0.8 mcg	1%
Zinc	0.7 mg	5%

*Percent Daily Values are based on a 2,000-calorie diet. Your daily values may be higher or lower depending on your caloric needs.

Black Bean and Spinach Soup

Say good-bye to wrinkles with this hearty and satisfying soup. Its combination of bell peppers, spinach, and garlic helps your skin fight wrinkles in a number of ways. Bell peppers contain lutein, which increases the skin's elasticity. Spinach is packed with antioxidants that stop free radicals from causing wrinkle-forming damage to your skin. Garlic inhibits inflammation that causes wrinkles. Plus, you'll get plenty of protein without high amounts of skin-aging saturated fat.

1 tablespoon (15 ml) canola oil

1 cup (160 g) diced onion

½ cup (75 g) diced bell pepper, green or red

1 garlic clove, finely minced

Three 15-ounce (425 g) cans black beans, rinsed and drained

5 cups (1.2 L) chicken or vegetable broth

2 to 3 allspice berries, or a dash of ground allspice

¼ teaspoon cumin seeds

¼ teaspoon dried oregano leaves

Pinch of ground cloves

½ teaspoon salt, or to taste

¼ teaspoon ground black pepper

1 tablespoon (15 ml) red wine vinegar, or to taste

4 cups (120 g) finely shredded fresh spinach leaves

Yield: 8 servings

1. Heat the oil in a large soup pot over moderate heat. Add the onion, bell pepper, and garlic. Sauté over low to medium heat until vegetables are tender, about 5 minutes.

2. Add the beans, broth, allspice, cumin, oregano, ground cloves, salt, and pepper. Simmer for about 40 minutes, or until the vegetables and beans are very tender. (If you can fish out the allspice berries at this point, do so, although it is fine to leave them in.)

3. Season the soup with vinegar, and more salt and pepper if necessary. Add the spinach and simmer for an additional 5 minutes, or until the sufficiently wilted and cooked. Serve in heated bowls.

Notes

- *If you already have cooked beans on hand, use 3 cups (516 g) in place of the canned beans.*

- *Allspice berries combine the flavors of several different spices, including cinnamon, clove, and nutmeg. They are the pea-sized berry of an evergreen pimento tree that is native to the West Indies and South America.*

- *If you can find callaloo, a delicious green that's popular throughout the West Indies, try it in place of the spinach. Note that using callaloo may increase the final cooking time slightly.*

- *If you like extra heat, add a whole habanero or Scotch bonnet pepper to the soup as it simmers.*

NUTRITIONAL ANALYSIS
_____

Each serving provides: 147 calories; 3 g total fat; 0.5 g saturated fat; 10 g protein; 21 g carbohydrate; 7 g dietary fiber; 0 mg cholesterol.

SUPERSKIN NUTRIENTS		% DAILY VALUE*
Vitamin A	1079.0 IU	22%
Vitamin B6	0.2 mg	10%
Vitamin C	14.4 mg	24%
Vitamin E	1.3 mg	7%
Magnesium	62.7 mg	16%
Manganese	0.7 mg	35%
Selenium	1.2 mcg	2%
Zinc	1.0 mg	7%

*Percent Daily Values are based on a 2,000-calorie diet. Your daily values may be higher or lower depending on your caloric needs.

INGREDIENT SPOTLIGHT

Spinach

There are more than a dozen different flavonoid compounds in spinach that function as antioxidants, which prevent damage to your skin caused by free radicals. Spinach is also packed with nutrients that can help with conditions in which inflammation plays a role, including asthma, arthritis, and wrinkles. Vitamins A and C, for instance, both found in spinach, have anti-inflammatory properties and thus help prevent free-radical formation.

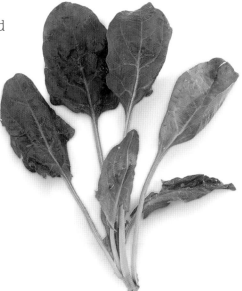

Roasted Tomato Soup

This soup is terrific on your tongue and even better for your skin. Cooked tomatoes are a great source of lycopene, which helps tighten your skin and protects it from the sun's damaging effects. Onions, celery, and leeks all offer your skin silica, your internal moisturizer.

1 tablespoon (15 ml) canola oil

1 cup (160 g) minced onion

¼ cup (25 g) minced celery

¼ cup (25 g) minced leeks (white portion only), optional

2 cups (475 ml) chicken or vegetable broth

2 cups (360 g) chopped plum tomatoes (fresh or canned)

1 cup (250 g) tomato purée

1 cup (206 g) Herb-Roasted Tomatoes (p. 210)

¼ cup (46 g) long grain white rice, uncooked

1 tablespoon (15 ml) balsamic vinegar

Salt and pepper to taste

Finely shredded fresh basil leaves or chives, optional

Yield: 6 servings

1. Heat the oil in a soup pot over medium high heat. Add the onion, celery, and leeks (if using). Cover the pot and cook for about 4 to 5 minutes, or until the vegetables start to release their juices.

2. Add the broth, plum tomatoes, tomato purée, and tomatoes. Simmer for 30 minutes.

3. Add the rice, and continue to simmer for another 15 minutes, or until the rice is cooked through. Purée the soup in a blender or with an immersion blender until very smooth.

4. Return the soup to the pot (if blender was used) and bring to a simmer. Season to taste with balsamic vinegar, salt, and pepper.

5. Garnish with basil or chives, if desired, and serve at once in heated bowls.

Note

- *If you don't have time to make the Herb-Roasted Tomatoes called for, simply substitute ⅓ cup (18 g) of chopped sun-dried tomatoes.*

NUTRITIONAL ANALYSIS

Each serving provides: 137 calories; 4 g total fat; 0.5 g saturated fat; 5 g protein; 23 g carbohydrate; 3 g dietary fiber; 0 mg cholesterol.

SUPERSKIN NUTRIENTS		% DAILY VALUE*
Vitamin A	1113.5 IU	22%
Vitamin B6	0.3 mg	15%
Vitamin C	29.1 mg	49%
Vitamin E	2.7 mg	14%
Magnesium	32.4 mg	8%
Manganese	0.5 mg	25%
Selenium	2.4 mcg	3%
Zinc	0.5 mg	3%

*Percent Daily Values are based on a 2,000-calorie diet. Your daily values may be higher or lower depending on your caloric needs.

INGREDIENT SPOTLIGHT

Onions

Vitamin C, quercetin, and isothiocyanates are three antioxidants found in onions that have anti-inflammatory effects on the skin and help to stop damage to collagen, the component that gives your skin structural support. What's more, onions also contain chromium, an important nutrient in the battle against acne.

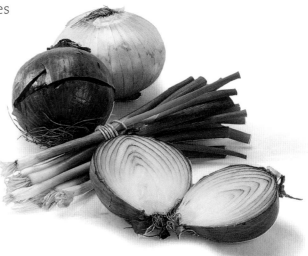

Chilled Cantaloupe Soup

Attack your wrinkles with the triple-action power of cantaloupe. This delicious melon is packed with vitamins A, C, and E, all of which help your skin prevent damage that leads to wrinkles. Enjoy this refreshingly cool soup on warm days and protect your skin from the wrinkling effects of the sun.

6 cups (930 g) diced cantaloupe (seeds and rind removed)

1 cup (230 g) plain reduced-fat yogurt, preferably Greek-style

½ cup (120 ml) water

1 tablespoon (15 ml) fresh lime juice

Pinch of salt

Lime zest, cut in strips, or lime wedges, optional

Yield: 4 servings

1. Combine all of the ingredients with the exception of the lime zest in a blender. Purée until very smooth.

2. Serve in chilled glasses or cups, garnished with a few thin strips of lime zest or a wedge of fresh lime, if desired.

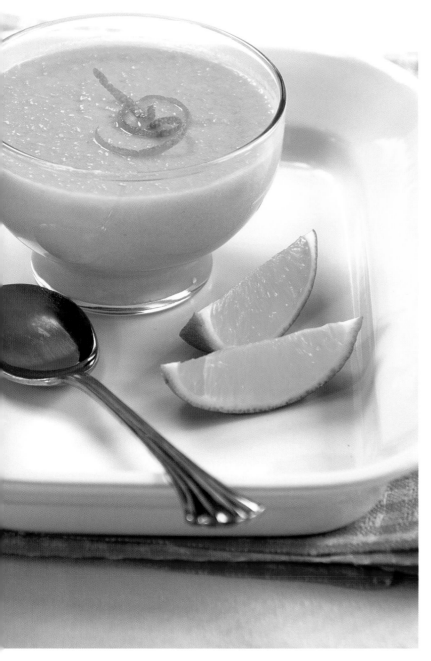

Note

This soup can also be served as a "cocktail." Dip the rim of a martini or wine glass first in water then in granulated sugar (a sanding sugar, found in the cake-decorating aisle, gives you color and texture options). Pour the soup into the glass and top with a bit of club soda.

NUTRITIONAL ANALYSIS

Each serving provides: 124 calories; 1.5 g total fat; 1 g saturated fat; 5 g protein; 25 g carbohydrate; 2 g dietary fiber; 4 mg cholesterol.

SUPERSKIN NUTRIENTS		% DAILY VALUE*
Vitamin A	7778.4 IU	156%
Vitamin B6	0.3 mg	15%
Vitamin C	102.9 mg	172%
Vitamin E	0.8 mg	4%
Magnesium	37.7 mg	9%
Manganese	0.1 mg	5%
Selenium	3.0 mcg	4%
Zinc	0.9 mg	6%

*Percent Daily Values are based on a 2,000-calorie diet. Your daily values may be higher or lower depending on your caloric needs.

Mango, Spinach, Sorrel, and Pistachio Salad

This colorful salad is armed with vitamins A and C, silica, and iron, all of which keep your skin beautiful. In fact, the nutrient combination of vitamin C (from the mango) and iron (from the spinach) work particularly well together, allowing for optimal nutrient absorption in the body.

2 garlic cloves, finely minced

Zest and juice of 1 lemon

2 tablespoons (30 g) walnut oil

Salt and pepper to taste

8 ounces (225 g) fresh spinach leaves, well-rinsed and dried

4 ounces (113 g) fresh sorrel leaves, well-rinsed and dried

1 ripe mango, peeled and cubed

¼ cup (31 g) shelled pistachios

Yield: 4 servings

1. For dressing, in a small bowl, whisk together the garlic, lemon zest and juice, and walnut oil. Season to taste with salt and pepper.

2. Tear the spinach and sorrel leaves into bite-sized pieces, and place in a salad bowl. Add the mango cubes.

3. Toss salad with dressing until lightly coated.

4. Sprinkle the salad with the pistachios, and serve on chilled plates.

Notes

- *Sorrel is a delicious, slightly tart salad green. If you can't find it, substitute another green such as arugula or watercress.*

- *The easiest way to cut a mango is as follows: Slice both large "cheeks" from either side of the narrow pit in the center of the mango. (It is easiest if you slice the mango from the narrower end toward the wider end.) Cut away any flesh that clings to the pit, and peel the skin from each slice. Cut the flesh into pieces.*

- *If you'd like to add a little dressing to your salad, try our Roasted Garlic and Mustard Vinaigrette on page 234.*

Each serving provides: 163 calories; 11.5 g total fat; 1 g saturated fat; 4 g protein; 15 g carbohydrate; 3 g dietary fiber; 0 mg cholesterol.

SUPERSKIN NUTRIENTS		% DAILY VALUE*
Vitamin A	6091.0 IU	122%
Vitamin B6	0.2 mg	10%
Vitamin C	69.5 mg	116%
Vitamin E	3.5 mg	18%
Magnesium	47.9 mg	12%
Manganese	0.2 mg	10%
Selenium	1.3 mcg	2%
Zinc	0.2 mg	1%

*Percent Daily Values are based on a 2,000-calorie diet. Your daily values may be higher or lower depending on your caloric needs.

INGREDIENT SPOTLIGHT

Mangoes

Mangoes contain vitamins A and C, two great protectors of your skin's tight, toned appearance. These antioxidants can stop free radicals from causing damage, thereby preventing droopy skin and keeping your skin fit and beautiful. And because vitamin A is fat-soluble and vitamin C is water-soluble, mangoes protect every part of your skin. Not only that, but they also contain silica, a nutrient that acts as an internal moisturizer, lubricating your joints and skin, helping you both look and feel younger.

Avocado, Grapefruit, Pomegranate, and Red Onion Salad

This delightful, fruity salad is bursting with flavor and nutrients to help your skin look its best. Avocados moisturize, grapefruit fights acne and psoriasis, onions prevent wrinkles, and pomegranate rids your skin of redness and puffiness. This perfect lunch or light dinner will awaken your taste buds and enhance your skin.

1 pomegranate

2 medium or 1 large grapefruit (pink or red)

1 ripe Haas avocado

3 cups (90 g) baby spinach leaves, well-rinsed and dried

½ red onion, peeled, sliced thin and separated into rings

Yield: 4 servings

1. Cut the pomegranate in half, pull back the tough outer peel, and pull out the segments of seeds. Continue cutting as necessary to expose all the seeds. Break the seeds up and remove any membrane. Set seeds aside in a small bowl.

2. Peel the grapefruit by cutting away the skin and pith. Cut the grapefruit into slices or sections. Set aside in a medium bowl.

3. Peel the avocado and remove the pit. Cut the avocado into ½-inch (1.25 cm) slices and fold them into the grapefruit (the juice from the grapefruit will help keep the avocado from turning brown).

4. Divide spinach among four plates; top each with the avocado and grapefruit mixture, then with rings of red onion and pomegranate seeds.

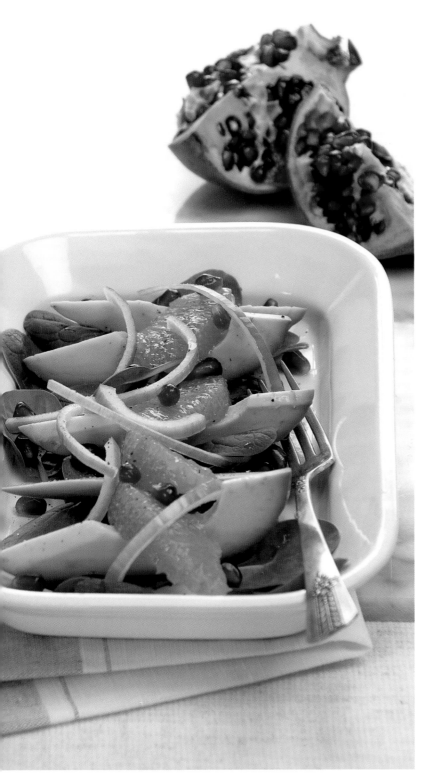

Note

If you have trouble removing the seeds from your pomegranate, try this easy trick: Cut off the crown of the pomegranate and slice the fruit into sections. Place the sections in a bowl of water and gently roll out the seeds with your fingers. The seeds will sink to the bottom and the membrane will float to the top.

NUTRITIONAL ANALYSIS

Each serving provides: 55 calories; 0.3 g total fat; 0 g saturated fat; 2 g protein; 13 g carbohydrate; 2 g dietary fiber; 0 mg cholesterol.

SUPERSKIN NUTRIENTS		% DAILY VALUE*
Vitamin A	1670.2 IU	33%
Vitamin B6	0.1 mg	5%
Vitamin C	32.3 mg	54%
Vitamin E	1.0 mg	5%
Magnesium	25.2 mg	6%
Manganese	0.5 mg	25%
Selenium	1.4 mcg	2%
Zinc	0.2 mg	1%

*Percent Daily Values are based on a 2,000-calorie diet. Your daily values may be higher or lower depending on your caloric needs.

Gazpacho Salad

Gazpacho is cool soup that makes a delicious and refreshing warm weather treat. Here, it's turned into a salad that can be prepared any time of year to give your skin a healthy boost of nutrients. Red peppers and tomatoes are wrinkle fighters, cucumbers can help reduce the puffiness of your skin, and olive oil is a natural moisturizer that will make you look luminous.

4 teaspoons (20 ml) balsamic vinegar

1 tablespoon (15 ml) extra-virgin olive oil

1 clove garlic, finely minced

¼ teaspoon Tabasco sauce

4 or 5 plum tomatoes, diced

1 cucumber, peeled, seeded, and diced

½ onion, sliced thin

2 scallions, minced

½ cup (75 g) diced red pepper

1 tablespoon (4 g) chopped fresh flat leaf parsley leaves

Yield: 4 servings

1. For dressing, whisk together vinegar, oil, garlic, and Tabasco sauce in a small mixing bowl.

2. Combine the remaining ingredients in a salad bowl and toss with dressing.

3. Allow the salad to sit at room temperature for 30 minutes before serving.

4. Serve in chilled bowls, lettuce cups, or over spinach.

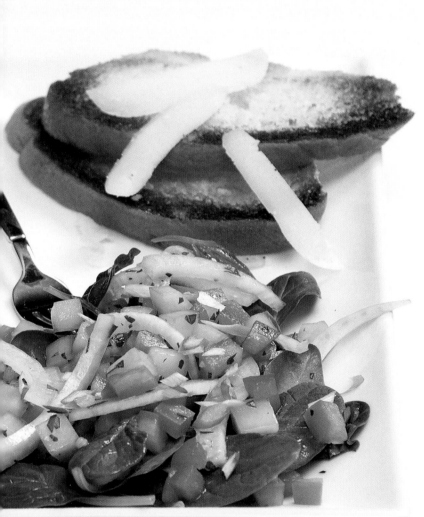

Notes

- *To make this gazpacho salad more substantial, turn it into panzanella, an Italian bread salad. Simply de-crust a few slices of leftover bread (preferably whole grain) and cut into large cubes. Place the cubes on a cookie sheet, mist with olive oil spray, and add seasonings such as salt, pepper, dried oregano or basil, and onion or garlic powder. Lightly toast in a 300°F (150°C, or gas mark 2) oven for about 10 to 12 minutes. Cool the croutons and toss with salad.*

- *For an even more sustaining supper, serve with a wedge of Manchego or a similar sharp-flavored, aged cheese.*

NUTRITIONAL ANALYSIS

Each serving provides: 63 calories; 4 g total fat; 0.5 g saturated fat; 1 g protein; 7 g carbohydrate; 2 g dietary fiber; 0 mg cholesterol.

SUPERSKIN NUTRIENTS		% DAILY VALUE*
Vitamin A	1599.0 IU	32%
Vitamin B6	0.2 mg	10%
Vitamin C	52.2 mg	87%
Vitamin E	1.3 mg	7%
Magnesium	16.9 mg	4%
Manganese	0.2 mg	10%
Selenium	0.5 mcg	1%
Zinc	0.2 mg	1%

*Percent Daily Values are based on a 2,000-calorie diet. Your daily values may be higher or lower depending on your caloric needs.

Roasted Garlic and Mustard Vinaigrette

Drizzle this dressing over baby spinach (or our Mango, Spinach, Sorrel, and Pistachio Salad on p. 228) for a super-powered, wrinkle-fighting dish. Garlic and spinach are full of free radical-fighting antioxidants—like vitamins A and C—that prevent inflammation and help your skin stay strong and tight. See the notes following this recipe to make a fresh garlic version, if you don't have roasted garlic on hand.

4 cloves Roasted Garlic
    (p. 208)
2 tablespoons (22 g) Dijon
    or coarse grain mustard
1 teaspoon (7 g) honey
Salt and pepper to taste
¾ cup (175 ml) canola or extra-
    virgin olive oil
¼ cup (60 ml) cider vinegar

Yield: 16 servings (about
    1 cup, or 270 ml, total)

1. Place the garlic cloves in a small mixing bowl and mash them together (using the back of a fork) with the mustard, honey, salt, and pepper.

2. Add the oil in a stream, whisking constantly.

3. Add the vinegar to the mixture, whisking constantly until well blended.

Notes

• *The vinaigrette may be stored in the refrigerator for up to 5 days. Before using, allow the dressing to return to room temperature. Whisk vigorously before serving to recombine all of the ingredients properly.*

• *This dressing is a good choice for salads made with assertive greens (e.g., romaine, arugula, radicchio) or as a marinade for grilled vegetables.*

• *Roasting tames and sweetens the flavor of garlic, but if you don't have roasted garlic on hand, this dressing is also great made with fresh garlic. Use just 1 clove of raw garlic to replace the 4 cloves of roasted garlic called for in recipe.*

NUTRITIONAL ANALYSIS

Each 1-tablespoon (17 g) serving provides: 96 calories; 10.5 g total fat; 0.5 g saturated fat; 0.2 g protein; 1 g carbohydrate; 0 g dietary fiber; 0 mg cholesterol.

SUPERSKIN NUTRIENTS		% DAILY VALUE*
Vitamin A	1.0 IU	0%
Vitamin B6	0.0 mg	0%
Vitamin C	0.3 mg	1%
Vitamin E	2.2 mg	11%
Magnesium	1.1 mg	0%
Manganese	0.0 mg	0%
Selenium	0.1 mcg	0%
Zinc	0.0 mg	0%

*Percent Daily Values are based on a 2,000-calorie diet. Your daily values may be higher or lower depending on your caloric needs.

INGREDIENT SPOTLIGHT

Honey

Honey contains antioxidants and flavonoids that function as antibacterial agents. Darker honeys, specifically honey from buckwheat flowers, sage, and tupelo, contain a greater amount of antioxidants than other honeys. Raw, unprocessed honey contains the widest variety of health-supportive substances, including an enzyme called glucose oxidase that, when combined with water, produces hydrogen peroxide, a mild antiseptic.

Spicy Thai-Style Salad Dressing

The zesty dressing will tighten and smooth your skin with its awesome antioxidant content, which comes mainly from the peanut powerhouses resveratrol and CoQ10. It's great on green salads and is equally delicious as a vinaigrette for grain or pasta salads—no matter how you use it, you'll spice up your menu and fight sagging skin.

2 tablespoons (30 g) smooth, natural peanut butter

1 tablespoon (15 g) brown sugar, tightly packed

2 teaspoons (10 g) roasted chili paste

¼ teaspoon red pepper flakes

½ teaspoon finely minced garlic

Salt and pepper to taste

5 tablespoons (75 ml) malt vinegar

¾ cup (180 ml) peanut oil

Yield: 16 servings (about 1 cup, or 300 g, total)

1. Blend the peanut butter, brown sugar, chili paste, red pepper flakes, garlic, salt, and pepper to a smooth paste in a small mixing bowl.

2. Whisk the vinegar into the mixture until evenly blended.

3. Add the peanut oil in a steady stream while whisking constantly until a smooth, lightly thickened dressing develops.

Notes

- *Natural peanut butter prepared without added sugar is the best choice for this vinaigrette.*

- *Chili paste is available in the Asian foods section of most grocery stores or in Asian markets.*

- *The dressing may be stored in the refrigerator for up to 5 days. Before using, allow the dressing to return to room temperature. Whisk vigorously before serving to recombine all of the ingredients properly.*

- *For an added punch, add chopped, dry-roasted or plain peanuts to your salad after it has been tossed with the dressing.*

NUTRITIONAL ANALYSIS

Each 1-tablespoon (19-g) serving provides: 107 calories; 11 g total fat; 2 g saturated fat; 0.5 g protein; 2 g carbohydrate; 0 g dietary fiber; 0 mg cholesterol.

SUPERSKIN NUTRIENTS		% DAILY VALUE*
Vitamin A	66.3 IU	1%
Vitamin B6	0.0 mg	0%
Vitamin C	0.7 mg	1%
Vitamin E	2.7 mg	14%
Magnesium	3.8 mg	1%
Manganese	0.1 mg	5%
Selenium	0.2 mcg	0%
Zinc	0.1 mg	1%

*Percent Daily Values are based on a 2,000-calorie diet. Your daily values may be higher or lower depending on your caloric needs.

INGREDIENT SPOTLIGHT

Peanuts

Peanuts contain monounsaturated fats, good fats that are very stable and not easily damaged (oxidized) by free radicals. When your diet contains such fats, free radicals that form from sunlight and toxins are less able to damage your skin cells.

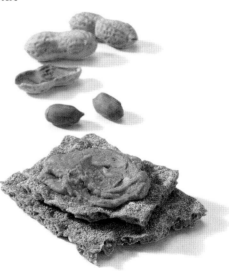

Free radicals are also targeted by the vitamin E in peanuts and other nuts. Vitamin E can help neutralize free radicals and prevent damage to your skin, which prevents signs of aging like wrinkles, spots, and sagging.

Tomato Herb Vinaigrette

This light vinaigrette has a heavy load of wrinkle-fighting nutrients. Tomatoes and olive oil are packed with nutrients, including lycopene, one of the toughest free radical scavengers around. Drizzle this dressing on your favorite salad, or use it as a dip for bread or veggies.

¾ cup (175 ml) tomato juice

¼ cup (60 ml) extra-virgin olive oil

2 tablespoons (30 ml) red wine vinegar (or more to taste)

2 tablespoons (12 g) minced scallions

2 tablespoons (5 g) chopped fresh herbs (suggestions: basil, dill, tarragon, chives, cilantro, thyme, and/or flat-leaf parsley)

Salt and pepper to taste

Yield: 16 servings (about 1 cup, or 285 g, total)

1. Combine all the ingredients in a blender, and blend on high speed until the oil has emulsified.

Notes

• *The vinaigrette should be refrigerated until ready to use (it will keep for up to 3 days). Before using, allow the dressing to return to room temperature. Whisk vigorously before serving to recombine all of the ingredients properly.*

• *Try this dressing with any of the following salad greens: romaine, watercress, Boston or bibb, arugula, oak leaf, or red leaf lettuce.*

Each 1-tablespoon (18-g) serving provides: 32 calories; 3.5 g total fat; 0.5 g saturated fat; 0 g protein; 0.5 g carbohydrate; 0 g dietary fiber; 0 mg cholesterol.

SUPERSKIN NUTRIENTS		% DAILY VALUE*
Vitamin A	79.2 IU	2%
Vitamin B6	0.0 mg	0%
Vitamin C	2.3 mg	4%
Vitamin E	0.5 mg	3%
Magnesium	1.7 mg	0%
Manganese	0.0 mg	0%
Selenium	0.1 mcg	0%
Zinc	0.0 mg	0%

*Percent Daily Values are based on a 2,000-calorie diet. Your daily values may be higher or lower depending on your caloric needs.

INGREDIENT SPOTLIGHT

Olive Oil

Olive oil has one of the highest concentrations of monounsaturated or "good" fat of any oil, with about 75 percent of its total fat makeup being monounsaturated. Because this type of fat also comprises about 25 percent of the fatty acids in the skin, such a concentration positively influences the fluidity of cell membranes—and when skin cells are more fluid, cell membranes can function more optimally, promoting the appearance of smooth, beautiful skin.

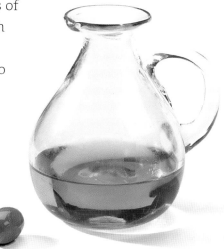

Brussels Sprouts with Mustard and Spicy Maple Pecans

Your kids will never complain about eating Brussels sprouts again, and you can sit back and smile, knowing that this side dish is packed with nutrients—vitamin A, vitamin C, magnesium, and fiber—that help your skin look its best.

Pinch of salt

1 pint or 2 cups (175 g) Brussels sprouts

1 tablespoon (15 ml) walnut oil

¼ cup (40 g) finely chopped onions

2 teaspoons (8 g) Dijon mustard

1 teaspoon (5 ml) red wine vinegar

Salt and pepper to taste

⅓ cup (33 g) Spicy Maple Pecans (p. 200)

Yield: 6 servings

1. Bring 2 quarts (1.9 L) of water to a boil in a saucepan. Add a generous pinch of salt.

2. Remove the outer leaves from the Brussels sprouts, and score each stem with an X.

3. Parboil the Brussels sprouts for about 8 to 10 minutes, or until tender. Drain the sprouts in a colander and let them cool slightly.

4. Heat the oil in a large skillet over medium heat. Add the onions and sauté, stirring occasionally, until they are limp and a light golden brown.

5. While the onions are sautéing, cut the Brussels sprouts into halves or quarters (they may be left whole if they are quite small).

6. Stir the mustard into the onions, then add the sprouts. Toss until they are lightly browned on the cut surfaces and heated through, 3 to 4 minutes.

7. Season the sprouts with the vinegar, salt, and pepper. Top with the Maple Toasted Pecans, and serve at once in a heated serving bowl.

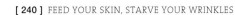

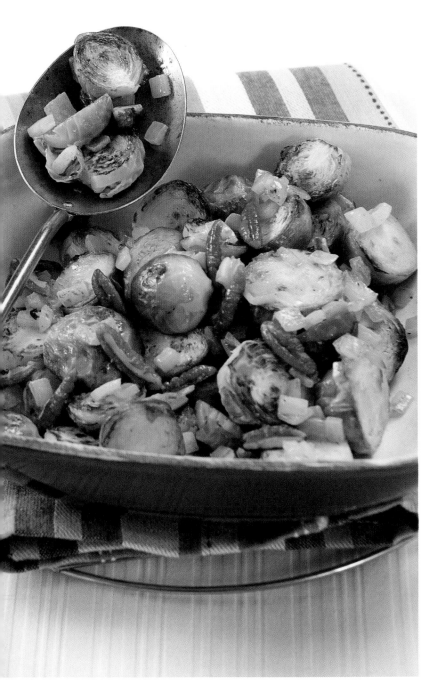

Notes

- To test the Brussels sprouts for doneness when parboiling, pierce the core of the largest one with the tip of a paring knife. The tip should slide in easily at first, with a little bit of resistance after it has gone in about ¼ inch (6.25 mm).

- Walnut oil gives the dish a nutty aroma and flavor. However, olive, light sesame, or peanut oil can be used instead.

- This dish makes an excellent accompaniment to a roasted turkey, chicken, pheasant, or Cornish game hen.

NUTRITIONAL ANALYSIS

Each serving provides: 91 calories; 7.5 g total fat; 1 g saturated fat; 2 g protein; 6 g carbohydrate; 2 g dietary fiber; 1 mg cholesterol.

SUPERSKIN NUTRIENTS		% DAILY VALUE*
Vitamin A	299.8 IU	6%
Vitamin B6	0.1 mg	5%
Vitamin C	25.6 mg	43%
Vitamin E	1.2 mg	6%
Magnesium	16.3 mg	4%
Manganese	0.5 mg	25%
Selenium	0.9 mcg	1%
Zinc	0.6 mg	4%

*Percent Daily Values are based on a 2,000-calorie diet. Your daily values may be higher or lower depending on your caloric needs.

Roasted Cauliflower and Peppers

This delicious side dish is a tastier alternative to steamed cauliflower and contains a host of valuable minerals, from both the cauliflower and the bell peppers. Cauliflower is rich in phytonutrients, fiber, and vitamin C, while peppers are packed with antioxidants like vitamin A, vitamin C, lutein, zeaxanthin, and lycopene—all of which keep your skin looking its best and brightest.

1 head cauliflower

2 tablespoons (30 ml) extra-virgin olive oil

½ teaspoon salt, or to taste

¼ teaspoon ground black pepper or to taste

½ cup (90 g) roasted red or yellow peppers (or a combination)

Yield: 6 servings

1. Preheat the oven to 400°F (200°C, or gas mark 6).

2. Remove the leaves from the cauliflower, trim the bottom, and slice the head in half. Lay the cut side on your work surface and cut the cauliflower into slices, about ¼-inch (6.25-mm) thick.

3. Rub a baking sheet with 1 tablespoon olive oil. Arrange the sliced cauliflower on the pan. (The slices should not overlap; use two baking sheets if necessary.) Brush the tops of the slices with remaining olive oil and season with salt and pepper.

4. Roast the cauliflower, uncovered, until the slices have a golden color (the edges may be a littler darker), about 25 minutes.

5. Sprinkle the roasted peppers over the slices and continue roasting for another 10 to 15 minutes. Serve hot.

Note

To roast your own peppers: Cut a pepper in half and remove stem and seeds. Place pepper halves skin-side up on a baking sheet and place under broiler for 5 to 7 minutes, or until skins are blistered and blackened. Place pepper halves in a bowl, cover, and allow to steam for 15 to 20 minutes. Discard skins and peppers are ready to use.

NUTRITIONAL ANALYSIS

Each serving provides: 47 calories; 2.5 g total fat; 0.5 g saturated fat; 2 g protein; 6 g carbohydrate; 2 g dietary fiber; 0 mg cholesterol.

SUPERSKIN NUTRIENTS		% DAILY VALUE*
Vitamin A	1347.9 IU	27%
Vitamin B6	0.0 mg	0%
Vitamin C	66.6 mg	111%
Vitamin E	0.4 mg	2%
Magnesium	1.8 mg	0%
Manganese	0.0 mg	0%
Selenium	0.0 mcg	0%
Zinc	0.0 mg	0%

*Percent Daily Values are based on a 2,000-calorie diet. Your daily values may be higher or lower depending on your caloric needs.

INGREDIENT SPOTLIGHT

Cauliflower

According to the latest research, the phytonutrients found in cauliflower and other cruciferous vegetables are even more powerful than typical antioxidants, in that they actually signal our genes to increase production of the enzymes involved in detoxification, the cleansing process through which our bodies eliminate harmful compounds. This ability may also help to explain why cruciferous vegetables appear to lower our risk of cancer more effectively than any other fruits or vegetables.

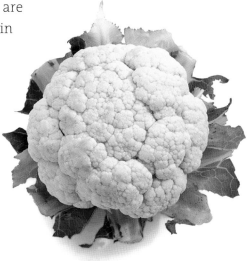

Asparagus with Anchovy, Garlic, and Lemon Sauce

Here's a lip-smackingly delicious way to get your omega-3s and reduce puffiness and redness in your skin. Asparagus can give you a natural face lift and contribute to the prevention of acne and psoriasis. It also contains silica, a nutrient that keeps your skin strong and wrinkle free. Serve this side dish often and enjoy beautiful skin.

1 pound (455 g) asparagus, washed

2 tablespoons (30 ml) extra-virgin olive oil

¼ teaspoon red pepper flakes

2 garlic cloves, peeled and thinly sliced

4 anchovy fillets, mashed

2 teaspoons (10 ml) freshly squeezed lemon juice

2 tablespoons (8 g) fresh flat leaf parsley, chopped

Salt and freshly ground black pepper to taste

Yield: 4 servings

1. Trim the ends from the asparagus, and lightly peel about halfway up the stalk. Slice the asparagus on the diagonal into pieces about 2-inches (5 cm) long.

2. Heat the olive oil in a large skillet over medium heat, and add the red pepper flakes and garlic. Lower the heat slightly and sauté the garlic until it turns a light golden brown. Add the anchovy fillets and cook for about 2 minutes, or until they have melted into the sauce.

3. Add the asparagus. Sauté, turning and rolling the asparagus frequently, until it is tender, 2 to 3 minutes.

4. Add the lemon juice, parsley, salt (if necessary, depending upon how salty the anchovies are), and pepper and serve.

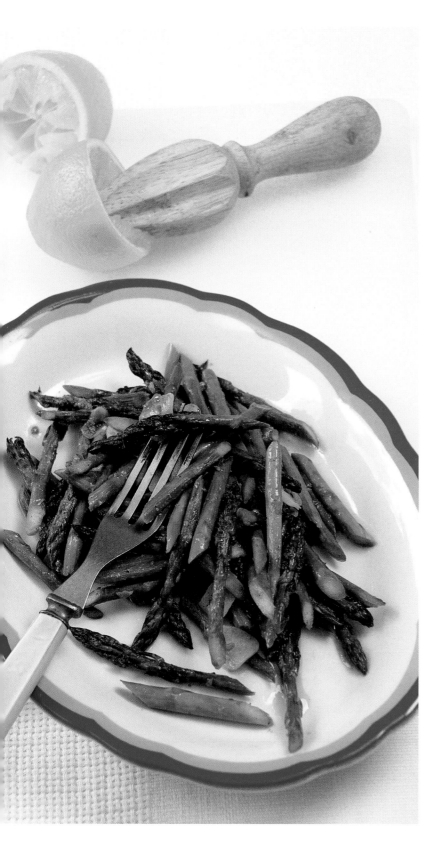

Notes

- *Here's an easy way to determine where to trim your asparagus stalk: Bend each stalk until it snaps—it will naturally break off at the woody tip, which can then be discarded. Fresh stalks should snap easily; if your stalks only bend, they may be past their prime.*

- *This dish can be served at room temperature or chilled as part of an antipasto platter. As a main dish, serve it hot on a bed of pasta, with roasted tomatoes, a drizzle of extra virgin olive oil, and plenty of freshly grated parmesan cheese.*

NUTRITIONAL ANALYSIS

Each serving provides: 102 calories; 7.5 g total fat; 1 g saturated fat; 4 g protein; 6 g carbohydrate; 3 g dietary fiber; 3 mg cholesterol.

SUPERSKIN NUTRIENTS		% DAILY VALUE*
Vitamin A	778.7 IU	16%
Vitamin B6	0.2 mg	10%
Vitamin C	19.1 mg	32%
Vitamin E	3.4 mg	17%
Magnesium	24.8 mg	6%
Manganese	0.3 mg	15%
Selenium	5.6 mcg	8%
Zinc	0.7 mg	5%

*Percent Daily Values are based on a 2,000-calorie diet. Your daily values may be higher or lower depending on your caloric needs.

Pickled Carrots

Fight wrinkles anytime and anywhere with the help of the carotenoids in these tantalizing carrots. As daily exposure to sunlight and environmental toxins constantly diminishes your body's level of carotenoids, it's important to seek out carotenoid-rich foods as often as you can. These carrots make an easy addition to your meal and are equally tasty as a quick snack.

3 cups (365 g) baby carrots

2 teaspoons (10 ml) Worcestershire sauce

2 teaspoons (12 g) salt

½ teaspoon black pepper

1 teaspoon (2 g) dried minced onion

¼ teaspoon garlic powder

¼ teaspoon dried red pepper flakes, optional

4 to 5 drops Tabasco sauce

2 cups (475 ml) cider vinegar

1 cup (235 ml) water

Yield: 12 servings (3 cups, or 1.3 L total)

1. Place the carrots in a nonreactive bowl or jar (a 1-quart canning jar is perfect). Add the Worcestershire sauce, salt, pepper, dried onion, garlic powder, red pepper flakes, and Tabasco sauce.

2. Pour the vinegar and water on top of the seasonings and stir to distribute as evenly as possible (or cover the jar and shake).

3. Tightly cover the jar or bowl and let the carrots "pickle" in the refrigerator for at least 8 hours.

Notes

- *The carrots will last for up to 2 weeks in the refrigerator.*

- *You can add other vegetables if you wish, such as cauliflower florets, mushroom caps, or chunks of celery.*

- *These make an unexpected and flavorful addition to any crudités platter; they are also a pungent and crunchy garnish for sandwiches or salads.*

NUTRITIONAL ANALYSIS

Each ¼-cup (109-g) serving provides: 27 calories; 0.1 g total fat; 0 g saturated fat; 0.6 g protein; 7 g carbohydrate; 1 g dietary fiber; 0 mg cholesterol.

SUPERSKIN NUTRIENTS		% DAILY VALUE*
Vitamin A	7579.2 IU	152%
Vitamin B6	0.1 mg	5%
Vitamin C	3.0 mg	5%
Vitamin E	0.0 mg	0%
Magnesium	15.1 mg	4%
Manganese	0.1 mg	5%
Selenium	0.1 mcg	0%
Zinc	0.0 mg	0%

*Percent Daily Values are based on a 2,000-calorie diet. Your daily values may be higher or lower depending on your caloric needs.

INGREDIENT SPOTLIGHT

Carrots

Carrots are rich in beta-carotene, an orange-colored nutrient that is associated with a reduction in skin wrinkling. Once consumed, beta-carotene is converted to vitamin A in the body, where it helps preserve and improve eyesight, fight free radicals, and stave off viral infections.

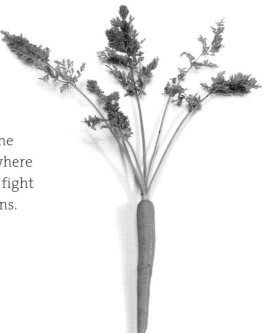

Mushrooms Stuffed with Barley, Kale, and Feta

A triple threat, this amazing side dish offers your skin three different beautifying benefits. Mushrooms are packed with B vitamins that help your complexion, kale fights wrinkles with vitamin A, and cheese contains probiotics that help tighten and smooth your skin. Beautiful skin never tasted so good!

2 teaspoons (10 ml) extra-virgin olive oil

½ cup (80 g) minced onions

2 teaspoons (6 g) minced garlic

½ cup (100 g) pearl barley

2 cups (475 ml) broth or water

¼ teaspoon salt

¼ teaspoon pepper

1 cup (67 g) chopped kale (see Note)

4 large portabello mushrooms, each about 3 inches (7.5 cm) in diameter

½ cup (75 g) crumbled feta cheese

Freshly squeezed lemon juice

Yield: 4 servings

1. Preheat oven to 350°F (180°C, or gas mark 4).

2. Heat the oil in a medium saucepan or soup pot over medium heat. Add the onions and garlic and cook, stirring frequently, until the onions are translucent and the garlic is aromatic, about 4 minutes. Add the pearl barley and continue to cook, stirring until the grains are coated with the oil.

3. Add the broth or water to the pan. Season with salt and pepper. Bring to a boil, stirring once or twice with a fork to separate the grains. Cover the pan and lower the heat, keeping the broth at a simmer. Cook the barley without stirring until it is tender, about 40 minutes.

4. Remove the pan from the heat, uncover, and fluff the barley with a fork to let the steam escape. Gently stir in the chopped kale. Taste and add more salt and pepper, if needed.

5. Prepare the mushrooms caps by cutting away the stems (these can be reserved to use in stock or broth recipes, if you wish). Scrape out the gills.

6. Set the caps in a baking dish and sprinkle with lemon juice. Fill each cap with the barley-kale mixture and top with the feta cheese (approximately ⅛ cup, or 19 g, for each cap). Cover the dish loosely with aluminum foil.

7. Bake the mushrooms until the caps and the barley are very hot, about 20 minutes. Remove the foil and continue to bake until the feta is very lightly browned, another 5 minutes. Serve at once.

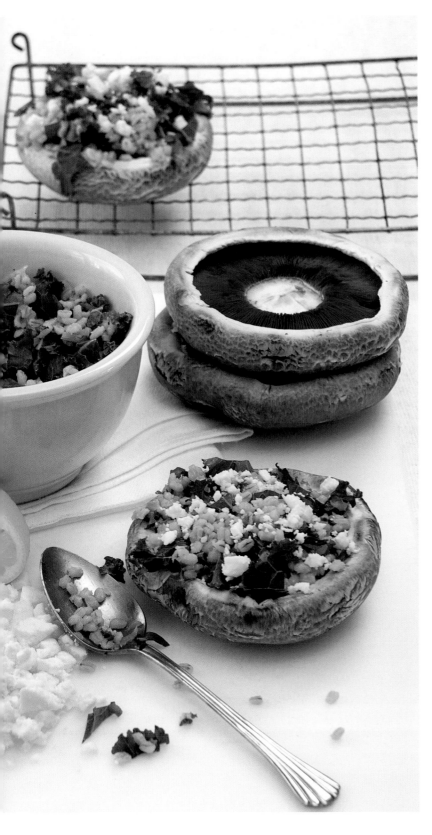

Note

If using frozen kale, let the kale thaw, then squeeze it well to remove as much water as possible. Chop the kale coarsely. To use fresh kale, trim the heavy stems from the leaves and discard; rinse and drain the leaves. Heat about ¼ inch (6.25 mm) of water in a large skillet. Bring to a boil, add the kale, stir to wilt the leaves, and cover the skillet to steam the kale for about 3 minutes. Drain in a colander. When it is cool enough to handle, squeeze the kale dry and chop coarsely.

NUTRITIONAL ANALYSIS

Each serving provides: 225 calories; 7.5 g total fat; 3.5 g saturated fat; 13 g protein; 31 g carbohydrate; 9 g dietary fiber; 17 mg cholesterol.

SUPERSKIN NUTRIENTS		% DAILY VALUE*
Vitamin A	1580.8 IU	32%
Vitamin B6	0.2 mg	10%
Vitamin C	22.6 mg	38%
Vitamin E	0.6 mg	3%
Magnesium	32.7 mg	8%
Manganese	0.6 mg	30%
Selenium	12.5 mcg	18%
Zinc	1.3 mg	9%

*Percent Daily Values are based on a 2,000-calorie diet. Your daily values may be higher or lower depending on your caloric needs.

Braised Lentils with Eggplant and Mushrooms

Satisfying mouthfuls of this dish will please your stomach while offering your complexion valuable nutrients; the olive oil and lentils help moisturize your skin while the eggplant and mushrooms help brighten and energize.

1 cup (192 g) green or brown lentils

4 cups (950 ml) broth or water

1 tablespoon (15 ml) extra-virgin olive oil

1 garlic clove, minced

1 teaspoon (3 g) grated fresh ginger root

1 yellow onion, diced

2 cups (164 g) diced eggplant

1 cup (70 g) quartered white or cremini mushrooms

2 teaspoons (4 g) curry powder

1 teaspoon (2 g) fresh lemon zest

Salt and pepper to taste

Yield: 6 servings

1. Simmer the lentils in the broth or water for 30 minutes, or until just tender. Remove from the heat.

2. Heat the oil in a large skillet over medium heat. Add the garlic, ginger, and onion. Sauté, stirring occasionally, until the onions are a light golden brown, about 6 to 8 minutes.

3. Add the eggplant, mushrooms, curry powder, and lemon zest. Continue to cook over medium heat, stirring occasionally, until the mushrooms begin to release some moisture, about 5 minutes.

4. Drain the lentils through a sieve set over a large bowl to catch the cooking liquid. Add the lentils to the eggplant mixture. Add enough of the reserved cooking liquid to moisten the mixture well. Cover the skillet and cook over low heat until the eggplant is very tender, about 30 minutes. Season with salt and pepper. Serve at once.

Notes

• *This dish can be prepared in advance and refrigerated for up to 3 days or frozen for up to 6 weeks. Reheat as is or place in a casserole dish, coat with a layer of fresh breadcrumbs, and drizzle with melted unsalted butter. Place the casserole in a 400°F (200°C, or gas mark 6) oven for about 20 minutes, or until the dish is heated through and the crust is crisp and brown. If the crust browns too quickly, cover the casserole with foil; remove the foil during the last 5 minutes of cooking.*

• *Leftover lentils can also be scooped into zucchini and yellow squash "boats." Simply hollow out a large slice of squash, fill the cavity with lentils, and bake at 325°F (170°C, or gas mark 3) until the squash is tender, about 30 to 40 minutes. Serve with tomato sauce.*

NUTRITIONAL ANALYSIS

Each serving provides: 140 calories; 2.5 g total fat; 0.5 g saturated fat; 8 g protein; 22 g carbohydrate; 6 g dietary fiber; 0 mg cholesterol.

SUPERSKIN NUTRIENTS		% DAILY VALUE*
Vitamin A	30.1 IU	1%
Vitamin B6	0.1 mg	5%
Vitamin C	2.7 mg	5%
Vitamin E	0.4 mg	2%
Magnesium	10.6 mg	3%
Manganese	0.1 mg	5%
Selenium	1.8 mcg	3%
Zinc	0.2 mg	1%

*Percent Daily Values are based on a 2,000-calorie diet. Your daily values may be higher or lower depending on your caloric needs.

INGREDIENT SPOTLIGHT

Lentils

Lentils are rich in folate and thiamin, two B vitamins involved in metabolism. Because the skin is a place of very active metabolism, it needs a steady intake of these vitamins to function properly. If the skin does not receive sufficient amounts, metabolism slows and the skin cannot maintain its moisture barrier or repair damage. Lentil eaters need not worry about any deficiency, however, as one cup (200 g) of cooked lentils provides nearly 90 percent of the recommended daily value of folate and 22 percent of thiamin.

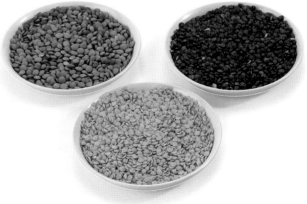

Smokey Black-Eyed Peas

Peas are a great source of folic acid, vitamin B6, and vitamin C, all of which are skin-beautifying nutrients that tighten and smooth. The black-eyed peas used in this dish are a wonderful, elegant-looking alternative to green peas.

1 strip bacon, chopped

½ cup (80 g) diced onion

2 garlic cloves, minced

¼ teaspoon red pepper flakes

1 red or green sweet bell pepper, seeded and diced

1 cup (235 ml) chicken broth

Two 15-ounce (425 g) cans
   black-eyed peas, rinsed and
   drained

1 bay leaf

1 sprig of fresh thyme, or ½
   teaspoon dried, ground
   thyme

Salt and pepper to taste

Hot pepper sauce to taste

Yield: 4 servings

1. Cook the bacon in a large saucepan over medium heat, stirring frequently, until the fat has rendered and the bacon bits are crisped. Remove with a slotted spoon and drain on a paper towel.

2. Pour off all but enough bacon fat to lightly coat the pan. Add the onion, garlic, and red pepper flakes. Sauté over medium heat, stirring occasionally, until the onions are golden brown. Add the diced bell pepper and sauté for 3 minutes, or until tender.

3. Add the chicken broth and bring to a boil. Add the black-eyed peas, bay leaf, and thyme. Cover the pot and cook over low heat for 35 to 40 minutes, or until the broth has nearly cooked away and the beans are extremely tender and flavorful.

4. Remove the cover and gently fold in the bacon pieces. Fish out the bay leaf and discard.

5. Season to taste with salt and pepper. Serve with hot sauce.

Notes

- *If you already have cooked peas on hand, use 3 cups (720 g) in place of the canned beans.*

- *Fresh black eyed peas, also known as "cowpeas" or "crowder peas," can also be substituted for the cooked peas. Fresh peas take only 10 minutes to cook, so there is no need to cook them separately in advance.*

- *This recipe can be made vegetarian by making the following changes: Replace the bacon with 1 to 2 tablespoons (15 to 30 ml) of extra-virgin olive or peanut oil; increase the garlic to 3 cloves; and use vegetable stock or water instead of chicken broth.*

NUTRITIONAL ANALYSIS

Each serving provides: 141 calories; 4 g total fat; 1.5 g saturated fat; 5 g protein; 21 g carbohydrate; 6 g dietary fiber; 4 mg cholesterol.

SUPERSKIN NUTRIENTS		% DAILY VALUE*
Vitamin A	2378.9 IU	48%
Vitamin B6	0.2 mg	10%
Vitamin C	60.2 mg	100%
Vitamin E	0.5 mg	3%
Magnesium	49.9 mg	12%
Manganese	0.7 mg	35%
Selenium	3.9 mcg	6%
Zinc	1.1 mg	7%

*Percent Daily Values are based on a 2,000-calorie diet. Your daily values may be higher or lower depending on your caloric needs.

INGREDIENT SPOTLIGHT

Black-Eyed Peas

In just one cup (170 g) of black-eyed peas, you get 23 percent of your daily recommended value of iron, which is used by your red blood cells to carry oxygen from your lungs to your skin and facial muscles. Iron also plays a vital role in the formation of the collagen scaffolding that keeps your skin tight, strong, and smooth.

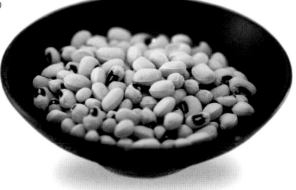

Quinoa Pilaf with Roasted Tomatoes and Pine Nuts

A great side dish to any meal, this pilaf offers your skin nutrients to help fight wrinkles and look radiant. Quinoa contains both manganese and copper, which are needed by one of your skin's best antioxidants, superoxide dismutase, in order to be functional. Serve this wholesome dish alongside grilled salmon and enjoy your reflection in the mirror even more.

¼ cup (35 g) pine nuts

⅔ cup (115 g) quinoa

1 tablespoon (15 ml) canola oil

¼ cup (40 g) minced onion

1½ cups (355 ml) chicken broth

1 bay leaf

1 sprig fresh thyme or ½ teaspoon dried thyme leaves

1 cup (255 g) Herb-Roasted Tomatoes (p. 210) or ⅓ cup (18 g) chopped sun-dried tomatoes

Salt and pepper to taste

Yield: 6 servings

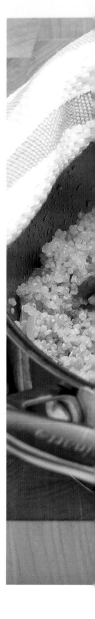

1. Toast the pine nuts by sautéing them in a dry skillet over medium high heat until barely golden. Immediately transfer them from the pan to a dish to cool.

2. Place the quinoa in a fine wire-mesh sieve and rinse well to remove any bitter coating that may remain on the grains.

3. Heat the oil in a saucepan over medium heat. Add the onion and sauté until it turns tender and very light golden brown, about 5 minutes.

4. Add the quinoa, broth, bay leaf, and thyme. Stir well, and bring the broth to a simmer over medium heat.

5. Reduce the heat to low, cover the pot, and simmer over low heat for about 15 minutes, or until the quinoa is tender and fluffy (the grain will open into tiny spirals once cooked). Remove from heat. (Note: If you are using sun-dried tomatoes in place of the herb-roasted tomatoes, place them in a small bowl, add enough hot water to barely cover, and let soak while the quinoa simmers to soften them.)

6. Remove and discard the bay leaf and thyme sprig. Fluff the grains with a fork to break up any clumps, and fold in the roasted or sun-dried tomatoes and pine nuts. Add salt and pepper to taste. Serve at once.

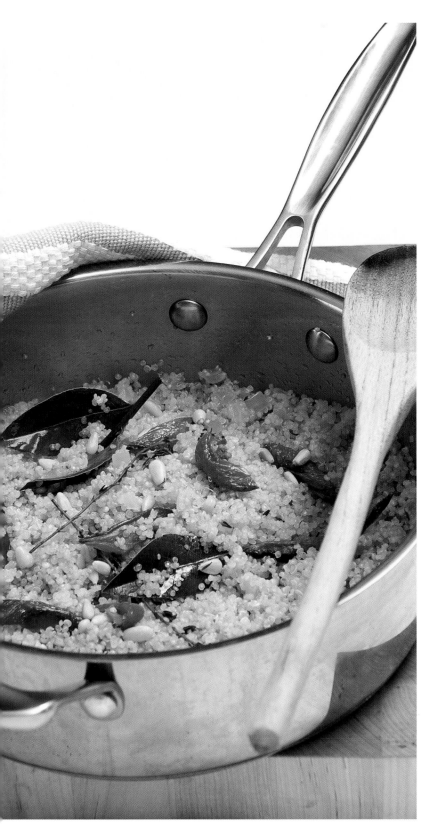

Note

Leftover quinoa can be combined with diced vegetables such as cucumbers, carrots, celery, avocado, and tomato and dressed with vinaigrette or salad dressing (such as any of those listed on pp. 234 to 238). Serve chilled as a salad or as the filling for a pita sandwich garnished with sunflower, alfalfa, or radish sprouts.

NUTRITIONAL ANALYSIS

Each serving provides: 153 calories; 7.7 g total fat; 1.1 g saturated fat; 6 g protein; 17 g carbohydrate; 2 g dietary fiber; 0 mg cholesterol.

SUPERSKIN NUTRIENTS		% DAILY VALUE*
Vitamin A	225.7 IU	5%
Vitamin B6	0.1 mg	5%
Vitamin C	7.1 mg	12%
Vitamin E	2.0 mg	10%
Magnesium	58.7 mg	15%
Manganese	0.8 mg	40%
Selenium	1.2 mcg	2%
Zinc	1.0 mg	7%

*Percent Daily Values are based on a 2,000-calorie diet. Your daily values may be higher or lower depending on your caloric needs.

Couscous

This skin-healthy pasta is a wonderful complement to any number of dishes. Couscous contains two key skin-beautifying minerals: manganese, which helps protect the skin from damage that can trigger inflammation and eventually lead to wrinkling, and selenium, which helps maintain skin elasticity and fight sag.

2 cups (475 ml) broth or water

¼ teaspoon salt

1 teaspoon (5 ml) oil or butter (5 g), optional

1 cup (175 g) couscous

Yield: 4 servings

1. Place the broth or water in a medium saucepan, and bring to a boil over high heat. Add the salt and the oil or butter (if desired).

2. Add the couscous and stir well with a fork to remove any lumps. Return to a boil, cover the pan with a tight-fitting lid, and remove from the heat. Let the couscous sit for about 10 minutes. Remove the lid and fluff the couscous with a fork to break up the clumps.

Note
Couscous makes a wonderful base for savory stews (see our Pumpkin and Chickpea Stew with Couscous on p. 268) and vegetables curries, or as a side dish with grilled lamb or pan-seared fish.

NUTRITIONAL ANALYSIS

Each serving provides: 173 calories; 1.5 g total fat; 0.1 g saturated fat; 6 g protein; 33 g carbohydrate; 2 g dietary fiber; 0 mg cholesterol.

SUPERSKIN NUTRIENTS		% DAILY VALUE*
Vitamin A	0.0 IU	0%
Vitamin B6	0.1 mg	5%
Vitamin C	0.0 mg	0%
Vitamin E	2.2 mg	11%
Magnesium	20.2 mg	5%
Manganese	0.3 mg	15%
Selenium	0.0 mcg	0%
Zinc	0.4 mg	3%

*Percent Daily Values are based on a 2,000-calorie diet. Your daily values may be higher or lower depending on your caloric needs.

INGREDIENT SPOTLIGHT

Couscous

In one cup (160 g) of cooked couscous, you'll get 7 percent of your recommended intake of the skin-savvy nutrient manganese. This mineral and trace element plays many essential roles in the body. It helps in the metabolism of food, functioning of the nervous system and thyroid, and production of sex hormones. It also works as an antioxidant and thus helps prevent damage in the skin caused by free radicals.

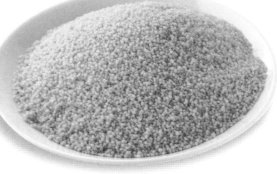

Rosemary Ginger Chicken with Orange-Honey Glaze

Beautiful skin is only a meal away with this delicious dish packed with skin-beautifying nutrients. Rosemary helps protect the collagen in your skin that keeps it tight and smooth, chicken contains the potent antioxidants selenium and CoQ10 that preserve your skin's healthy glow, and oranges help prevent the appearance of sunspots.

Four 5-ounce (140 g) boneless, skinless chicken breasts

Salt and pepper

For the marinade:

½ cup (120 ml) orange juice

2 tablespoons (30 ml) red wine vinegar

2 tablespoons (12 g) minced fresh ginger

2 tablespoons (20 g) minced shallots or onion

2 teaspoons (6 g) minced garlic

1 teaspoon (1.2 g) minced rosemary

½ cup (120 ml) canola oil

For the glaze:

3 tablespoons (45 ml) orange juice concentrate

¼ cup (85 g) honey

1 tablespoon (15 ml) red wine vinegar

2 teaspoons (4 g) finely minced fresh ginger

Yield: 4 servings

1. Trim any visible fat from the chicken breasts. Season breasts with salt and pepper.

2. Combine the marinade ingredients in a large resealable bag or a nonreactive dish or container. Add the chicken. Turn the bag or the chicken pieces to coat evenly. Place chicken in the refrigerator for at least 3 and up to 12 hours before baking.

3. Preheat oven to 375°F (190°C, or gas mark 5).

4. While the oven is preheating, combine all the glaze ingredients in a small pan and bring to a simmer. Keep the glaze warm while the chicken is baking.

5. Remove the chicken from the marinade and place into a baking dish (use a rack if you have one to keep the pieces from sitting directly on the pan). Bake the chicken, brushing with the glaze every 5 minutes, until the meat is thoroughly cooked, about 20 to 25 minutes.

6. Serve on heated plates.

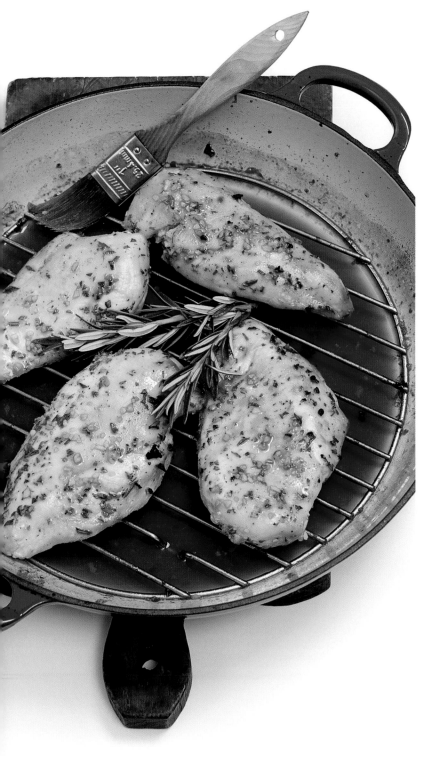

Note

If you find you have leftover ginger, consider using it in the Iced Minted Green Tea recipe on page 272. Add ½ to 1 teaspoon minced ginger with the tea bags (step 3) and allow to steep. You can remove the ginger along with the bags, or leave in—it's up to you.

NUTRITIONAL ANALYSIS

Each serving provides: 636 calories; 33.5 g total fat; 3.5 g saturated fat; 54 g protein; 29 g carbohydrate; 0.5 g dietary fiber; 146 mg cholesterol.

SUPERSKIN NUTRIENTS		% DAILY VALUE*
Vitamin A	726.2 IU	15%
Vitamin B6	1.1 mg	55%
Vitamin C	31.4 mg	52%
Vitamin E	6.5 mg	33%
Magnesium	61.3 mg	15%
Manganese	0.1 mg	5%
Selenium	47.8 mcg	68%
Zinc	1.9 mg	13%

*Percent Daily Values are based on a 2,000-calorie diet. Your daily values may be higher or lower depending on your caloric needs.

Escabeche of Tuna

Escabeche refers to a dish of poached or fried fish that has been covered with a spicy marinade. It is a popular dish in Spain (where its name originates from) and for good reason—the good fats in fish reduce inflammation that can give your skin a red, puffy appearance and cause wrinkles to form.

2 tablespoons (30 ml) freshly squeezed lime juice

1 tablespoon (15 ml) extra-virgin olive oil

4 teaspoons (5 g) chopped fresh cilantro or parsley

1 teaspoon (3 g) minced jalapeno

1 garlic clove, minced

½ teaspoon salt, or to taste

¼ teaspoon ground black pepper, or to taste

½ pound (225 g) tuna fillet

½ cup canola oil

½ cup flour

Yield: 4 servings

1. Combine the lime juice, olive oil, cilantro (or parsley), jalapeno, garlic, salt, and pepper to taste in a bowl and whisk to blend well. Set aside in a large shallow bowl.

2. Trim the tuna if necessary, and cut in large cubes. Season lightly with salt and pepper.

3. In large skillet with tall sides, pour enough oil to come to a depth of ¼ inch (6.25 mm). Heat the oil over high heat until the surface is hazy and ripples lightly.

4. Spread flour out onto a large plate, and dredge the tuna pieces in the flour, shaking off any excess. Carefully add them to the hot oil, adding only a few pieces to the pan at a time and allowing a good amount of space around each piece. Cook just long enough to stiffen the exterior of the fish, 1 to 2 minutes on each side.

5. Add the tuna pieces to the lime juice mixture while the fish is still hot, and toss to coat evenly.

6. Place the pieces into a bowl, cover, and refrigerate for about 8 hours (or overnight) before serving.

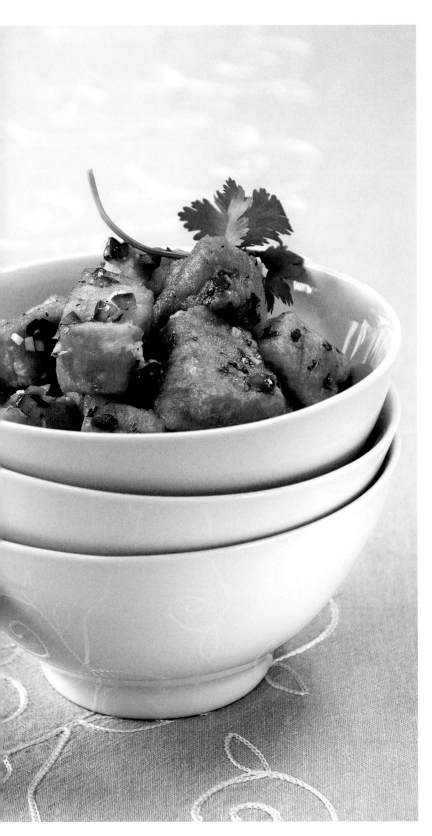

Notes

- *Other seafood, such as scallops, shrimp, swordfish, squid, or monkfish, can be substituted for the tuna. The important point is to select fish that is as fresh as possible.*

- *Serve with wedges of fresh tomato, sliced avocado, scallions, and diced red onion on a bed of baby greens or spinach.*

NUTRITIONAL ANALYSIS

Each serving provides: 197 calories; 8 g total fat; 1 g saturated fat; 18 g protein; 13 g carbohydrate; 0.5 g dietary fiber; 34 mg cholesterol.

SUPERSKIN NUTRIENTS		% DAILY VALUE*
Vitamin A	56.2 IU	1%
Vitamin B6	0.6 mg	30%
Vitamin C	3.2 mg	5%
Vitamin E	2.1 mg	11%
Magnesium	29.3 mg	7%
Manganese	0.1 mg	5%
Selenium	32.0 mcg	46%
Zinc	0.7 mg	5%

*Percent Daily Values are based on a 2,000-calorie diet. Your daily values may be higher or lower depending on your caloric needs.

Sesame-Crusted Salmon Bake

This delectable dish delivers one of the best anti-inflammatory nutrients on earth—omega-3 fatty acids. These healthy fats relieve inflammation, fight acne and psoriasis, improve your complexion, and give your skin a healthy glow. Served alongside vitamin B–rich mushrooms and cartenoid-laden carrots, this is one "bake" that won't leave your skin parched and dry.

¼ cup (60 ml) rice wine vinegar

2 tablespoons (30 ml) soy or tamari sauce, divided

½ cup (35 g) sliced cremini or shiitake mushrooms

½ cup (55 g) thinly sliced or coarsely grated carrots

¼ cup (31 g) thinly sliced red onion

1½ cups (105 g) thinly shredded bok choy

½ cup (75 g) sesame seeds (white), or as needed

1¼ pounds (½ kg) fresh, skinless salmon fillet (center cut, if possible)

Salt and pepper

Yield: 4 servings

1. Preheat oven to 400°F (200°C, or gas mark 6).

2. Place the rice wine vinegar and 1 tablespoon (15 ml) of soy sauce in a shallow baking dish. Add the mushrooms, carrots, onion, and bok choy, and toss to coat all ingredients evenly. Set aside.

3. Place the sesame seeds in a shallow pan for dredging.

4. Lay the salmon fillet on a plate and brush both sides with the remaining soy or tamari sauce. Season generously with salt and pepper. Dredge one side of the salmon in the sesame seeds, pressing gently to form a crust.

5. Carefully place the salmon on top of the vegetables with the crusted side facing up. Cover the dish loosely with foil and bake for about 10 minutes, or until the salmon is almost cooked through. (If you press on the salmon gently with a fork, it should fall apart into flakes that are slightly translucent near the center.)

6. Remove the foil from the salmon and set the oven to broil. Move the salmon under the broiler and toast just long enough to barely color the sesame seeds, about 1 minute. Serve at once.

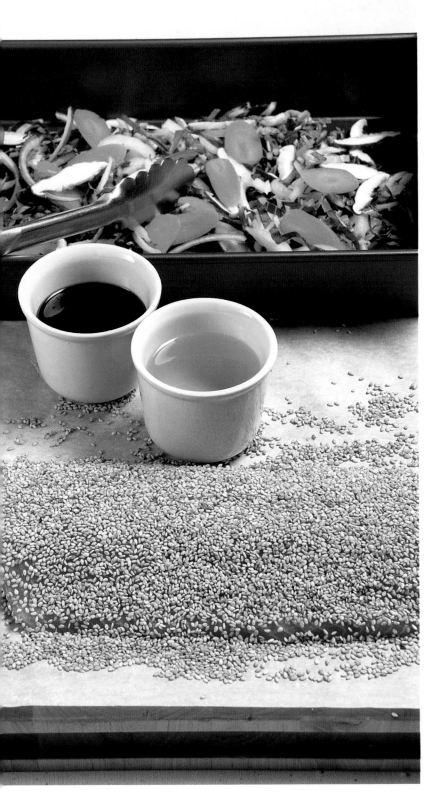

Note

Concerns about mercury, PCBs and other contaminants as of late have raised concerns about fish consumption. Nutritional experts agree, however, that the benefits of eating at least two servings of fish a week far outweigh any potential, underlying risk from contaminants.

NUTRITIONAL ANALYSIS

Each serving provides: 331 calories;
18 g total fat; 2.5 g saturated fat; 33 g protein;
10 g carbohydrate; 4 g dietary fiber;
80 mg cholesterol.

SUPERSKIN NUTRIENTS		% DAILY VALUE*
Vitamin A	4713.7 IU	94%
Vitamin B6	1.4 mg	70%
Vitamin C	13.9 mg	23%
Vitamin E	2.5 mg	13%
Magnesium	117.4 mg	29%
Manganese	0.6 mg	30%
Selenium	57.6 mcg	82%
Zinc	2.7 mg	18%

*Percent Daily Values are based on a 2,000-calorie diet. Your daily values may be higher or lower depending on your caloric needs.

Whole Wheat Pasta with Clams and Toasted Bread Crumbs

Tighten up your skin with this yummy clam pasta. Hidden inside these tasty shells are vitamins and minerals that help your skin stay firm and beautiful. Whole grains are also packed with nutrients, including iron, fiber, and B vitamins, all of which work to brighten your complexion.

1 pound (455 g) whole wheat pasta (spaghetti, linguini, or fettuccini)

Salt

1 cup (110 g) fresh bread crumbs (see Notes)

3 tablespoons (45 ml) extra-virgin olive oil

4 garlic cloves, peeled and sliced as thinly as possible

½ cup (50 g) thinly sliced scallions

2 anchovy fillets, optional

¼ cup (60 ml) dry white wine or dry vermouth

2 cups (455 g) shucked clams and their juices (see Notes)

Salt and pepper to taste

Yield: 4 servings

1. Cook the pasta according to package instructions. While the pasta is cooking, you should be able to finish making the sauce.

2. Heat a dry skillet over medium-high heat. Add the bread crumbs to the pan and cook, stirring frequently, until they are toasted, about 3 minutes. Pour the bread crumbs into a bowl and set aside.

3. In the same pan, heat the olive oil. Add the garlic slices and the scallions and cook until the scallions are bright green, about 2 minutes. Add the anchovies (if using), and smash them into the mixture until they dissolve.

4. Add the wine or vermouth and simmer until the liquid has nearly cooked away, about 5 minutes. Add the clams and their juices to the pan. Continue to simmer gently until the edges of the clams begin to curl, about 8 to 9 minutes. Season with salt and pepper.

5. As the sauce finishes cooking, prepare the cooked pasta. Drain it well and transfer to a large heated bowl or individual serving dishes.

6. Pour the clams and sauce over the pasta. Sprinkle with the toasted bread crumbs. Serve immediately.

Note

• *To make fresh bread crumbs, leave a few slices of sturdy, peasant-style bread—preferably whole-grain—out on a plate for about 4 hours (or pop them into the freezer for 30 minutes or so). Once the bread has hardened, grate it or break into pieces and pulse into crumbs in a blender or food processor.*

NUTRITIONAL ANALYSIS

Each serving provides: 735 calories; 14.5 g total fat; 2.5 g saturated fat; 43 g protein; 112 g carbohydrate; 16 g dietary fiber; 56 mg cholesterol.

SUPERSKIN NUTRIENTS		% DAILY VALUE*
Vitamin A	509.7 IU	10%
Vitamin B6	0.4 mg	20%
Vitamin C	21.1 mg	35%
Vitamin E	5.4 mg	27%
Magnesium	194.1 mg	49%
Manganese	4.6 mg	230%
Selenium	134.1 mcg	192%
Zinc	5.3 mg	35%

*Percent Daily Values are based on a 2,000-calorie diet. Your daily values may be higher or lower depending on your caloric needs

INGREDIENT SPOTLIGHT

Clams

Iron can help your skin regain a rosy, healthy glow. Involved in energy metabolism, iron acts as an oxygen carrier in hemoglobin, which carries oxygen in your red blood cells from the lungs to every cell in your body. Because the cells in your skin are far away from your lungs and need lots of oxygen due to their high rate of metabolism, your skin needs a steady supply of iron to get the job done. Thankfully, clams can provide you with all the iron you need—just one 3-ounce (84 g) serving provides you with more than 100 percent of your daily iron requirement.

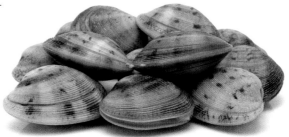

Broccoli Sauté with White Beans and Orecchiette

This dish is a deliciously unique way to enjoy broccoli, one of your skin's best defenses against redness and puffiness. Rich in protein and vitamin C and low in saturated fat, this meal is a great choice for your skin—and your taste buds.

3 cups (215 g) fresh broccoli florets

2 tablespoons (30 ml) extra-virgin olive oil

2 or 3 garlic cloves, peeled and sliced very thin

2 cups (230 g) cooked orecchiette pasta, al dente

½ cup (125 g) cooked or canned cannellini beans, rinsed and drained

Salt and pepper

Freshly grated parmesan or Romano cheese

Yield: 4 servings

1. Lightly blanch broccoli florets to give the broccoli better texture and flavor. To do this, bring a large pot of water to a rolling boil. Add a generous pinch of salt, then the florets. Cook uncovered for about 2 minutes. Drain in a colander, rinse under cold water until the florets are cool, and drain well.

2. Heat the olive oil in a skillet over medium heat. Add the garlic and sauté until garlic turns soft and translucent, but has not taken on any color, about 2 minutes.

3. Add the broccoli florets and cook, stirring occasionally, until they are very hot, 3 to 4 minutes.

4. Add the cooked orecchiette and beans and toss to combine everything together. Continue to sauté until heated through, about 5 minutes. Drizzle with a little additional olive oil if necessary to lightly coat all of the ingredients. Season with salt and pepper.

5. Serve hot with grated cheese.

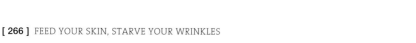

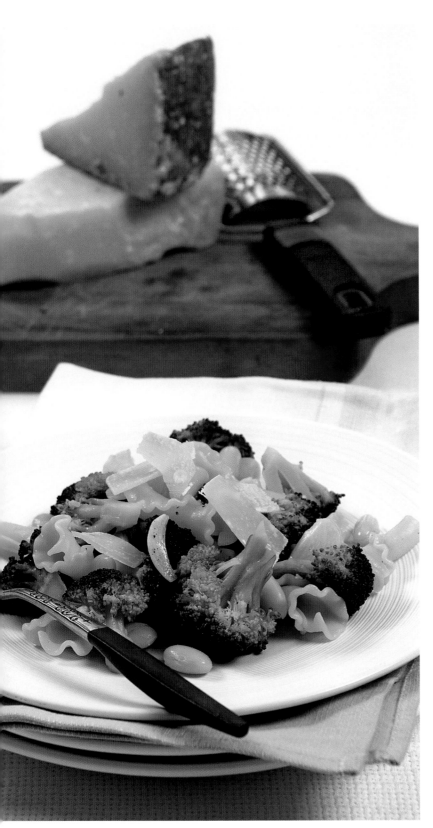

Notes

- *Feel free to use whatever pasta shape you prefer—other options include penne, elbows, radiatore, bowties, or shells—and look for whole-grain pasta if you can.*

- *For a more mellow flavor, replace the raw garlic with Roasted Garlic (see recipe on p. 208). Follow the recipe directions, but in step 2, only sauté the garlic for about 30 seconds to get it soft and hot.*

NUTRITIONAL ANALYSIS

Each serving provides: 212 calories; 9.5 g total fat; 2 g saturated fat; 8 g protein; 24 g carbohydrate; 4 g dietary fiber; 5 mg cholesterol.

SUPERSKIN NUTRIENTS		% DAILY VALUE*
Vitamin A	865.1 IU	17%
Vitamin B6	0.1 mg	5%
Vitamin C	50.1 mg	84%
Vitamin E	1.8 mg	9%
Magnesium	27.3 mg	7%
Manganese	0.3 mg	15%
Selenium	15.7 mcg	22%
Zinc	0.7 mg	5%

*Percent Daily Values are based on a 2,000-calorie diet. Your daily values may be higher or lower depending on your caloric needs.

Pumpkin and Chickpea Stew with Couscous

This stew's rich orange color will draw raves, but your guests will be all the more thrilled when you tell them that it contains beta-carotene, a nutrient that will protect their skin from aging and dryness, and manganese, an antioxidant that helps protect cells from free-radical damage.

1 tablespoon (15 ml) extra-virgin olive oil

1 cup (160 g) diced onion

¼ teaspoon ground ginger powder

1 teaspoon (2 g) curry powder

½ cup (58 g) diced pumpkin, butternut squash, or Hubbard squash (fresh, or frozen and thawed)

½ cup (82 g) cooked or canned chickpeas, rinsed and drained

1 teaspoon (2 g) freshly grated orange zest

2 cups (475 ml) vegetable broth

1 cup (124 g) diced zucchini

Salt and pepper to taste

Prepared couscous (p. 256)

For garnish:

2 tablespoons (14 g) toasted slivered almonds

2 tablespoons (18 g) dried currants or dark raisins

2 tablespoons (6 g) snipped fresh chives

Hot pepper sauce (see Note)

Lemon wedges

Yield: 4 servings

1. Heat oil in a Dutch oven or flameproof casserole. Add the onion and cook over medium heat until the onion is tender and light golden in color, 3 to 4 minutes. Add the ginger and curry powders and stir until the spices are evenly distributed.

2. Add pumpkin, chickpeas, and orange zest to the pan, and enough of the broth to barely cover the vegetables. Simmer until the pumpkin is tender and cooked through, about 20 to 30 minutes.

3. Stir in the zucchini and continue to simmer until the zucchini is tender, about 10 to 12 minutes. Season with salt and pepper and simmer for an additional 5 minutes.

4. Serve on a bed of couscous with your choice of garnishes.

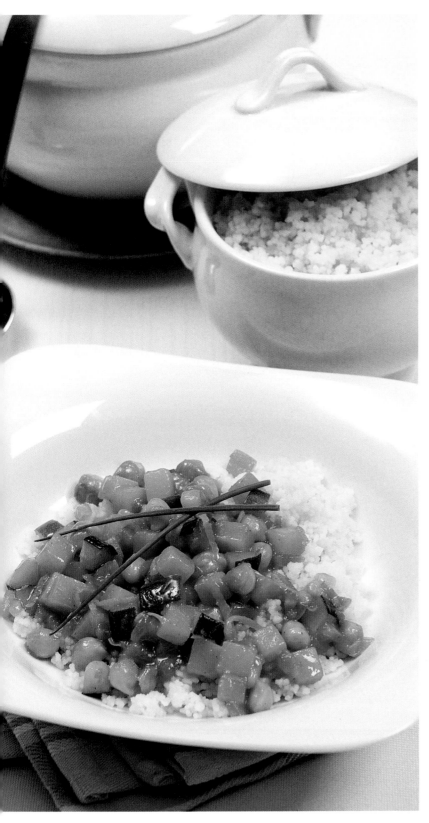

Note

Harissa, a fiery Tunisian-style hot sauce made from pungent dried chiles, is traditional in this dish. You can find prepared harissa in markets that feature Italian, Middle Eastern, or Mediterranean foods. You may want to dilute the sauce with a little water to tame its intense heat.

NUTRITIONAL ANALYSIS

Each serving provides: 306 calories; 8.5 g total fat; 1 g saturated fat; 10 g protein; 50 g carbohydrate; 6 g dietary fiber; 0 mg cholesterol.

SUPERSKIN NUTRIENTS		% DAILY VALUE*
Vitamin A	840.2 IU	17%
Vitamin B6	0.1 mg	5%
Vitamin C	10.1 mg	17%
Vitamin E	3.9 mg	20%
Magnesium	43.5 mg	11%
Manganese	0.5 mg	25%
Selenium	0.5 mcg	1%
Zinc	0.7 mg	5%

*Percent Daily Values are based on a 2,000-calorie diet. Your daily values may be higher or lower depending on your caloric needs.

Ratatouille

Easy to make and bursting with wrinkle-fighting power, this dish is a perfect meal. Olive oil is nourishing and moisturizing for your skin and the combination of tomatoes, eggplant, and bell peppers provides an entire rainbow of antioxidants to fight wrinkles. Serve hot or cold, either as a side dish or as an appetizer with bread or crackers.

2 tablespoons (30 ml) extra-virgin olive oil

2 garlic cloves, minced

1 red onion, sliced thin

2 tablespoons (32 g) tomato paste

1 cup (180 g) sliced zucchini

1 cup (150 g) diced bell pepper (green or red)

2 cups (164 g) diced eggplant

1 cup (113 g) sliced yellow squash

3 canned plum tomatoes, seeded and chopped

Chicken or vegetable broth, or water, as needed

2 tablespoons (2 g) chopped fresh herbs (choose from chives, parsley, tarragon, chervil, basil, oregano, and rosemary)

½ teaspoon salt

¼ teaspoon freshly ground black pepper

Yield: 6 servings

1. Heat the olive oil in a large skillet over medium heat. Add the garlic and red onion. Sauté, stirring occasionally, for about 5 to 6 minutes, or until the onions are tender and translucent. Add the tomato paste and cook briefly until the mixture has a slight rusty color and a sweet aroma.

2. Add the zucchini, bell pepper, eggplant, squash, and tomatoes. Stir to combine.

3. Reduce the heat to a gentle simmer. Cook the vegetables until they are very tender, about 25 to 30 minutes. Add a bit of broth or water if the stew seems too dry as it cooks. Note, however, that it should never appear soupy.

4. Add the fresh herbs, salt, and pepper. Serve at once.

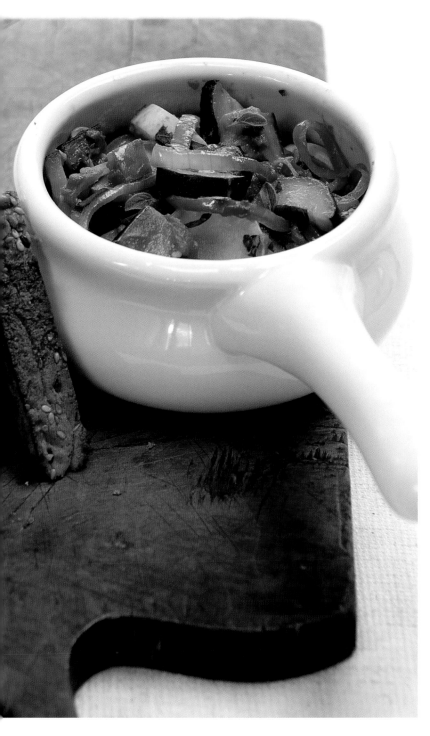

Notes

- With this stew, it is perfectly permissible to add a little more of this, a little less of that, or to include whatever is at the peak of its season at the market. Cooking the garlic, onion, and tomato paste until aromatic is the flavor base that determines the success of the dish.

- To lend the dish a richer flavor, add a handful of chopped sun-dried tomatoes, and top the dish with crumbled goat cheese.

- This stew also can stand as the basis of a vegetarian meal. Serve on a bed of couscous (p. 256), noodles, rice, or other grains.

NUTRITIONAL ANALYSIS

Each serving provides: 83 calories; 5 g total fat; 0.5 g saturated fat; 2 g protein; 9 g carbohydrate; 3 g dietary fiber; 0 mg cholesterol.

SUPERSKIN NUTRIENTS		% DAILY VALUE*
Vitamin A	674.2 IU	13%
Vitamin B6	0.2 mg	10%
Vitamin C	35.9 mg	60%
Vitamin E	1.5 mg	8%
Magnesium	24.4 mg	6%
Manganese	0.3 mg	15%
Selenium	0.7 mcg	1%
Zinc	0.3 mg	2%

*Percent Daily Values are based on a 2,000-calorie diet. Your daily values may be higher or lower depending on your caloric needs.

Iced Minted Green Tea

If you're looking for a refreshing way to jazz up your green tea, look no further. The green tea in this tasty drink increases the skin's elasticity and contains the powerful antioxidant EGCG, which prevents inflammation that causes puffy, red, and wrinkled skin.

1 cup (200 g) sugar
  (see Notes)
1 cup (235 ml) water
1 bunch fresh mint
4 cups (950 ml) boiling water
5 green tea bags
Additional mint for garnish,
  optional

Yield: 4 servings (4 cups,
  or 950 ml)

1. To prepare the sugar syrup, combine the sugar and water in a small saucepan over medium heat, stirring as the sugar dissolves. Simmer for 3 to 4 minutes, then remove the pan from the heat.

2. Rinse and dry the mint. Gather the mint sprigs in your hand and crush and bruise them. Add the mint to the syrup, and let the mixture cool to room temperature. Strain through a sieve to remove the mint and pour the syrup into a jar or bottle. Discard the mint.

3. To make the iced tea, place the tea bags in a large pot or pitcher. Cover with the boiling water and let them steep for 4 or 5 minutes. (Because you will be serving this over ice, and the ice will dilute the flavor of the tea, let it brew a little longer than you normally would for a cup of hot tea. It should be a little stronger than hot tea.)

4. Remove the tea bags and let the tea cool to room temperature. If possible, chill the tea before sweetening it with the mint syrup.

5. To serve, add enough of the mint syrup to sweeten and flavor the tea to your taste. (Leftover simple syrup can be stored at room temperature indefinitely and used to sweeten cold or iced drinks.) Pour the tea over ice cubes in large glasses and garnish with a leaf or two of fresh mint, if desired.

Note

• *In place of sugar, use stevia or honey to sweeten the tea—your skin will thank you for it. (Note that stevia and honey are much sweeter than sugar, so you'll need less. Use about half as much honey as you would sugar, or just a few teaspoons of stevia.)*

NUTRITIONAL ANALYSIS

Each serving provides: 194 calories; 0 g total fat; 0 g saturated fat; 0 g protein; 50 g carbohydrate; 0 g dietary fiber; 0 mg cholesterol.

SUPERSKIN NUTRIENTS		% DAILY VALUE*
Vitamin A	34.0 IU	1%
Vitamin B6	0.0 mg	0%
Vitamin C	0.3 mg	1%
Vitamin E	0.0 mg	0%
Magnesium	3.6 mg	1%
Manganese	0.0 mg	0%
Selenium	0.3 mcg	0%
Zinc	0.1 mg	1%

*Percent Daily Values are based on a 2,000-calorie diet. Your daily values may be higher or lower depending on your caloric needs.

INGREDIENT SPOTLIGHT

Green Tea

Green tea is among the top ten most antioxidant-rich foods on earth. Antioxidants stop free radicals from damaging collagen, elastin, and skin cells. Epigallocatechin-3-gallate (EGCG) is the active compound in green tea thought to be responsible for its amazing antioxidant ability. EGCG appears to prevent the movement of white blood cells into the skin, protecting skin from the damaging oxidizing products that they release and thus preventing wrinkle formation.

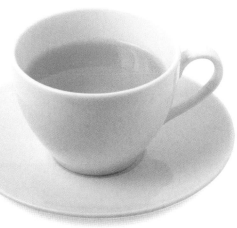

Watermelon Punch

Delight your guests with this pretty pink punch. Be sure to tell them that watermelon is a natural skin moisturizer, and they're sure to come back for seconds. You can also mention this refreshing fruit is packed with some of nature's most effective antioxidants, including vitamins A and C, which neutralize free radicals in every part of the skin.

½ cup (120 ml) water

½ cup (100 g) sugar (see Notes)

4 cups (600 g) watermelon chunks, dark seeds removed

2 tablespoons (30 ml) fresh lime juice, or to taste

Club soda, optional

For garnish:

Lime wedges

Skewers of watermelon cubes, grapes, or other fresh fruit

Yield: 4 servings

1. Combine water and sugar in a small pan over medium heat. Bring to a simmer as you stir. Simmer for 3 to 4 minutes, then remove the pan from the heat. Pour the syrup into a clean jar or pitcher (see Notes).

2. Purée the watermelon in a blender or food processor until smooth. Strain the watermelon pulp through a strainer lined with a coffee filter into a glass jar or pitcher. Discard the pulp.

3. Chill the watermelon juice for at least 2 hours, or until very cold.

4. Once the watermelon juice is chilled, measure out ⅓ cup (80 ml) of the simple syrup. Add half of the syrup and half of the lime juice to the watermelon juice and stir to combine. Taste, and add more of each, if necessary, to suit your taste. (Note: Because you have the option of adding club soda, take that into account as you evaluate the flavor of your cooler. The soda will dilute the flavors somewhat, so you may want to add a bit more syrup and lime juice than you would with a non-carbonated punch.)

5. Serve the punch chilled, over ice, or as a cooler. To make a cooler, add ice cubes to a tall glass and fill halfway with punch. Top with club soda and garnish with a lime wedge or fruit skewer, if desired.

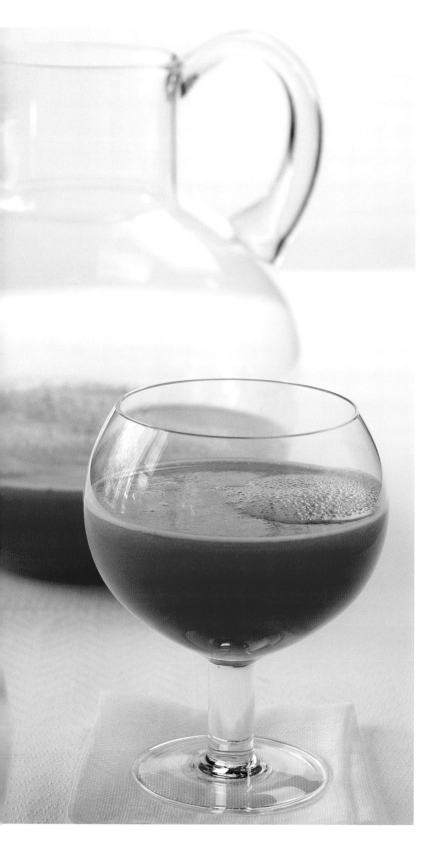

Notes

- *In place of sugar, use stevia or honey to sweeten the punch—your skin will thank you for it. (Note that stevia and honey are much sweeter than sugar, so you'll need less. Use about half as much honey as you would sugar, or just a few teaspoons of stevia.)*

- *Simple syrup can be stored at room temperature indefinitely and used to sweeten cold or iced drinks.*

NUTRITIONAL ANALYSIS

Each serving provides: 197 calories; 1 g total fat; 0 g saturated fat; 1 g protein; 49 g carbohydrate; 1 g dietary fiber; 0 mg cholesterol.

SUPERSKIN NUTRIENTS		% DAILY VALUE*
Vitamin A	742.8 IU	15%
Vitamin B6	0.3 mg	15%
Vitamin C	22.5 mg	38%
Vitamin E	0.3 mg	2%
Magnesium	23.3 mg	6%
Manganese	0.1 mg	5%
Selenium	0.4 mcg	1%
Zinc	0.2 mg	1%

*Percent Daily Values are based on a 2,000-calorie diet. Your daily values may be higher or lower depending on your caloric needs.

Spiced Hot Cocoa

Cuddle up with a cup of this wrinkle-fighting cocoa on a cold night, and feel young again. Cocoa has more antioxidants than red wine or green tea—doesn't get much sweeter than that!

1 cup (200 g) sugar

⅓ cup (26 g) premium un-
   sweetened cocoa

1 tablet or about ¾ ounce
   (21 g) Mexican chocolate,
   grated (see Note)

1 teaspoon (2 g) ground cinnamon

½ teaspoon ground cardamom

⅛ teaspoon ground cloves

⅛ teaspoon cayenne pepper

Pinch of salt

Almond, rice, soy, or skim milk

Yield: 24 servings (1½ cups,
   or 250 g, dry mix)

1. Combine all the ingredients except the milk in a bowl and whisk until blended. Transfer the mixture to a jar or tin with a tight-fitting lid.

2. For each serving, blend two tablespoons (28 g) of the dry mix with two tablespoons (15 ml) of milk in a mug. If making multiple servings, combine the appropriate amount of mix and milk in a small saucepan. Stir until the mixture is wet and smooth.

3. Add ¾ cup (175 ml) of milk for each serving and heat the liquid until very hot. Taste, and adjust with additional cocoa mix if necessary.

Note
You can find Mexican chocolate in many supermarkets in the ethnic or international foods aisle, or in Latin markets. It is made by grinding dark bitter chocolate with sugar and cinnamon. Some varieties include nuts and chiles, which would give this hot chocolate a richness and subtle spice. If you cannot find Mexican chocolate, substitute high-quality bittersweet chocolate and a touch more cinnamon than called for in the recipe.

NUTRITIONAL ANALYSIS

Each serving (including skim milk) provides: 124 calories; 1 g total fat; 0.5 g saturated fat; 9 g protein; 22 g carbohydrate; 0 g dietary fiber; 4 mg cholesterol.

SUPERSKIN NUTRIENTS		% DAILY VALUE*
Vitamin A	504.2 IU	10%
Vitamin B6	0.1 mg	5%
Vitamin C	2.5 mg	4%
Vitamin E	0.1 mg	1%
Magnesium	34.9 mg	9%
Manganese	0.1 mg	5%
Selenium	5.4 mcg	8%
Zinc	1.1 mg	7%

*Percent Daily Values are based on a 2,000-calorie diet. Your daily values may be higher or lower depending on your caloric needs.

INGREDIENT SPOTLIGHT

Dark Chocolate

Dark chocolate is an excellent source of flavonoids, powerful antioxidants that protect the skin from free radical damage and inflammation. In fact, studies have found that the flavonoids in cocoa-based drinks improve blood flow to skin cells, improve the hydration and texture of the skin, and prevent free radical damage to the fatty components of skin cells.

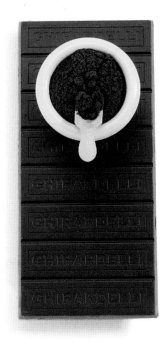

Chocolate Yogurt Mousse

This dessert is as elegant and beautiful as your skin will be, thanks to the probiotics in yogurt and the antioxidants in chocolate. Yes, chocolate is good for you—it helps fight wrinkles! Enjoy this dessert after dinner, and your skin will enjoy a good morning without puffy eyes.

1¼ cups (290 g) plain low fat yogurt

1½ ounces (42 g) dark chocolate

¼ cup (22 g) cocoa powder, sifted twice

4 egg whites, at room temperature

3 tablespoons (40 g) sugar

Yield: 6 servings

1. A day in advance, line a colander or strainer with a cheesecloth or a clean linen or cotton cloth or napkin. Place the yogurt in the lined colander, and set the colander in a larger bowl. Place in the refrigerator and allow the yogurt to drain for 24 hours.

2. Remove the drained yogurt from the colander and place it in a mixing bowl. Let it come to room temperature while melting the chocolate.

3. Heat the chocolate or over low heat or in a microwave at 50 percent power until just melted. Remove chocolate from the heat, and allow it to cool to room temperature, but not harden.

4. Add the chocolate and cocoa powder to the yogurt and gently stir until blended.

5. Using an electric mixer, whip the egg whites and sugar until medium peaks form. By hand, gently fold half of the beaten egg whites into the chocolate-yogurt mixture. Gradually fold in the remaining whites.

6. Spoon the mousse into serving dishes or molds, and chill for at least 4 hours, or overnight, before serving.

Notes

- *It is important to have all of the ingredients at room temperature before mixing the mousse together so that they combine evenly and have a light, creamy texture.*

- *The yogurt can be drained a few days in advance, then transferred to a container and covered until you are ready to prepare the mousse. You can also make a double batch of the strained yogurt— also known as Greek yogurt—and enjoy some on its own, topped with fresh fruit and granola.*

NUTRITIONAL ANALYSIS

Each serving provides: 115 calories; 3.5 g total fat; 2 g saturated fat; 6 g protein; 16 g carbohydrate; 2 g dietary fiber; 3 mg cholesterol.

SUPERSKIN NUTRIENTS		% DAILY VALUE*
Vitamin A	35.8 IU	1%
Vitamin B6	0.0 mg	0%
Vitamin C	0.4 mg	1%
Vitamin E	0.2 mg	1%
Magnesium	37.4 mg	9%
Manganese	0.2 mg	10%
Selenium	6.3 mcg	9%
Zinc	0.8 mg	5%

*Percent Daily Values are based on a 2,000-calorie diet. Your daily values may be higher or lower depending on your caloric needs.

INGREDIENT SPOTLIGHT

Yogurt

Yogurt is a good source of riboflavin, with one cup providing you with 30 percent of your recommended daily value. This B vitamin helps protect cells from oxygen damage and supports cellular energy production. It also plays a role in maintaining adequate supplies of its fellow B vitamins (of which there are seven).

Apple, Pear, and Dried Fruit Strudel

Full of fall's best flavors, this dessert will enhance any dinner table while enhancing your complexion. Apples offer your skin quercetin, a powerful wrinkle-fighting antioxidant, pears work to keep red, puffy skin away, and dried fruit tightens, smoothes, and prevents sagging.

½ cup (75 g) chopped dried fruits (raisins, apricots, figs, prunes, dates, etc.)

2 tablespoons (30 ml) brandy or dark rum

¼ cup (60 ml) boiling water

2 Red Delicious apples, cored, peeled, and diced

2 Fuji apples, cored, peeled, and diced

2 pears, cored, peeled, and diced

5 teaspoons (25 g) brown sugar, packed

2 tablespoons (15 g) chopped toasted pecans or walnuts

¼ teaspoon ground nutmeg

¾ teaspoon ground cinnamon

8 sheets phyllo dough

5 teaspoons (25 ml) melted butter

½ cup (40 g) graham cracker crumbs

Yield: 8 servings

1. Place the dried fruit in a small bowl. Add the brandy (or rum) and boiling water and allow the fruit to plump for about 30 minutes.

2. Preheat the oven to 425°F (220°C, or gas mark 7).

3. Combine the apples, pears, brown sugar, chopped nuts, nutmeg, and cinnamon in a large bowl and toss until the fruit is well coated. Add the dried fruit and its soaking liquid and toss until blended.

4. Lay two sheets of phyllo—one layered on top of the other—on a flat work surface and brush lightly with 1 teaspoon (5 ml) of the melted butter. Sprinkle with a quarter (⅛ cup, or 10 g) of the graham cracker crumbs. Top with another two sheets of phyllo, and again brush with butter and sprinkle with graham cracker crumbs. Repeat until all the phyllo sheets are stacked up. Your final layer should be graham cracker crumbs.

5. Mound the fruit filling along one of the long sides of the dough, and then roll the strudel up tightly. Place seam side down on a baking sheet.

6. Brush the finished strudel with the remaining teaspoon of butter. Use a sharp knife to very lightly score the top of the strudel (see photo).

7. Bake the strudel for about 25 minutes, or until the dough is a golden brown. Let the strudel cool slightly before slicing and serving.

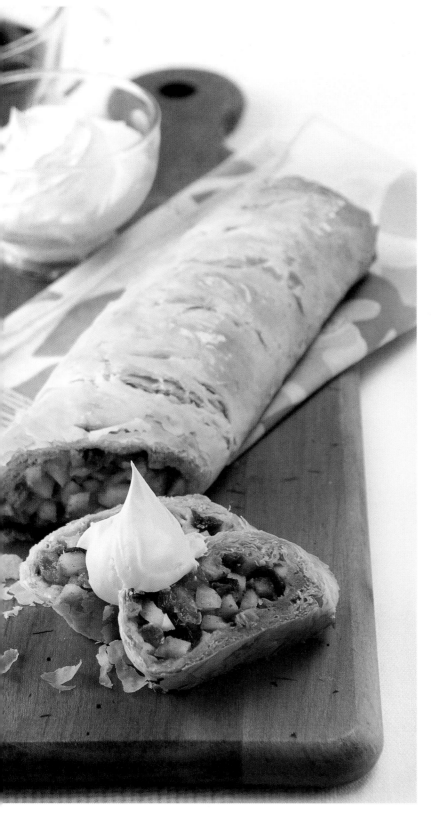

Notes

- *The strudel can be prepared through step 6 and then wrapped and frozen. It can be baked without thawing as follows: Bake the strudel at 375°F (190°C, or gas mark 5) for 30 minutes, then increase the heat to 425°F (220°C, or gas mark 7) and bake for 10 more minutes.*

- *Whipped cream or vanilla ice cream is the perfect accompaniment to this dessert. If you prefer to avoid the calories and extra fat, serve with nonfat frozen yogurt.*

NUTRITIONAL ANALYSIS

Each serving provides: 213 calories;
5.5 g total fat; 1.5 g saturated fat; 3 g protein;
40 g carbohydrate; 4 g dietary fiber;
5 mg cholesterol.

SUPERSKIN NUTRIENTS		% DAILY VALUE*
Vitamin A	298.1 IU	6%
Vitamin B6	0.0 mg	0%
Vitamin C	5.5 mg	9%
Vitamin E	0.7 mg	4%
Magnesium	21.2 mg	5%
Manganese	0.1 mg	5%
Selenium	8.0 mcg	11%
Zinc	0.5 mg	3%

*Percent Daily Values are based on a 2,000-calorie diet. Your daily values may be higher or lower depending on your caloric needs.

Armagnac Prunes

Dried fruit like prunes are terrific sources of nutrients such as beta-carotene, B vitamins, vitamin C, and potassium, all of which serve to tighten, smooth, and fight sagging. With the added benefit of the inflammation-fighting powers of maple syrup, your skin will love this dessert as much as your mouth will.

¾ cup (175 ml) Armagnac

2 cups (350 g) pitted prunes

3 tablespoons (45 ml) maple syrup

2 cups (475 ml) water

2 tablespoons (12 g) fresh orange zest

Yield: 4 servings (2 cups, or 1052 g, total)

1. Place the prunes in a jar or bowl and pour Armagnac over them. Cover, and let steep for at least 8 and up to 24 hours.

2. In a saucepan, combine the prunes and Armagnac with the maple syrup, enough water to barely cover the prunes, and orange zest. Bring to a gentle simmer over low heat and cook until the prunes are extremely tender and the cooking liquid is lightly thickened, about 20 minutes. Transfer to a bowl or a clean jar.

3. For serving ideas, see below.

Notes

• *Serve the prunes on their own, as a compote, or as a topping for the Cottage Cheese Pancakes on page 198 in place of the blueberry syrup. You can also use the prunes to stuff baking apples. Dot each with a bit of butter and bake, covered, at 325°F (170°C, or gas mark 3) for 45 minutes.*

• *If you don't have Armagnac on hand, try substituting brandy, cognac, dark rum, scotch, or bourbon.*

• *Look for grade B maple syrup, which has a slightly stronger, smokier flavor than regular grade syrup, as it is a perfect match for the Armagnac.*

NUTRITIONAL ANALYSIS

Each serving provides: 342 calories; 0.5 g total fat; 0 g saturated fat; 2 g protein; 64 g carbohydrate; 6 g dietary fiber; 0 mg cholesterol.

SUPERSKIN NUTRIENTS		% DAILY VALUE*
Vitamin A	1701.6 IU	34%
Vitamin B6	0.2 mg	10%
Vitamin C	6.9 mg	12%
Vitamin E	2.1 mg	11%
Magnesium	42.2 mg	11%
Manganese	0.7 mg	35%
Selenium	2.1 mcg	3%
Zinc	1.1 mg	7%

*Percent Daily Values are based on a 2,000-calorie diet. Your daily values may be higher or lower depending on your caloric needs.

INGREDIENT SPOTLIGHT

Prunes

Prunes are a good source of beta-carotene, a fat-soluble antioxidant that helps eliminate free radicals that would otherwise cause damage to cells and cell membranes. Studies show beta-carotene to be helpful in the prevention of a variety of diseases, including atherosclerosis, diabetic heart disease, and colon cancer. It is also useful in reducing the severity of inflammatory conditions like asthma, osteoarthritis, and rheumatoid arthritis.

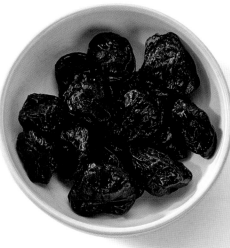

Polenta Soufflé with Caramel and Pear

Detox your skin by way of dessert with this elegant and delicious souf-flé. Due to their high fiber content, pears are a great detoxifier for your skin, and they also contain copper to help prevent inflammation that leads to redness and puffiness. How sweet beautiful skin can be!

Vegetable oil spray or veg-etable oil

¾ cup (150 g) sugar, divided, plus 3 tablespoons (39 g) sugar

1¼ cups (295 ml) skim milk

1 strip orange peel, approximately 1 × 2 inch (2.5 × 5 cm)

5 tablespoons (45 g) cornmeal

¼ cup (59 ml) pear juice (or apple juice, apple cider, or water)

1 tablespoon (14 g) unsalted butter

2 ripe pears, cored, peeled, and diced

Pinch of cinnamon

3 egg whites

Yield: 4 servings

1. Preheat oven to 400°F (200°C, or gas mark 6). Prepare a 1-quart (946-ml) soufflé mold by spraying it lightly with a vegetable oil spray or rubbing vegetable oil over the interior with a paper towel. Scatter the 3 tablespoons (39 g) of sugar over the sides and bottom of the mold. Rotate the mold until the inside is evenly coated with sugar. Tap the mold gently to release excess sugar and shake it out.

2. Place the skim milk and orange peel in a large saucepan. Heat to a simmer and add ¼ cup (50 g) sugar. Stir until the sugar is completely dissolved. Add the cornmeal in a thin stream, stir-ring constantly. Simmer the polenta, stirring frequently, until it is thickened and soft, about 15 to 20 minutes. Remove from the heat and let cool. Remove and discard the orange peel.

3. Combine ¼ cup (50 g) sugar, pear juice, and butter in a skillet. Cook over medium heat until the sugar dissolves and the mixture turns a deep caramel brown, 1 to 2 minutes. Add the diced pears and cinnamon. Cook over medium heat until the pears are ten-der, 8 to 10 minutes. Fold into the polenta mixture and set aside.

4. Using an electric mixer, whip the egg whites to a heavy foam and add the remaining ¼ cup (50 g) sugar. Continue to beat until the egg whites form medium peaks (see Note).

5. Fold half of the egg white mixture into the polenta mixture. Gradually add the remaining eggs whites, folding just until in-corporated. Pour the mixture into the sugar-coated soufflé mold.

6. Place the mold into a baking dish with sides and place in the oven. Working carefully, add about ¼ inch (6.25 mm) of hot wa-ter to the baking dish. Bake the soufflé for about 35 minutes, or until it has risen and the top is golden. Remove the soufflé from the oven, and serve immediately.

Note

You'll know you've reached medium-peak stage with your egg whites when the top of your "peak" folds over itself a little, but doesn't fall completely.

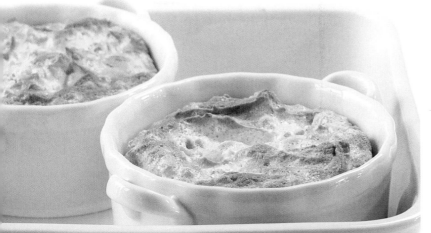
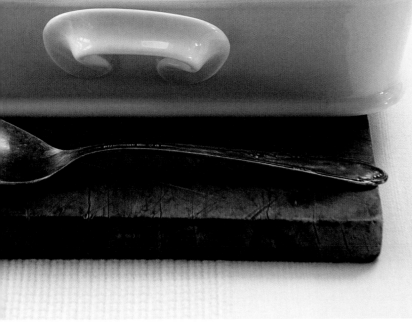

NUTRITIONAL ANALYSIS
Each serving provides: 307 calories; 3.5 g total fat; 2 g saturated fat; 7 g protein; 65 g carbohydrate; 3 g dietary fiber; 9 mg cholesterol.

SUPERSKIN NUTRIENTS		% DAILY VALUE*
Vitamin A	333.4 IU	7%
Vitamin B6	0.1 mg	5%
Vitamin C	24.3 mg	41%
Vitamin E	0.7 mg	4%
Magnesium	21.2 mg	5%
Manganese	0.1 mg	5%
Selenium	8.0 mcg	11%
Zinc	0.5 mg	3%

*Percent Daily Values are based on a 2,000-calorie diet. Your daily values may be higher or lower depending on your caloric needs.

Glacéed Grapes

Grapes are known to help reduce the risk of heart disease, but few people appreciate how effective they are at fighting inflammation in your skin. Get in on the secret with this special dessert that turns grapes into sparkly, sweet gems.

½ cup (100 g) sugar

1 large egg white

4 cups (600 g) fresh grapes, rinsed and dried

Yield: 8 servings

1. To prepare, place the sugar in a shallow dish or plate and line a cookie sheet with waxed paper.

2. In a mixing bowl, whisk the egg white until it forms a loose foam.

3. Drop the grapes a few at a time into the beaten egg white, and lift them from the bowl with a slotted spoon, allowing any excess egg white to drain away.

4. Gently roll the grapes in the sugar until they are coated. Transfer the grapes to the cookie sheet. Continue this process until all the grapes have been coated.

5. Place the tray in the freezer and freeze at least 2 hours.

6. Once frozen, the grapes are ready to serve. If storing for a longer period, transfer to a freezer container or bag.

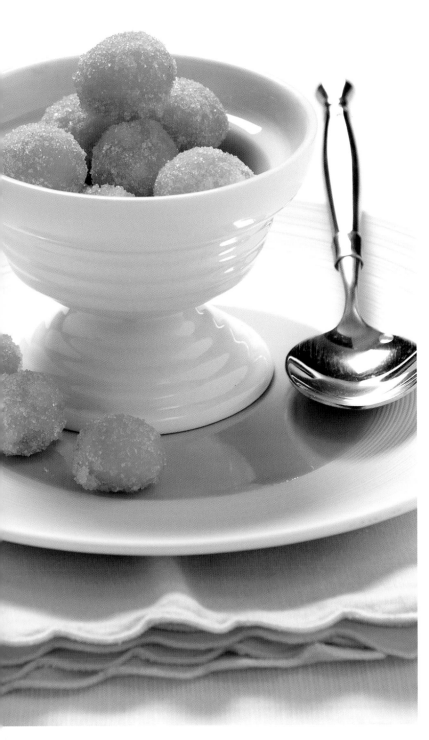

Notes

- *Glacéed grapes make for a delicious treat on their own, but also go great with ice cream or yogurt.*

- *Grapes aren't the only fruit that can be glacéed; cranberries, whole strawberries, and orange segments work well too.*

NUTRITIONAL ANALYSIS

Each ½-cup (97 g) serving provides:
107 calories; 0.5 g total fat; 0.2 g saturated fat; 1 g protein; 27 g carbohydrate; 1 g dietary fiber; 0 mg cholesterol.

SUPERSKIN NUTRIENTS		% DAILY VALUE*
Vitamin A	58.4 IU	1%
Vitamin B6	0.1 mg	5%
Vitamin C	8.6 mg	14%
Vitamin E	0.6 mg	3%
Magnesium	5.3 mg	1%
Manganese	0.1 mg	5%
Selenium	1.0 mcg	1%
Zinc	0.0 mg	0%

*Percent Daily Values are based on a 2,000-calorie diet. Your daily values may be higher or lower depending on your caloric needs.

Lemon Ice

What should you do when life gives you lemons? Cleanse your palate and your skin! Lemons contain limonins, regarded as the longest-lasting antioxidant in your skin and an ever-lasting protector against damage.

1 cup (200 g) sugar

3½ cups (825 ml) water

2 tablespoons (12 g) finely grated lemon zest

1 cup (235 ml) fresh lemon juice

Yield: 6 servings

1. Combine the sugar and water in a saucepan and bring to a boil over medium high heat. When the syrup has reached a full boil, add the lemon zest. Immediately remove the syrup from the heat and let it cool to room temperature.

2. Once cooled, stir in the fresh lemon juice and pour into a shallow pan (a glass baking dish is best). Place the pan in the freezer, uncovered.

3. Freeze the lemon ice for 3 hours before serving. As it freezes, use a serving spoon to stir and scrape the ice every 10 to 15 minutes to create a light, soft texture in the finished dessert.

4. Once fully frozen, scoop into chilled dishes (or paper cups for an authentic Italian ice experience).

Note
This ice can be prepared with a variety of other citrus fruits, such as lime, grapefruit, orange, or a blend of several citrus juices to create your own special flavor.

NUTRITIONAL ANALYSIS

Each serving provides: 140 calories; 0 g total fat; 0 g saturated fat; 0.2 g protein; 37 g carbohydrate; 0 g dietary fiber; 0 mg cholesterol.

SUPERSKIN NUTRIENTS		% DAILY VALUE*
Vitamin A	9.1 IU	0%
Vitamin B6	0.0 mg	0%
Vitamin C	21.3 mg	36%
Vitamin E	0.1 mg	1%
Magnesium	4.1 mg	1%
Manganese	0.0 mg	0%
Selenium	0.3 mcg	0%
Zinc	0.1 mg	1%

*Percent Daily Values are based on a 2,000-calorie diet. Your daily values may be higher or lower depending on your caloric needs.

INGREDIENT SPOTLIGHT

Lemons

Antioxidants known as limonins, which are found in lemons and other citrus fruits, have been shown in clinical trials to fight skin and other types of cancer. These antioxidants are present in citrus fruits in the same amount as vitamin C and stay in the blood stream longer than other antioxidant compounds. In fact, in a study conducted by the U.S. Agricultural Research Service, researchers found that traces of limonin were still present in some volunteers 24 hours after consumption. The phenols in green tea and chocolate, on the other hand, remain active for only 4 to 6 hours.

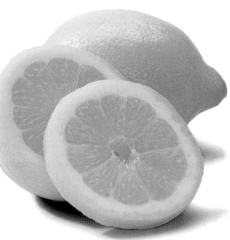

READING LIST

Interested in learning more? The following is a list of recommended titles that offer additional information on food and herbs and how they relate to skin and health:

Barnes, J., L.A. Anderson, and J.D. Phillipson. 1996. *Herbal Medicine: A Guide for Healthcare Professionals.* Pharmaceutical Press: London, UK.

Blumenthal, M., et al. 2003. *The ABC Clinical Guide to Herbs.* American Botanical Council: Austin, TX.

Bowden, J. 2007. *The 150 Healthiest Foods on Earth: The Surprising Unbiased Truth About What You Should Eat and Why.* Fair Winds Press: Beverly, MA.

Department of Health and Human Services. *More Than Skin Deep! Skin Health Activity Handbook.* National Institutes of Health: Washington, D.C.

Ensminger, A.H., et al. 1986. *Food for Health: A Nutrition Encyclopedia.* Pegus Press: Clovis, CA.

Haas, E.M. 1992. *Staying Healthy with Nutrition.* Celestial Arts Publishing Company: Berkeley, CA.

Larson-Duyff, R. 2006. *American Dietetic Association Complete Food and Nutrition Guide.* John Wiley & Sons, Inc.: Hoboken, NJ.

Mateljan, G. 2006. *The World's Healthiest Foods: Essential Guide for the Healthiest Way of Eating.* George Mateljan Foundation: New York, NY.

Murray, M., L. Pizzorono, and J. Pizzorono. 2005. *The Encyclopedia of Healing Foods.* Atria Books: New York, NY.

Perricone, N. 2004. *The Clear Skin Prescription: The Perricone Program to Eliminate Problem Skin.* Harper Collins: New York, NY.

Purba, M. et al. 2001. "Skin Wrinkling: Can Food Make a Difference?" *Journal of the American College of Nutrition,* 20 (1): 71¬80.

Shulman, J. 2005. *The Natural Makeover Diet: A 4-step Program to Looking and Feeling Your Best from the Inside Out.* John Wiley & Sons, Inc.: Hoboken, NJ.

Stradler-Mitrea, L. 2005. *Pathology and Nutrition: A Guide for Professionals.* CSNN Publishing: Toronto, Canada.

Tannis, A. 2008. *Probiotic Rescue: How You Can Use Probiotics to Fight Cholesterol, Cancer, Superbugs, Digestive Complaints and More.* John Wiley & Sons, Inc.: Hoboken, NJ.

Tannis, A. 2005. *Vitality: Quest for a Healthy Diet in the Wake of the Low Carb Craze.* Volumes: Kitchener, Ontario.

Unknown. 1999. *The Review of Natural Products by Facts and Comparisons.* Wolters Kluwer Co.; St. Louis, MO.

Vanderhaeghe, L.R. and K. Karst. 2003. *Healthy Fats for Life: Preventing and Treating Common Health Problems with Essential Fatty Acids.* John Wiley & Sons, Inc.: Hoboken, NJ.

Wolpowitz, D. and B.A. Gilchrest. 2006. "The Vitamin D Question: How Much Do You Need and How Should You Get It?" *Journal of the American Academy of Dermatology,* 54 (2): 301–317.

GLOSSARY

A

Acne—a skin disorder caused by inflammation of the skin glands and hair follicles; marked by pimples, especially on the face and back.

Allergic reactions—sensitivities to a specific substance, called an allergen. Allergens are contacted through the skin, inhaled into the lungs, swallowed, or injected.

Anti-inflammatory—any agent that counteracts inflammation in the skin cells. Vitamins C and E are well known for their anti-inflammatory properties.

Antioxidant—a substance capable of bonding with and thus neutralizing hazardous free-radicals within the body. Antioxidants inhibit oxidation and the deleterious effects it causes.

B

Bioflavonoids—biologically active flavonoids (such as hesperidin and quercetin) derived from plants and primarily found in fruits and vegetables. Bioflavonoids have numerous health benefits, including improving the absorption of vitamin C in the body. Also called flavonoids.

C

Collagen—an insoluble fibrous protein that is the chief constituent of connective tissue in the skin, tendons, and bones. Collagen provides skin with its structural support.

D

Dermis—the layer of skin beneath the epidermis that consists of connective tissue and cushions the body from stress and strain.

Detox—to remove or be freed from an intoxicating or addictive substance.

E

Elastin—a protein similar to collagen that is the chief constituent of elastic fibers. Elastin is responsible for the skin's ability to retain in its shape.

Enzyme—complex proteins that are produced by living cells and that catalyze specific biochemical reactions in the body. Enzymes work by dissolving the dead skin cells on the top layer of skin.

Epidermis—the outermost layer of the skin that forms a waterproof, protective wrap over the body's surface.

Epithelial tissue—a membranous cellular tissue that covers a free surface or lines a tube or cavity of an animal body (e.g., skin, intestinal lining). Epithelial tissue serves to enclose and protect the other parts of the body, to produce secretions and excretions, and to function in assimilation.

Essential fatty acids (EFAs)—the basic building block of the cellular membrane, vital in preventing cellular water loss. Includes omega-3 and omega-6 fatty acids.

Extracellular matrix—the materials produced by cells and secreted into the surrounding medium.

F

Fibroblasts—cells that make up the structural fibers and ground substance of connective tissue.

Flavonoids—a class of water-soluble pigments found in plants that are beneficial to health. Flavonoids strengthen capillaries and other connective tissue, and some function as anti-inflammatory, antihistaminic, and antiviral agents. Also called bioflavonoids.

Free radicals—unstable molecules found naturally in the body and in the environment. Free radicals react with certain chemicals in the body, and in the process, interfere with the cells' ability to function normally. Free radicals are a main cause of aging and skin damage.

H

Hair follicle—part of the skin that grows hair by packing old cells together.

Humectant—a substance that draws water to the surface of the skin.

Hyaluronic acid—an acid that helps retain the skin's natural moisture. It can hold 1000 times its weight in water.

Hypodermis—the thin layer of loose fatty connective tissue underlying the skin and binding it to the parts beneath.

I

Immune cells—cells in the body capable of reacting with a specific antigen and preventing disease. Also called lymphocytes.

Inflammation—a response to injury or damage that is marked by the dilation of capillaries (small blood vessels), leukocytic (white blood cell) infiltration, redness, heat, pain, and swelling. Serves as a mechanism to remove harmful agents and damaged tissue.

Intracellular laminar lipids—fats in the skin that are involved in maintaining moisture levels.

K

Keratin—an extremely strong protein, made of amino acids, which is a major component of skin, hair, nails, and teeth.

Keratinocytes—epidermal cells that produce keratin.

L

Langerhans cells—specialized immune cells found in the skin.

M

Melanin—a substance that gives the skin and hair its natural color and helps protect the skin from ultraviolet radiation.

Melanocytes—cells located in the bottom layer of the skin's epidermis that produce melanin.

Metabolism—the chemical changes in living cells by which energy is provided for vital processes and activities and new material is assimilated.

Monounsaturated fat—an oil, fat, or fatty acid containing one double or triple bond per molecule. Considered a healthy fat for its ability to lower cholesterol and possibly reduce heart disease, it is found in greatest amounts in plant-based food, especially canola and olive oil.

N

Natural moisturizing factor (NMF)—also called hygroscopic agents, a group of compounds in the skin that promote moisture.

O

Omega-3 fatty acids—polyunsaturated fatty acids found in leafy green vegetables, vegetable oils, and fish such as salmon and mackerel capable of reducing serum cholesterol levels and having anticoagulant properties. Must be consumed in the diet daily as the human body cannot manufacture or store these fats.

Omega-6 fatty acids—polyunsaturated fatty acids found chiefly in vegetable oils, nuts, beans, seeds, and grains that contribute to cellular health. Must be consumed in the diet daily as the human body cannot manufacture or store these fats.

Organelle—a specialized subunit within a cell that has a specific function, and is separately enclosed within its own lipid membrane.

Oxidation—a process in which oxygen combines with an atom or molecule, altering its structure and changing or destroying its normal function.

P

Phenolic compounds—molecular substances found in fruits and vegetables that are essential for the growth and reproduction of plants. When consumed by the human body, these compounds help prevent against oxidative damage. Also called phenols.

Photoaging—damage to the skin caused by the sun or ultraviolet rays.

Phytochemicals—compounds found in fruits and vegetables that act as free radical scavengers to help eliminate oxidation. Phytochemicals are known for their antioxidant properties.

Phytonutrients—plant-based compounds that provide health benefits through their antioxidant and anti-inflammatory abilities.

Phytosterols—fats found in plants that are a natural constituents of the human diet. Also called plant sterols.

Pigmentation—coloration with or deposition of pigment (color).

Proliferation—rapid and repeated production of new parts or offspring (such as cell proliferation).

Psoriasis—a chronic skin disease characterized by circumscribed red patches covered with white scales.

S

Seborrhea—severe oiliness in the skin.

Sebum—oil in the skin.

Stratum corneum—the outermost layer of the skin.

U

Ultraviolet rays—invisible rays that are part of the energy that comes from the sun and that cause damage to cells.

V

Vitamin A—increases collagen production, and acts as a wrinkle fighter and exfoliant. Although it's only found in foods of animal origin, some fruits and vegetables contain compounds, called cartenoids, that can be converted into vitamin A by your body.

Vitamin B complex—group of twelve water-soluble vitamins that function as co-enzymes and have wide range of functions, including increasing blood circulation and tissue repair.

Vitamin C—known for its antioxidant and healing properties, this vitamin helps protects cells from free radical damage, aids in the regeneration of vitamin E, and improves iron absorption.

Vitamin E—serves the body as an antioxidant by preventing cell damage from free radicals. Also protects your skin from ultraviolet light and allows your cells to communicate effectively.

Vitamin K—helps reduce skin redness and also acts an antioxidant to prevent oxidative damage.

ABOUT THE AUTHOR

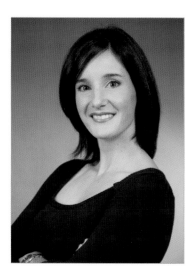

Allison Tannis, M.S., R.H.N. is a nutritional scientist and leading health educator in nutrition and natural medicine. A registered holistic nutritionist with a practice based in Ontario, Canada, her specialty is helping people discover how to arm themselves with the tools they need to live healthier lives.

Allison is also the host of the popular radio show *Healthy Living* and the author of *Vitality: Quest for a Healthy Diet* and *Probiotic Rescue: How You Can Use Probiotics to Fight Cholesterol, Cancer, Superbugs, Digestive Complaints and More*. She holds a Master's degree in the field of Human Biology and Nutritional Sciences from the University of Guelph in Ontario.

ACKNOWLEDGMENTS

We can all be radiant and enjoy more beautiful skin thanks to several amazing people:

A big thanks to Mary D. Donovan, the creator of these delicious recipes, for making healthy skin such an easy and tasty pursuit. These dishes are not only delicious—they're also packed with nutrients that feed and fortify our skin.

Thanks to Jill and the entire Fair Winds Press team for such a fun adventure in the world of food. I would also like to thank Nicole for her help.

Last, but certainly not least, thank you Chris, for all of your love and support, and for your great sense of humor. Meals are much more fun with your "manly" jokes like, "Oh, no, honey— we can't eat that. It's not good for my skin."

INDEX

triglycerides, 24
triiodothyronine, 88
Tropical Flavors Snack Mix, 206–207
Tropical Fruit Smoothie, 192–193
Tufts University, 36
tuna, *40*, 72–73, 137, 177, 260–261
turkey, *150*, 153, 215
turkey sausage, 214–215

U

ubiquinone (CoQ10). *See* CoQ10
ultraviolet radiation, 11, 23, 25, 27, 31, 34, 35, 38, 42, 52–53, 79, 130, 146, 149, 165, 168, 293. *See also* sun exposure
ultraviolet rays, 293. *See also* ultraviolet radiation
uneven complexions, 25
University of Glasgow, 45
U.S. Agricultural Research Service, 184
U.S. Food and Drug Administration (FDA), 93
UVA radiation, 22, 25, 149
UVB radiation, 22, 25, 45, 54, 70, 72, 149
UVC radiation, 149

V

vascular system, 122
vegetables, 36, 38, *40*, 53–63, 76, 79, 100, 176. *See also specific vegetables*
vitamin A, *13*, 31, 43, 49, 52, 54, 56–57, 60, 62, 88, 89, 90, 95, 102, 105, 108, 112, 116–117, 122, 131–132, 135, 151, 163, 167, 176, 185, 293
  toxicity of, 57
vitamin B12, *13*, 88, 122, 137
vitamin B1 (thiamin), 43, 44, 71–72, 89, 95, 102, 110, 116, 127, 130, 136, 157, 179
vitamin B2 (riboflavin), *13*, 43, 44, 102, 116, 130, 133, 162
vitamin B3 (niacin), *13*, 43, 44, 73, 102, 106, 116, 130, 139–140, 167, 179. *See* vitamin B3 (niacin)
vitamin B5, 130
vitamin B6 (pyridoxine), *13*, 50, 73, 95, 102, 116, 118, 130, 136, 137, 168, 169, 176

vitamin B complex, *13*, 293. *See also* B vitamins
vitamin C, 10, 11, *13*, 20, 22, 31, 36, 43, 44, 46, 49, 50, 51, 54, 58–59, 60–63, 80, 88, 90, 95, 98, 100, 102–103, 105, 107, 108, 112, 116, 117, 124, 131, 132, 135, 141, 143, 150, 152, 159, 167, 168, 176, 179, 182, 183–184, 185, 186, 293
vitamin D, 131, 161–162
vitamin E, *13*, 31, 36, 39, 47, 50, 63, 65, 67, 68, 76, 79, 82, 85, 86, 88, 98, 100, 105, 106, 108, 110, 124, 128, 136, 142, 150, 158, 176, 178, 186, 293
vitamin K, 62, 82, 116, 293
vitamins, 11, 38, 39, 41, 46, 50, 56, 88, 103, 122, 134. *See also* B vitamins; *specific vitamins*

W

walnuts, 206–207
water, 55, 76, 79, *80*, 80, 93–94, 101, 116–117
watermelon, *80*, 94–95, 274–275
Watermelon Punch, 274–275
wheat, 128–129
wheat bran, 128
wheat germ, *125*, 128, 136
white beans, 266–267
white blood cells, 24, 103
white button mushrooms, 129, 131
white grapes, 105
whiteheads, 172
white tea, 70
WHO. *See* World Health Organization (WHO)
Whole Wheat Pasta with Clams and Toasted Bread Crumbs, 264–265
wolfberries. *See* goji berries
World Health Organization (WHO), 93
wrinkles, 15, 23, 25, 27, 47, 63, 69, 149
  carotenoids and, 57
  causes of, 34–35
  environmental factors, 34–35
  foods that fight wrinkles, 33–73, *40*
  menopause and, 35
  new wrinkle cure, 35–39

oily skin and, 24
vitamin C and, 43
wrinkle preventers, 19–23

X

xanthone gamma-mangoestin, 138

Y

yeast infections, 127
yeasts, 23, 24. *See also* Brewer's yeast
yogurt, *150*, 162–163, 278–288

Z

Zante grapes, 105
zeaxanthin, 50, 54
zinc, *13*, 88, 89, 98, 102, 112, 116, 128, 131, 132, 134, 135, 136, 142, 176, 184–185
zucchini, *80*, 90–91